volume 42 2006

Essays in Biochemistry

The Biochemical Basis of the Health Effects of Exercise

Edited by A.J.M. Wagenmakers

Portland Press

Essays in Biochemistry is published by Portland Press Ltd on behalf of the Biochemical Society

Portland Press Limited
Third Floor, Eagle House
16 Procter Street
London WC1V 6NX
U.K.
Tel.: +44 (0)20 7280 4110
Fax: +44 (0)20 7280 4169
email: editorial@portlandpress.com
www.portlandpress.com

British Library Cataloguing-in-Publication Data
A catalogue record for this book is available from the British Library
ISBN-10 1 85578 159 X
ISBN-13 978 1 85578 159 7
ISSN   0071 1365

Typeset by TechBooks, Delhi, India
Printed in Great Britain by Information Press Ltd, Oxford

Essays in Biochemistry

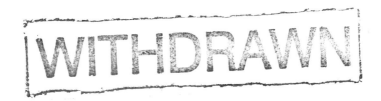

Other recent titles in the Essays in Biochemistry series

Essays in Biochemistry volume 41: The Ubiquitin–Proteasome System
edited by R.J. Mayer and R. Layfield
2005 ISBN-10 1 85578 153 0
      ISBN-13 978 1 85578 153 5

Essays in Biochemistry volume 40: The Nuclear Receptor Superfamily
edited by I.J. McEwan
2004 ISBN-10 1 85578 150 6
      ISBN-13 978 1 85578 150 4

Essays in Biochemistry volume 39: Programmed Cell Death
edited by T.G. Cotter
2003 ISBN-10 1 85578 148 4
      ISBN-13 978 1 85578 148 1

Essays in Biochemistry volume 38: Proteases in Biology and Medicine
edited by N.M. Hooper
2002 ISBN-10 1 85578 147 6
      ISBN-13 978 1 85578 147 4

Essays in Biochemistry volume 37: Regulation of Gene Expression
edited by K.E. Chapman and S.J. Higgins
2001 ISBN-10 1 85578 138 7
      ISBN-13 978 1 85578 138 2

Essays in Biochemistry volume 36: Molecular Trafficking
edited by P. Bernstein
2000 ISBN-10 1 85578 131 X
      ISBN-13 978 1 85578 131 3

Essays in Biochemistry volume 35: Molecular Motors
edited by G. Banting and S.J. Higgins
2000 ISBN-10 1 85578 103 4
      ISBN-13 978 1 85578 103 0

Contents

1 Signalling mechanisms in skeletal muscle: role in substrate selection and muscle adaptation

John A. Hawley, Mark Hargreaves and Juleen R. Zierath

2 Control of gene expression and mitochondrial biogenesis in the muscular adaptation to endurance exercise

Anna-Maria Joseph, Henriette Pilegaard, Anastassia Litvintsev, Lotte Leick and David A. Hood

3 **Effects of acute exercise and training on insulin action and sensitivity: focus on molecular mechanisms in muscle**
Jørgen F.P.Wojtaszewski and Erik A. Richter

4 **Lipid metabolism, exercise and insulin action**
Arend Bonen, G. Lynis Dohm and Luc J.C. van Loon

5 **Resistance exercise, muscle loading/unloading and the control of muscle mass**
Keith Baar, Gustavo Nader and Sue Bodine

6 Resistance training, insulin sensitivity and muscle function in the elderly
Flemming Dela and Michael Kjaer

7 Fatty acid metabolism in adipose tissue, muscle and liver in health and disease
Keith N. Frayn, Peter Arner and Hannele Yki Järvinen

8 The anti-inflammatory effect of exercise: its role in diabetes and cardiovascular disease control
Bente Klarlund Pedersen

9 Vascular nitric oxide: effects of physical activity, importance for health

Richard M. McAllister and M. Harold Laughlin

10 Muscle metabolism and control of capillary blood flow: insulin and exercise

Stephen Rattigan, Eloise A. Bradley, Stephen M. Richards and Michael G. Clark

11 Vascular function in the metabolic syndrome and the effects on skeletal muscle perfusion: lessons from the obese Zucker rat

Jefferson C. Frisbee and Michael D. Delp

12 Microvascular dysfunction: causative role in the association between hypertension, insulin resistance and the metabolic syndrome?

Erik H. Serné, Renate T. de Jongh, Etto C. Eringa, Richard G. Ijzerman, Michiel P. de Boer and Coen D.A. Stehouwer

13 Exercise, genetics and prevention of type 2 diabetes

Gang Hu, Jesús Rico-Sanz, Timo A. Lakka and Jaakko Tuomilehto

14 Integration of the metabolic and cardiovascular effects of exercise

Anton J.M. Wagenmakers, Natal A.W. van Riel, Michael P. Frenneaux and Paul M. Stewart

Preface

As recently pointed out in an excellent review by Chakravarthy and Booth [1], man in prehistoric times had a high daily energy expenditure, while the availability of food was irregular and restricted. Most of the men were hunters and most of the women food gatherers. Both activities required a disciplined lifestyle involving regular training sessions to practice the typical hunting skills (the equivalent to speed, strength and resistance training) or long days with heavy physical labour (equivalent to moderate-intensity endurance training). In order to develop successful survival strategies and earn the respect of fellow tribe members, individuals always had to maintain high fitness levels and a strong, lean and healthy constitution. Children followed the example of their parents and were carefully prepared and conditioned for their later tasks in life. It was in this period (50000–10000 BC) that evolution via the 'survival of the fittest' principle selected the genes that most of us still carry today [1].

Since the middle of the 20th Century, major and rapid changes have occurred in the mean physical activity of mankind; the introduction of automobiles, television, machines that take over manual labour in agriculture and industry, and the introduction of computers, computer games and the World Wide Web have grossly reduced the mean number of hours in which people are physically active. Children, until the 1960s, walked or cycled to school, had more hours of physical education (PE) at school than today and were heavily involved in post-school physical activities (both for fun and physical work). In urban areas, rapid increases in car use and traffic density since the 1960s and 1970s made walking and cycling into activities regarded to be increasingly dangerous by most of the parents [2]. Therefore, most parents bring their children by car to school and to all post-school activities, often not realizing how detrimental the lack of exercise is for the health of their children [3–6]. PE has nearly disappeared in the last two decades both from primary and secondary schools worldwide as academic learning is given higher priority. Many children have a minimal involvement in post-school sport and playing activities. Most of their time is spent watching television, behind a computer screen playing computer games or surfing the Internet. The American Paediatric Association recommends 60 minutes of moderate to vigorous exercise at least 5 days a week for school-aged children and fear that very few achieve this [3].

In addition to the decrease in physical activity, food and drinking habits have changed in recent decades and many children, adolescents and adults consume far too many calories for their low physical activity level. Excessive exposure to affluent amounts of energy-rich, but low-quality, food (e.g. via vending machines in schools, stations, public buildings and sport clubs) has greatly increased the consumption of snacks between the three traditional main meals. Too little exercise and the consumption of too many calories are regarded as the main causes of the current epidemic increase in the frequency of obesity, type 2 diabetes and cardiovascular disease, both by expert committees [7] and the World Health Organization [8]. It is clear that the genes that we inherited from our prehistoric ancestors cannot cope with this abrupt change in lifestyle. Obesity, type 2 diabetes and atherosclerosis were regarded until recently as diseases of the elderly, but today frequently occur in children below the age of 10 years [4,5]. The increase in healthcare costs and reduction in quality of life of those affected and their families are already high and expected to increase much further when the present generation of obese children have reached adulthood [6,8].

This volume of *Essays in Biochemistry* could not have been more timely, with the current epidemic increases in obesity, Type 2 diabetes and cardiovascular disease [7,8]. Each essay has been written by leading experts with complimentary expertise in human physiology and biochemistry. Both the metabolic impairments that occur in the human body as a result of inactivity and disease, and the beneficial effects of exercise in correcting these mechanisms and improving health, are described. Together, the essays give clear mechanistic insight into the multitude of enzymes, signalling pathways, tissues and bodily functions that benefit from relatively modest increases in physical activity. The volume compiles the hard, experiment-based evidence that shows how exercise improves human health and well-being. It covers the mechanisms that operate in muscle (endurance exercise in Chapters 1–4 and resistance exercise in Chapters 5 and 6), the metabolic interaction between muscle, liver and adipose tissue (Chapter 7), the effect of cytokines and inflammation (Chapter 8), the mechanisms that operate in the endothelium of the vascular wall (Chapters 9–12), the genetic differences between subjects in acquiring chronic diseases and the therapeutic effect of exercise upon it (Chapter 13). Finally. Chapter 14 integrates the metabolic effects in muscle and the cardiovascular effects of exercise.

Originally, it was my intention to aim this volume primarily at final-year undergraduate and postgraduate students and their teachers in the biological and medical sciences; however, I expect that the diversity of the topics covered also makes it interesting and stimulating reading for colleagues already active in the field. Finally, I do hope that it also will be an important and accessible source of information for the current generation of medical doctors, health professionals, dieticians and policymakers in public health. The quantity and diversity of the therapeutic effect of exercise seems to illustrate the acute need for active interference of governments and health agencies to make the current and future world populations as least as physically active as people were 100 years ago.

I would like to express my sincere thanks to all my colleagues for their excellent contributions and discussing their individual areas of expertise in a clear and erudite manner. I am also grateful to the many reviewers for their constructive comments and helpful suggestions for improvement of the submitted manuscripts. My thanks also go to Mike Cunningham and his colleagues at Portland Press Ltd for their hard work and diligence in ensuring the high quality of this book.

Anton J.M. Wagenmakers
Birmingham, UK
October 2006

References

1. Chakravarthy, M.V. & Booth, F.W. (2004) Eating, exercise, and 'thrifty' genotypes: connecting the dots toward an evolutionary understanding of modern chronic diseases. *J. Appl. Physiol.* **96**, 3–10

2. Furedi, F. (2001) *Paranoid Parenting*, Allen Lane, London

3. Strong, W.B., Malina, R.M., Blimkie, C.J.R., Daniels, S.R., Dishman, R.K., Gutin, B., Hergenroeder, A.C., Must, A., Nixon, P.A., Pivarnik, J.M., et al. (2005) Evidence based physical activity for school-aged youth. *J. Pediatr.* **146**, 732–737

4. Ehtisham, S., Hattersley, A.T., Dunger, D.B. & Barrett, T.G. (2004) First UK survey of paediatric type 2 diabetes and MODY. *Arch. Dis. Child.* **89**, 526–529

5. Iannuzzi, A., Licenziati, M.R., Acampora, C., Salvatore, V., Auriemma, L., Romano, M.L., Panico, S., Rubba, P. & Trevisan, M. (2004) Increased carotid intima-media thickness in obese children. *Diabetes Care* **27**, 2506–2508

6. Srinivasan, S., Bao, W., Wattigney, W.A. & Berenson, G.S. (1996) Adolescent overweight is associated with adult overweight and related multiple cardiovascular risk factors: The Bogalusa Heart Study. Metab., Clin. Exp. **45**, 235–240

7. World Health Organization (2003) Diet, nutrition and the prevention of chronic diseases. *WHO Technical Report Series* no. 916, World Health Organization, Geneva (http://www.fao.org/docrep/005/ac911e/ac911e00.htm)

8. World Health Organization (2006) Global strategy on diet, physical activity and health: Diabetes. World Health Organization, Geneva (http://www.who.int/dietphysicalactivity/publications/facts/diabetes/en/index.html)

Authors

John A. Hawley is currently Head of the Exercise Metabolism Research Group and Professor of Exercise Metabolism in the School of Medical Sciences at RMIT University, Melbourne, Australia. His research interests include the interaction of exercise training and dietary manipulations on glucose and lipid regulation in skeletal muscle, with a special interest in Type 2 diabetes; the regulation of carbohydrate and fat metabolism in skeletal muscle during exercise; and the molecular basis of training adaptation. He has published over 130 original research papers and review articles and has authored numerous book chapters for sports medicine/exercise biochemistry texts. In 1994, he became the first New Zealand researcher to be elected as a Fellow of the American College of Sports Medicine. Currently he holds editorial positions with several leading scientific journals. **Mark Hargreaves** is Professor in Physiology at The University of Melbourne, Australia. His research interests focus on the regulation of skeletal muscle carbohydrate metabolism in response to acute and chronic exercise, with a particular emphasis on GLUT4 expression. He has authored over 100 peer-reviewed articles and has editorial roles with the *Journal of Applied Physiology, Exercise and Sport Sciences Reviews* and *Medicine and Science in Sports and Exercise*. **Juleen R. Zierath** is head of the Section of Integrative Physiology, Department of Molecular Medicine at the Karolinska Institutet, Stockholm, Sweden. Her research focuses on cellular mechanisms underlying the development of insulin resistance in type 2 diabetes and she and has published over 140 original research papers and review articles. In 2001, Professor Zierath was awarded the prestigious Minkowski Prize from the European Association for the Study of Diabetes, and in 2005 she was a recipient of a Strategic Research Grant from the Foundation for Strategic Research, Sweden. In 2006, she was appointed to the Nobel Assembly at the Karolinska Institutet. She currently holds editorial positions with several leading scientific journals.

    Anna-Maria Joseph is a fourth-year PhD student in the Biology Department at York University in Toronto, Canada. She completed her BSc and MSc degrees in Kinesiology and Health Science, also at York University, Toronto. **Anastassia Litvintsev** is a first-year PhD student in Kinesiology and Health Science at York University, Toronto; she also completed her BSc and MSc degrees in the same programme. **Henriette Pilegaard** is an Assistant Professor at the Institute of Molecular Biology and Physiology at University of Copenhagen. She has an MSc degree in biology (major) and exercise (minor) and did her PhD at the University of Copenhagen. The main focus of her current research is on the regulation of adaptive gene responses and substrate choice within skeletal muscle. **Lotte Leick** is a first-year PhD student at the Institute of Molecular Biology and Physiology at the University of Copenhagen. She holds an MSc degree in biology (major) and exercise (minor). **David A. Hood** is a Professor in the School of Kinesiology and Health Science at York University, Toronto, and is cross-appointed in the university's Department of Biology. He holds a Canada Research Chair in Cell Physiology, with an emphasis on the study of mitochondrial biogenesis in muscle, and the role of exercise.

Jørgen F.P. Wojtaszewski received his PhD from the University of Copenhagen in 1997. Postdoctoral positions at Joslin Diabetes Center and the Copenhagen Muscle Research Centre followed. In 2003, he obtained the prestigious Hallas Møller Research Stipend from the Novo Nordisk Foundation and in 2004 he also was appointed Associate Professor at the Copenhagen Muscle Research Centre, Institute of Exercise and Sports Science. He has published more than 60 original research papers and many reviews. **Erik A. Richter** is Professor of Physiology and Exercise Physiology at the Copenhagen Muscle Research Centre, Institute of Exercise and Sport Sciences, University of Copenhagen. He was one of the founders of the Copenhagen Muscle Research Centre and is currently head of the Department of Human Physiology, Institute of Exercise and Sport Sciences, University of Copenhagen. He has published more than 200 original research papers and many reviews.

Arend Bonen holds the Canada Research Chair in Metabolism and Health, and is a Professor in the Department of Human Health and Nutritional Sciences at the University of Guelph, Guelph Ontario, Canada. Work in his laboratory focuses on the molecular regulation of substrate transport and metabolism in skeletal muscle during exercise and in obesity and Type 2 diabetes. His research is supported by the Canadian Institutes of Health Research, the Heart and Stroke Foundation of Ontario and the Natural Sciences and Engineering Research Council of Canada. **G. Lynis Dohm** is a Distinguished Research Professor of Physiology at the Brody School of Medicine, East Carolina University, Greenville, NC. His research focuses on the metabolic changes that occur in skeletal muscle in response to exercise, obesity and diabetes. His research group has identified factors that lead to the increase in muscle glucose transport and GLUT4 glucose transporter protein in response to exercise, and has worked towards an understanding the causes of muscle insulin resistance in obesity. His work has been supported by the National Institutes of Health (USA). **Luc van Loon** is an Assistant Professor in the Department of Movement Sciences at Maastricht University, The Netherlands. His research focuses on human skeletal muscle metabolism, namely the adaptation to endurance and resistance exercise and the use of combined physical activity and/or dietary interventions to improve health in chronic metabolic diseases. He is also scientific co-ordinator of the Stable Isotope Research Center (SIRC) at the Academic Hospital Maastricht. His research is supported by The Netherlands Organization for Scientific Research (NWO), the Dutch Diabetes Research Foundation (DFN) and several industrial-research grants.

Keith Baar is the Director of the Functional Molecular Biology Laboratory and a lecturer in the Division of Molecular Physiology at the University of Dundee, Scotland, U.K. He received his PhD in Physiology from the University of Illinois Medical Center in Chicago before completing postdoctoral work at Washington University in St. Louis, University College London and the University of Michigan. His primary research goal is to understand how muscle size and phenotype are regulated and use this information to engineer functional heart and skeletal muscle *ex vivo*. **Gustavo Nader** is Research Associate in the Research Center for Genetic Medicine at the Children's National Medical Center (CNMC) in Washington D.C. He received his PhD in Kinesiology from the University of Illinois, Chicago, and post-doctoral education in genomics at CNMC. His primary research interest is to develop a physiological genomics approach to understand skeletal muscle adaptation, specifically the mechanisms controlling ribosome biogenesis during skeletal muscle growth. **Sue Bodine** is a Professor in the Section of Neurobiology, Physiology and Behavior at the University of California, Davis. She returned to academia in 2003 after spending 7 years in the biotechnology industry at Regeneron Pharmaceuticals, Inc and Elixir Pharmaceuticals, Inc, pursuing the development of drugs to treat muscle atrophy. She received her PhD in Muscle Biology from the University of California, Los Angeles and began her academic career in the Department of Orthopedics at the University of California, San Diego. Her primary research interests are in understanding the mechanisms that regulate skeletal muscle size under growth and atrophy conditions.

Michael Kjaer received an MD from the University of Copenhagen in 1984, after which his doctoral thesis (1988) investigated hormonal regulation during exercise. He has been Professor of Sports Medicine at the University of Copenhagen since 1998 and is head of a research group investigating the responses of muscle and connective tissue to exercise. **Flemming Dela** MD, DMSCi. is Professor in the Pathophysiology section at the Department of Medical Physiology, University of Copenhagen, Denmark. He has published 67 peer-reviewed original papers and 11 book chapters. Keywords to his main field of research are: exercise physiology, metabolism, diabetes, skeletal muscle and mitochondria.

Keith Frayn is Professor of Human Metabolism at the University of Oxford. He graduated from the University of Cambridge and studied for his PhD at St Bartholomew's Medical College, London, before working with the MRC Toxicology Unit and later the MRC Trauma Unit. He has been in Oxford since 1986, where he leads a research group with interests in fat metabolism in humans, studying both basic physiology and the pathophysiology of obesity, insulin resistance and Type 2 diabetes. Professor Frayn is author of the textbooks *Lipid Biochemistry: an Introduction* (5th edition, with M.I. Gurr and J.L. Harwood, Blackwell Science, 2002) and *Metabolic Regulation: a Human Perspective* (2nd edition, Blackwell Publishing 2003). **Peter Arner** is Professor of Medicine at Karolinska Institutet, from where he also graduated and studied for his PhD. He received specialist training as an MD at Karolinska University Hospital, Stockholm, Sweden, where he currently is senior physician in endocrinology and deputy chairman at the Department of Medicine. He has been at the Karolinska Institutet since 1963, and he leads a research group with interest in human adipose tissue, studying both basic mechanisms and pathophysiology of obesity, insulin resistance, Type 2 diabetes and dyslipidaemia. Professor Arner has published over 300 original research articles and is one of the most cited scientists in the obesity field according to the Institute of Scientific Information. **Hannele Yki-Järvinen** is Professor of Medicine at the Department of Medicine, University of Helsinki. She leads a research group with interest in causes and consequences of insulin resistance in humans. She has received several major international science awards and published over 200 original research articles and is author of textbook chapters in *International Textbook of Diabetes Mellitus* (3rd edition, John Wiley & Sons, 2004) and in *Textbook of Diabetes* (3rd edition, Blackwell Publishing, 2003).

Bente Klarlund Pedersen is a Professor at the University of Copenhagen. and senior consultant at Rigshospitalett, Copenhagen. She is the director of The Danish National Research Foundation Centre of Inflammation and Metabolism (CIM), where the main area of research is the molecular mechanisms involved in physical activity and how these benefit human health. Professor Pedersen has written more than 350 scientific articles and books, and appears as guest professor all over the world. She is President of the Research Council of Rigshospitalet, University of Copenhagen, leader of the Muscle Cluster at the Faculty of Health Sciences, University of Copenhagen and Chair of the National Council for Public Health.

Richard M. McAllister earned his BSc in Kinanthropology from the University of Ottawa, Ontario, Canada, his MA in Exercise Physiology from Ball State University in Muncie, IN, USA, and his PhD in Physiology from the State University of New York Health Science Center in Syracuse, NY, USA. After post-doctoral training at the University of Missouri, he moved to Kansas State University, where he attained the rank of Associate Professor in the Departments of Kinesiology and of Anatomy and Physiology. He then returned to the University of Missouri, where he is currently a Research Associate Professor in the Department of Biomedical Sciences.

M. Harold Laughlin earned his BA in Biology and Chemistry from Simpson College in Indianola, IA, USA and his PhD in Physiology and Biophysics from the University of Iowa College of Medicine in Iowa City. After post-doctoral training at the University of Iowa, he moved to the US Air Force School of Aerospace Medicine in San Antonio, TX. He then moved to Oral Roberts University in Tulsa, OK, where he attained the rank of Associate Professor of Physiology. He subsequently moved to the University of Missouri, where he is currently Professor and Chair of the Department of Biomedical Sciences.

Stephen Rattigan earned his degrees in biochemistry from the University of Western Australia, Perth. He then worked as a post-doctoral fellow at the Commonwealth Scientific and Industrial Research Organisation's (CSIRO) Division of Human Nutrition in Adelaide, South Australia, before moving to the Biochemistry Department, University of Tasmania, Hobart, as a research fellow. He spent three years as a visiting research scientist at the University of Virginia, Charlottesville, USA, and after returning to the University of Tasmania is now an Associate Professor and Australian Heart Foundation Career Fellow in Hobart. **Eloise Bradley** earned her degree at the University of Tasmania, where she is presently a research associate and post-graduate student. **Stephen M. Richards** earned his degrees in biochemistry from the University of Tasmania. He then worked as a post-doctoral fellow at the Baker Heart Research Institute and The Alfred Hospital in Melbourne, INSERM Unit 390 in Montpellier, France, and returned to Australia under a National Health and Medical Research Council (Australia) Howard Florey Centenary Research Fellowship, joining the Department of Physiology, University of Melbourne. He returned to University of Tasmania to take up a tenured lectureship in 1999. **Michael G. Clark** earned his degrees in biochemistry from the University of New South Wales. He then worked at the University of Wisconsin, Madison, as postdoctoral fellow before returning to Australia, first as Senior Lecturer at Flinders Medical School, Adelaide, then as Section Head of the CSIRO Division of Human Nutrition, Adelaide. He is currently the Professor and Head of the Biochemistry, University of Tasmania, and has been in this role since 1985.

Jefferson C. Frisbee is an Assistant Professor in the Department of Physiology and Pharmacology and is a core member of the Center for Interdisciplinary Research in Cardiovascular Sciences at West Virginia University School of Medicine. His research is currently funded by the National Institutes of Health and the American Heart Association, and focuses on the evolving impairments to vascular structure and function in the metabolic syndrome, the mechanistic bases of these myriad dysfunctions and how these impact the integrated regulation of blood flow control. His most recent work focuses on the regulation of microvessel density in the metabolic syndrome. **Michael D. Delp** is a Professor in the Division of Exercise Physiology and the Center for Interdisciplinary Research in Cardiovascular Sciences at West Virginia University School of Medicine. His research, funded by NASA and NIH, has focused on how physical deconditioning associated with old age, microgravity and diabetes alters smooth muscle and endothelial cell function of resistance arteries and, correspondingly, control of arterial pressure and tissue perfusion. In addition, the effects of how exercise training alters vascular cell signaling mechanisms to improve endothelial function and tissue blood flow are being investigated.

Gang Hu is a Senior Researcher and Docent at the Department of Epidemiology and Health Promotion of the National Public Health Institute, Helsinki, Finland, and at the Department of Public Health, University of Helsinki. **Timo A. Lakka** is a Professor of Medical Physiology, a Specialist in Internal Medicine and an Academy Research Fellow at the Institute of Biomedicine, Department of Physiology, University of Kuopio, Finland. He is also an Adjunct Associate Professor at Pennington Biomedical Research Center, Louisiana State University, USA. **Jaakko Tuomilehto** is a Professor at the Department of Epidemiology and Health Promotion, National Public Health Institute, Helsinki, and Professor of Public Health at the Department of Public Health, University of Helsinki. **Jesús Rico-Sanz** is an Associate Professor at the School of Human Performance and Recreation, School of Health of the University of Southern Mississippi. He obtained a BS in Exercise Physiology and MS in Exercise Science at the University of California at Davis, USA. His PhD in exercise physiology is from the August Krogh Institute, University of Copenhagen, Denmark. After completing his PhD, he held research positions at the Hammersmith Hospital, Imperial College London, UK, the University Autonoma of Barcelona, Spain, Pennington Biomedical Research Center in Louisiana, USA, the National Public Health Institute in Helsinki and the Department of Medicine at University of Kuopio. During the past 5 years, Dr Rico-Sanz has been involved in human genetic studies. He has performed genome scans on exercise capacity phenotypes as well as association studies of candidate genes with metabolic and disease marker phenotypes. His current research interests are the interactions of genes and exercise on the development of Type 2 diabetes, obesity and the metabolic syndrome.

In 1993, **Erik Serné** obtained his MD at the Vrije Universiteit in Amsterdam. He finished his thesis 'Essential hypertension and insulin resistance: role for microcirculatory function? in 2001' at the Vrije Universiteit Medical Centre (VUmc). He completed his specialization in internal medicine in 2006 and is presently working as a staff member of the Department of Internal Medicine. His field of expertise is the microvasculature and its role in the metabolic syndrome and cardiovascular disease. **Renate de Jongh** studied medicine at the Vrije Universiteit in Amsterdam, from where she graduated with honours in 2001. The subject of her subsequent research is microvascular function as a possible link in relationships among obesity, hypertension and insulin resistance, under the supervision of Coen Stehouwer at the VUmc. In 2004, she began her training in internal medicine. **Etto Eringa** studied biology at the University of Groningen, The Netherlands, graduating in 1999. Afterwards he worked at the Institute for Cardiovascular Research, Vrije Universiteit in Amsterdam, on insulin signalling in vascular endothelium and rat models of insulin resistance. In 2004, he was awarded a PhD by Vrije Universiteit for his thesis on 'Selective insulin resistance in the microcirculation: a new concept for studying microvascular function and insulin sensitivity'. Since then he has worked as a junior researcher in the Laboratory for Physiology at the same institute on physiological regulation of insulin signalling in vascular endothelium and regulation of blood pressure by phosphatidylinositol 3-kinase. **Richard G. Ijzerman** studied at the Vrije Universiteit in Amsterdam and he acquired his MD with honours in 1997. In 2004, he obtained a PhD at VUmc, the subject of which was 'Birth weight, microvascular function and cardiovascular risk factors'. In 2004, he started his residency in internal medicine at the VUmc. His particular field of interest relates to the subject of his thesis and also consists of the study of the role of genetic and/or intrauterine factors in cardiovascular risk factors. **Michiel de Boer** studied medicine at the Vrije Universiteit in Amsterdam and received his MD in 2003. Subsequently, he worked as a house officer in pulmonology at the Medical Center in Alkmaar, The Netherlands, and in internal medicine at the Westfries Gasthuis Hospital in Hoorn, The Netherlands. In 2005, he started research for a PhD on insulin's actions on skin and muscle microcirculation in hypertensive, obese and healthy subjects: a role for endothelin-1? **Coen Stehouwer** obtained his MD with honours at the Erasmus University in Rotterdam in 1985. After registering as an internist in 1990, he was awarded a PhD at VUmc in 1992 for his thesis 'Albuminuria and endothelial function in diabetes'. He was appointed Professor of Medicine at VUmc in 2000. From 1992 to 2004, he led the Diabetes and Vascular Medicine Research Programme at VUmc's Institute of Cardiovascular Research. In 2004, he was appointed Professor and Chair of Medicine at the University Hospital in Maastricht. His field of expertise is in the vascular complications of metabolic diseases, with particular emphasis on diabetes, hypertension and hyperhomocysteinaemia.

Anton Wagenmakers is Professor of Exercise Biochemistry in the School of Sport and Exercise Sciences, University of Birmingham, UK and occupies a chair at Eindhoven University of Technology to work on integrative mathematical models of metabolic regulation mechanisms. His main scientific interests are the therapeutic effect of exercise and lifestyle changes on metabolism and cardiovascular physiology in chronic diseases. He serves on the Executive Committee of the International Research Group of the Biochemistry of

Exercise and is member of the Scientific Board of the European College of Sport Sciences. **Natal van Riel** is Assistant Professor in the Department of Biomedical Engineering at Eindhoven University of Technology. He leads the Bioregulation and Systems Biology research programme, which is an inter-departmental programme involving the Departments of Biomedical Engineering and Electrical Engineering. He is a principal investigator with the Eindhoven Biomedical Systems Biology Platform. **Michael Frenneaux** is British Heart Foundation Chair of Cardiovascular Medicine at the University of Birmingham UK. He is a clinical cardiovascular physiologist whose main research focus on heart failure and heart-muscle diseases. His current research interests include cardiac energetic impairment in heart failure and insulin resistance, the consequences of metabolic modulation in heart failure, cardiomyopathies and insulin resistance, diastolic ventricular interaction, the physiological control of capacitance vessels, the pathophysiology of heart failure with normal left ventricular ejection fraction, and the mechanisms responsible for increased cardiovascular risk in depression. **Paul Michael Stewart** is Professor of Medicine in the Department of Medicine, joint director of The Wellcome Trust Clinical Research Facility and Associate Dean for Clinical Research at the University of Birmingham's Medical School. His research specialties include reproductive endocrinology, steroid hormone metabolism, mineralocorticoids, glucocorticoids and endocrine hypertension. Specifically, Professor Stewart is head of a research group that explores the hypothesis that altered cortisol metabolism might underpin diverse diseases, including hypertension, obesity-glucose tolerance, glaucoma, malignancy and bone disease, and may cause foetal problems, such as growth restriction. Professor Stewart serves on committees for the Medical Research Council, The Wellcome Trust and the British Heart Foundation.

Abbreviations

ACC	acetyl-CoA carboxylase
ACE	angiotensin I-converting enzyme
ADR	adrenergic receptor
AGE	advanced glycation end-products
AICAR	5-aminoimidazole-4-carboxamide-1-β-D-ribonucleoside
Akt/PKB	protein kinase B
AMPK	AMP-activated protein kinase
ANF	atrial natriuretic factor
APS	adaptor proteins
AS160	Akt substrate of 160 kDa
ATGL	adipose triglyceride lipase
BAT	brown adipose tissue
BH_4	tetrahydrobiopterin
BMI	body mass index
BNF	brain natriuretic factor
CaMK	calcium/calmodulin-dependent protein kinase
CAP	c-Cbl associated protein
CARDIA Study	Coronary Artery Risk Development in Young Adults
cdk	cyclin-dependent protein kinase
CEU	contrast-enhanced ultrasound
COX	cytochrome c oxidase
CPT	carnitine palmitoyltransferase
CRE	cAMP response element
CREB	cAMP response element-binding protein
CRP	C-reactive protein
DDP	deafness/dystonia peptide
DNL	*de novo* lipogenesis
DPP	Diabetes Prevention Program
DPS	Diabetes Prevention Study
Drp-1	dynamin-related protein 1
4E-BP	eIF4E binding protein
E1	ubiquitin-activating enzyme
E2	ubiquitin-conjugating enzyme
E3	ubiquitin ligase
EDHF	endothelium-derived hyperpolarizing factor

EGP	endogenous glucose production
eIF	eukaryotic initiation factor
eNOS	endothelial NOS
ERK	extracellular signal-related kinase
ET	endothelin
FABP	fatty acid binding protein
FABPpm	fatty acid binding protein in the plasma membrane
FAT	fatty acid translocase
FATP	fatty acid transport protein
Fis-1	mitochondrial fission protein
FOXO	forkhead transcription factor
GAP	GTPase-activating protein
GH	growth hormone
GLUT4	glucose transporter 4
GMEB	glucocorticoid modulatory element binding protein
GS	glycogen synthase
GSK3	glycogen synthase kinase 3
HbA1c	haemoglobin A1c
HDL	high-density lipoprotein
HK	hexokinase
HL	hepatic lipase
HSL	hormone-sensitive lipase
IGF-1	insulin-like growth factor-1
IL	interleukin
IL-6R	IL-6 receptor
IL-1ra	interleukin-1 receptor antagonist
IMCL	intra-myocellular lipid
iNOS	inducible NOS
IR	insulin receptor
IRS-1	insulin receptor substrate-1
IκK	IκB kinase
JNK	c-Jun N-terminal kinase
LAR	leukocyte antigen related phosphatase
LDL	low-density lipoprotein
LEPR	leptin receptor
L-NAME	N^{ω}-nitro-L-arginine methyl ester
LPL	lipoprotein lipase
MAFbx	muscle atrophy F-box protein/atrogen-1
MAPK	mitogen-activated protein kinase
MEF2	myocyte enhancer factor 2
Mfn	mitofusin
MGF	mechano growth factor

MHC	myosin heavy chain
mtDNA	mitochondrial DNA
mTOR	mammalian target of rapamycin
MuRF	muscle ring finger protein
1-MX	1-methylxanthine
NEFA	non-esterified fatty acid
NF-κB	nuclear factor-κB
NHANES	National Health and Nutrition Examination Survey
nNOS	neuronal NOS
NO	nitric oxide
NOS	nitric oxide synthase
NRF	nuclear respiratory factor
OZR	obese Zucker rat
PCr	phosphocreatine
PDK	phosphoinositol-dependent protein kinase
PGC-1α	peroxisome proliferator activated receptor γ coactivator-1α
PGH	prostaglandin H_2
PI3K	phosphatidylinositol 3-kinase
PIP3	phosphatidylinositol-3,4,5-trisphosphate
PKA	protein kinase A
PKB	protein kinase B
PKC	protein kinase C
PPAR	peroxisome-proliferator-activated receptor
PS	capillary permeability-surface area product
PTEN	phosphatase and tensin homologue deleted on chromosome 10
PTP	protein tyrosine phosphatase
ROS	reactive oxygen species
S6K1	ribosomal S6 protein kinase
SH2	Src (Sarcoma virus protein) homology-2
SHIP	SH2-containing inositol phosphatase 2
siRNA	small interfering RNA
SRF	serum response factor
sTNF-R	soluble TNF-α-receptor
T2D	type 2 diabetes
TEA	tetraethylammonium chloride
Tfam	mitochondrial transcription factor A
TFB	mitochondrial transcription factor B
TG	triacylglycerol
TIM	translocases of the inner membrane
TNF	tumour necrosis factor

TOM	translocases of the outer membrane
5′TOP	5′ terminal oligopyrimidine tract
TORC	mTOR complex
TR	thyroid receptor
TxA_2	thromboxane A_2
TZD	thiazolidinedione
UBF	upstream binding factor
UCP1	uncoupling protein 1
VCAM-1	vascular cell adhesion molecule-1
VDR	vitamin D receptor
VLDL	very-low-density lipoprotein
VNTR	variable number of tandem repeats
VSM	vascular smooth muscle
WAT	white adipose tissue

1

Signalling mechanisms in skeletal muscle: role in substrate selection and muscle adaptation

John A. Hawley[*][1], Mark Hargreaves[†] and Juleen R. Zierath[‡]

Exercise Metabolism Group, School of Medical Sciences, RMIT University, Bundoora 3083, Australia, †Department of Physiology, The University of Melbourne, 3010, Australia, and ‡Karolinska Institute, Department Molecular Medicine and Surgical Sciences, Section of Integrative Physiology, Stockholm, Sweden.

Abstract

Exercise produces a multitude of time- and intensity-dependent physiological, biochemical and molecular changes within skeletal muscle. With the onset of contractile activity, cytosolic and mitochondrial [Ca^{2+}] levels are rapidly increased and, depending on the relative intensity of the exercise, metabolite concentrations change (i.e. increases in [ADP] and [AMP], decreases in muscle creatine phosphate and glycogen). These contraction-induced metabolic disturbances activate several key kinases and phosphatases involved in signal transduction. Important among these are the calcium-dependent signalling pathways that respond to elevated Ca^{2+} concentrations (including Ca^{2+}/calmodulin-dependent kinase, Ca^{2+}-dependent protein kinase C and the Ca^{2+}/calmodulin-dependent phosphatase calcineurin), the 5′-adenosine monophosphate-activated protein kinase, several of the mitogen-activated

[1]*To whom correspondence should be addressed email (john.hawley@rmit.edu.au).*

protein kinases and protein kinase B/Akt. The role of these signal transducers in the regulation of carbohydrate and fat metabolism in response to increased contractile activity has been the focus of intense research efforts during the past decade.

Introduction

Skeletal muscle ATP stores are small and would be consumed in several seconds of maximal contraction if not rapidly replenished. Without a rapid resynthesis of ATP, skeletal muscle would be incapable of initiating any further contraction. Hence, the metabolic pathways that synthesize ATP must have the capacity to respond immediately to an increased demand for ATP that can increase 100-fold above resting requirements during intense physical activity. In most situations a precise matching of ATP demand and resynthesis is accomplished to maintain skeletal muscle ATP concentrations. To accomplish this, marked changes in metabolism occur in skeletal muscle including increased glycogen breakdown, glycolysis, glucose uptake and fatty acid oxidation. A fundamental goal of exercise biochemistry is to understand the mechanism(s) by which perturbations in energy status are monitored inside contracting muscle cells and to identify molecules that are regulated to increase fuel substrate supply in order to maintain ATP levels. In addition, many of these (acute) signals initiate responses that form the basis of the metabolic adaptations to regular exercise training. This chapter will focus on the cellular and molecular mechanisms governing fuel utilization and metabolic adaptations in human skeletal muscle during and after endurance exercise.

Integration of the metabolic responses to exercise

Important intramuscular metabolic signals responsible for the activation and coordination of the various energy-producing pathways during exercise include alterations in $[Ca^{2+}]$, changes in the concentrations of metabolites related to the cytoplasmic phosphorylation potential of the muscle cell and the mitochondrial reduction/oxidation (redox) state of [NAD]/[NADH] [1]. Ca^{2+} release plays an essential role in initiating muscle contraction and activating metabolism via a 'feed-forward' mechanism. Calcium provides the trigger for force development and ATP hydrolysis and contributes to the activation of glycogenolysis and possibly oxidative phosphorylation. A rise in intracellular $[Ca^{2+}]$ levels also contributes to the regulation of glucose uptake during muscle contraction, by activating a signal transduction pathway leading to GLUT-4 (glucose transporter 4) translocation. Several other contraction-induced signalling intermediates [i.e. PKC (protein kinase C)] and the MAPK (mitogen-activated protein kinase) cascades] are also sensitive to changes in $[Ca^{2+}]$ and are likely to mediate exercise-induced responses, that may include glucose and lipid metabolism or gene regulatory events.

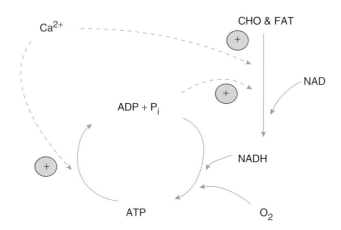

Figure 1. The major metabolic signals in the activation and coordination of the various energy-producing pathways in skeletal muscle during exercise
CHO, carbohydrate; P_i, inorganic phosphate. Reprinted from [33]. © 2002 Lippincott Williams & Wilkins; reproduced with permission.

Whilst Ca^{2+}-activated signals are important for early events in excitation–contraction coupling and the stimulation of metabolic pathways, the concentrations of metabolites related to the cytoplasmic phosphorylation potential of skeletal muscle (i.e. [ATP]/[ADP][P_i]) provide feedback signals necessary to balance ATP production with ATP consumption (Figure 1). Changes in the concentrations of metabolites in the phosphagen pool provide the main stimulus for increased oxidative phosphorylation and are necessary (but not sufficient) for full activation of glycolytic ATP synthesis during intense (≥85% of maximal aerobic power [V_{O_2}max]) sustained exercise. The redox state of the skeletal muscle activates numerous reactions in substrate/product or activator/inhibitor capacities. All three types of signal are important in coordinating the expression of enzymes that are vital for ATP production in mitochondrial and cytoplasmic compartments during exercise [1]. Along with systemic factors, such as increased blood flow leading to increased delivery of oxygen and hormonal factors, intramuscular and extramuscular substrate availability and the local release of growth factors and cytokines from contracting muscle, these signals provide the framework in which fuel mobilization and utilization are increased and intracellular signal transduction to the transcriptional machinery in the nucleus is enhanced, thereby modulating gene expression and ultimately protein turnover.

Signalling pathways during exercise

The relative importance of various putative signalling pathways in the acute regulation of metabolism in response to exercise and chronic metabolic adaptations to exercise training has been the focus of considerable research

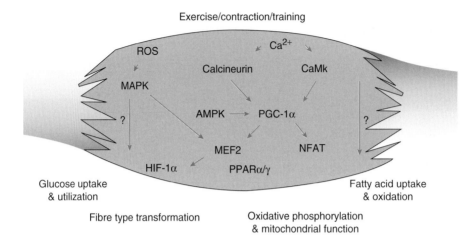

Figure 2. Putative cellular and molecular mechanisms governing fuel utilization and metabolic adaptations in human skeletal muscle during and after endurance exercise
HIF, hypoxia inducible factor; MEF2, myocyte enhancer factor 2; NFAT, nuclear factor of activated T-cells; PGC-1α, peroxisome-proliferator-activated receptor-γ coactivator-1α; PPAR, peroxisome-proliferator-activated receptor; ROS, reactive oxygen species. Reprinted from [36].

efforts in recent years. Some of the major pathways are summarized in Figure 2 and are discussed subsequently.

There has also been much interest in the interactions between the insulin and contraction-signalling pathways within skeletal muscle. Whilst these pathways independently activate metabolic processes (e.g. GLUT4 protein translocation and glucose uptake, Figure 3), enhanced insulin action is a well described effect of acute and chronic exercise, suggesting communication between these pathways. Further work is required to elucidate the underlying mechanisms to explain such phenomena.

Calcium-dependent signalling

The increase in sarcoplasmic [Ca^{2+}] levels during exercise has a fundamental role in excitation–contraction coupling, stimulation of ATP-generating metabolic pathways and activation of transcriptional responses (Figure 4). Calcium-dependent signalling pathways include CaMK (Ca^{2+}/calmodulin-dependent kinase), PKC (Ca^{2+}-dependent protein kinase C) isoforms and the Ca^{2+}/calmodulin-dependent phosphatase calcineurin. A number of CaMK isoforms have been identified, but CaMK II appears to be the dominant isoform expressed in skeletal muscle [2]. Exercise increases CaMK II activity in human skeletal muscle [3], with the magnitude of the increase during very high-intensity (approx. 100% VO$_2$max) exercise being greater than that during moderately high-intensity (approx. 75% VO$_2$max) exercise. Early studies in rat muscle demonstrated increased PKC activity with electrical stimulation, consistent with activation of conventional and novel PKC isoforms

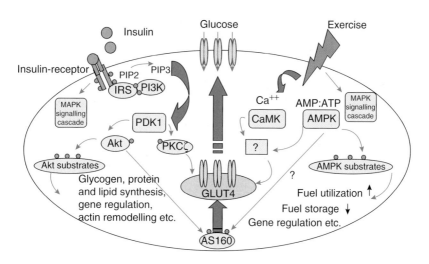

Figure 3. Insulin and exercise signalling in skeletal muscle control pathways governing fuel utilization and storage and gene expression
AS160, Akt substrate of 160 kDa; IRS, insulin receptor substrate; PDK, phosphoinositide dependent kinase; PI3K, phosphoinositide 3-kinase.

by contraction-induced increases in Ca^{2+} and diacylglycerol [4]. Recent studies in humans suggest that the increase in total PKC activity in skeletal muscle following exercise may be the result of activation of the atypical PKC isoforms [5,6]. We are unaware of any studies that have examined the effects of exercise on calcineurin activity in skeletal muscle.

Calcium binds directly to and activates phosphorylase kinase, which in turn transforms phosphorylase to an active form, thereby contributing to enhanced glycogenolysis in skeletal muscle during exercise. Further stimulation of glycogenolysis is provided by increases in inorganic phosphate, AMP and ADP. Calcium has long been recognized to also increase glucose uptake, although the specific signalling intermediates are unresolved [7]. Inhibition of CaMK reduced glucose uptake by approx. 50% during contraction of epitrochlearis muscles *in vitro* [8] and completely abolished the increase in glucose uptake during tetanic contractions in soleus muscle [9]. The PKC inhibitor calphostin C attenuates the contraction-induced increase in skeletal muscle glucose uptake [4]. In addition, PKC is believed to regulate the activation of HSL (hormone-sensitive lipase), a key enzyme in the degradation of intramuscular triglyceride [10]. Finally, increased Ca^{2+} results in transcriptional activation of numerous genes involved in mitochondrial biogenesis and muscle hypertrophy [2]. All of the Ca^{2+}-dependent signalling pathways are believed to be involved in metabolic and gene regulatory events to some extent. For example, CaMK inhibition abolishes Ca^{2+}-induced mitochondrial biogenesis [11], PKC has been implicated in increased cytochrome c expression following Ca^{2+} stimulation [2] and calcineurin has a role in determining skeletal muscle fibre type [12].

AMP-activated protein kinase

A key pathway in skeletal muscle that responds to changes in the concentrations of metabolites related to the cytoplasmic phosphorylation potential is AMPK (AMP-activated protein kinase). This kinase appears to be a key sensor of skeletal muscle energy status [13]. AMPK exists as a heterotrimer consisting of α, β and γ subunits. The α subunit of AMPK, of which there are two known isoforms (α1 and α2), contains the catalytic domain that transfers a high-energy phosphate from ATP to serine and threonine residues on a number of different target proteins. In addition, the α subunit contains a specific threonine residue (Thr[172]) that functions as an activating phosphorylation site for several upstream kinases. The α2 isoform is abundant in skeletal muscle and is more sensitive to changes in AMP than the α1 isoform. The β and γ regulatory subunits are essential for full enzymatic activity and multiple isoforms of β (β1 and β2) and γ (γ1, γ2 and γ3) exist. Submaximal exercise in humans primarily increases AMPK α2 activity in skeletal muscle [14,15], although intense exercise can increase AMPK α1 activity [16]. The increased AMPK activity during exercise is attenuated by elevated pre-exercise muscle glycogen availability [17], further emphasizing the role of AMPK as a fuel/energy sensor.

There has been considerable interest in the potential role of AMPK in stimulating muscle glucose uptake during exercise/contractions [4,7,18]. Such interest arises from observations that AICAR (5-aminoimidazole-4-carboxamide riboside), a compound taken up by skeletal muscle and metabolized to ZMP (an analogue of AMP), which is an activator of AMPK, enhances glucose transport in rat skeletal muscle [7,8]. AICAR has been used as a pharmacological tool to activate the 'exercise-responsive' pathway to glucose transport. Approaches in functional genomics reveal that AMPK is necessary and sufficient for AICAR induced glucose transport [18]. Ablation of either the AMPK α2 or γ3 subunit, or overexpression of a kinase dead AMPK α2 mutant rendered skeletal muscle insensitive to AICAR on glucose uptake [18]. Consistent with this, skeletal muscle specific deletion of LKB1, the putative upstream AMPK kinase, largely abolished the contraction-induced increase in AMPK activation and glucose uptake [13]. However, contraction-induced glucose transport was only reduced approx. 40% in skeletal muscles from transgenic mice with the kinase dead AMPK α2 mutant and was normal in both α1 and α2 whole-body knockout mice [13] and AMPK γ3 knockout mice [18] despite complete abolition of the AICAR response in all models. Finally, in rats AMPK was shown not to be necessary for slow twitch soleus muscle glucose transport during contractions *in vitro* [9]. Collectively, these results suggest that there are factors in addition to AMPK that regulate skeletal muscle uptake during exercise.

AMPK promotes fatty acid oxidation in skeletal muscle during exercise by inhibiting ACC-β (acetyl-CoA carboxylase) and activating malonyl-CoA, thus removing inhibition of mitochondrial fatty acyl-CoA translocation by

CPT-1 (carnitine palmitoyltransferase-1). A number of studies have reported that these exercise-induced effects on ACC-β and malonyl-CoA are closely paralleled by activation of AMPK [19,20] especially the α2 isoform when isoform-specific activity has been determined [20]. Effects of exercise intensity on AMPK signalling and whole-body rates of fat oxidation in humans have been determined [21]. With low- (approx. 40% V_{O_2}max) to moderate- (approx. 60% V_{O_2}max) intensity cycling, AMPK α1 (1.5-fold) and AMPK α2 (5-fold) activities were increased, with a further increase in AMPK α2 activity during high-intensity compared with moderate-intensity exercise. Rates of whole-body fat oxidation increased from rest to low intensity exercise and paralleled the increases in ACC-β phosphorylation. As expected, rates of fat oxidation declined during high-intensity exercise, despite a further increase in AMPK activity and ACC-β phosphorylation [21]. AMPK opposes the adrenergic stimulation of skeletal muscle HSL activity during exercise, but HSL activity is dissociated from intramuscular triglyceride hydrolysis, suggesting the possible involvement of other skeletal muscle lipases [10]. Following short-term exercise training, there remains a robust increase in glucose uptake and fat oxidation during exercise, despite an almost complete blunting of the increase in AMPK α2 activity [22]. These findings challenge the role of AMPK in the regulation of carbohydrate and fat metabolism during exercise in humans.

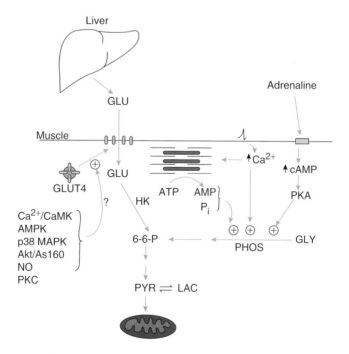

Figure 4. Overview of putative metabolic signals regulating carbohydrate metabolism in skeletal muscle during exercise
AS160, Akt substrate of 160 kDa; GLU, glucose; GLY, glycogen; HK, hexokinase; LAC, lactate; PHOS, glycogen phosphorylase; PYR, pyruvate.

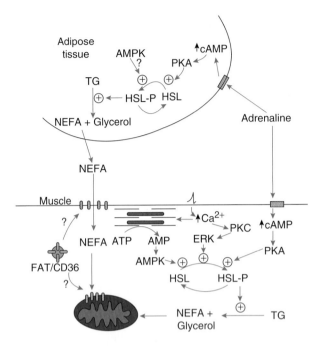

Figure 5. Overview of putative metabolic signals regulating lipid metabolism in adipose tissue and skeletal muscle during exercise
FAT/CD36, fatty acid translocase/CD36; NEFA, non-esterified fatty acid; TG, triglyceride.

Pharmacological activation of AMPK by AICAR increases protein expression of GLUT4, hexokinase and several oxidative enzymes, as well as mitochondrial density and muscle glycogen content [23,24]. However, the exercise-induced increase in transcription or mRNA abundance of selected metabolic genes was unchanged between α-AMPK knockout mice and wild-type mice [25], suggesting that AMPK is insufficient and that other pathways also contribute to transcriptional activation by exercise (e.g. CaMK, MAPK).

MAPKs

The MAPK signal transduction cascade has been identified as a candidate system that converts contraction-induced biochemical perturbations into appropriate intracellular responses [1,26]. Exercise is a powerful and rapid activator of several MAPK isoforms including the ERK (extracellular signal-regulated kinases)1/2 and the two stress-activated protein kinases, p38 MAPK and JNK (c-Jun NH_2-terminal kinase) [27]. Local and systemic factors mediate phosphorylation of MAPK signalling cascades [27] that are implicated in exercise metabolism and transcriptional regulation of important genes [26]. The p38 MAPK pathway has been implicated in the contraction-induced activation of muscle glucose uptake, whilst the role of ERK is equivocal [4]. Increased ERK activity may contribute to increased skeletal muscle HSL activity during exercise [10]. Exercise-induced activation of the p38 MAPK pathway has recently been demonstrated to play a role in skeletal muscle adaptation by promoting specific co-activators involved in mitochondrial biogenesis and slow muscle fibre formation [28]. MAPK activation can result not only in the production of transcription factors mediating gene expression, but can also stimulate the activity of the translational stage of protein synthesis.

PKB/Akt

The protein kinase B/Akt is a serine/threonine kinase with three isoforms (Akt1, Akt2 and Akt3) that share >80% homology. Akt 1 and Akt 2 are the predominant isoforms expressed in skeletal muscle. This protein kinase family has been implicated as an important target for mediating insulin action on glycogen synthesis, GLUT4 translocation and glucose transport and gene regulatory responses [29]. Many, but not all studies have reported that skeletal muscle contraction increases Akt activity or phosphorylation [7]. The time course of contraction-stimulated glucose transport and Akt activation are similar, suggestive of a role for Akt in signalling glucose transport into exercising muscle. However, when contraction-stimulated Akt phosphorylation and activity are inhibited, glucose transport is unaffected, suggesting that Akt does not function to increase contraction-induced glucose transport [7]. Several Akt substrates have been identified as putative links between insulin signalling and metabolic or gene regulatory responses. A novel 160 kDa signalling-protein has been identified and characterized as an Akt substrate (AS160) in 3T3-L1 adipocytes and skeletal muscle. AS160 is phosphorylated in rat skeletal muscle in response to contraction [30] and also in human skeletal muscle in response to exercise [31]. Whilst contraction-induced AS160 phosphorylation in isolated skeletal muscle was completely abolished by wortmannin [30], glucose uptake was not inhibited by this agent. Future studies are warranted to identify and characterize the multiple exercise-responsive Akt substrates in skeletal muscle.

Adrenergic signalling

The increase in sympathoadrenal activity that occurs during exercise, particularly at higher exercise intensities, has an important role in substrate mobilization and utilization (Figure 5). Adrenaline stimulates muscle glycogenolysis [32] and HSL activity [10] via the β-adrenergic receptor and activation of protein kinase A. The importance of adrenaline and sympathetic noradrenergic activity in the mobilization of liver glycogen during exercise is equivocal, but they are crucial for adipose tissue lipolysis and the mobilization of fatty acids into the blood stream [33]. A blunting of sympathoadrenal activity during exercise is a key factor mediating altered substrate metabolism following exercise training [34]. Adrenergic blockade is associated with increased fatigue and reduced exercise tolerance, but does not appear to prevent the training-induced increase in muscle oxidative capacity [35].

Conclusion

One fundamental goal of exercise biochemistry is to characterize the mechanism(s) by which changes in energy status are monitored in skeletal muscle during periods of increased demand and to identify the specific molecular pathways (and downstream targets) that are regulated to increase fuel provision and maintain ATP levels. Linking specific signalling cascades to defined metabolic responses and changes in gene expression that occur after exercise will be complicated because there is a high degree of cross-talk between many of these pathways, with feedback regulation, transient activation and redundancy.

Summary

- *The main intramuscular metabolic signals responsible for the activation and coordination of the various energy-producing pathways during exercise are alterations in [Ca^{2+}], changes in the concentrations of metabolites related to the cytoplasmic phosphorylation potential of the muscle cell and the mitochondrial reduction/oxidation (redox) state of [NAD]/[NADH].*
- *Calcium-dependent signalling pathways include CaMK, PKC isoforms and the Ca^{2+}/calmodulin-dependent phosphatase calcineurin. A number of CaMK isoforms have been identified, but CaMK II appears to be the dominant isoform expressed in skeletal muscle.*
- *A key pathway in skeletal muscle that responds to changes in the concentrations of metabolites related to the cytoplasmic phosphorylation potential is AMPK. This kinase appears to be a key sensor of skeletal muscle energy status.*
- *Submaximal exercise in humans increases AMPK α2 activity in skeletal muscle whereas intense exercise also increases AMPK α1 activity.*
- *Exercise is a powerful and rapid activator of several MAPKs including ERK1/2 and the two stress-activated protein kinases, p38 MAPK and JNK. Local and systemic factors mediate phosphorylation of MAPK signalling cascades implicated in exercise metabolism and transcriptional regulation of important genes.*
- *The protein kinase B/Akt is a serine/threonine kinase with two isoforms (Akt1 and Akt2) that have been implicated as an important target for mediating insulin action on glycogen synthesis, GLUT4 translocation and glucose transport and gene regulatory responses in skeletal muscle.*

References

1. Hawley, J.A. & Zierath, J.R. (2004) Integration of metabolic and mitogenic signal transduction in skeletal muscle. *Exerc. Sport Sci. Rev.* **32**, 4–8
2. Chin, E.R. (2005) Role of Ca^{2+}/calmodulin-dependent kinases in skeletal muscle plasticity. *J. Appl. Physiol.* **99**, 414–423

3. Rose, A.J. & Hargreaves, M. (2003) Exercise increases Ca^{2+}/calmodulin-dependent kinase II activity in human skeletal muscle. *J. Physiol.* **553**, 303–309

4. Richter, E.A., Nielsen, J.N., Jørgensen, S.B., Frøsig, C. & Wojtaszewski, J.F.P. (2003) Signalling to glucose transport in skeletal muscle during exercise. *Acta Physiol. Scand.* **178**, 329–335

5. Perrini, S., Henriksson, J., Zierath, J.R. & Widegren, U. (2004) Exercise-induced protein kinase C isoform-specific activation in human skeletal muscle. *Diabetes* **53**, 21–24

6. Rose, A.J., Michell, B.J., Kemp, B.E. & Hargreaves, M. (2004) Effect of exercise on protein kinase C activity and localization in human skeletal muscle. *J. Physiol.* **561**, 861–870

7. Jessen, N. & Goodyear, L.J. (2005) Contraction signalling to glucose transport in skeletal muscle. *J. Appl. Physiol.* **99**, 330–337

8. Wright, D.C., Hucker, K.A., Holloszy, J.O. & Han, D.H. (2004) Ca^{2+} and AMPK both mediate stimulation of glucose transport by muscle contractions. *Diabetes* **53**, 330–335

9. Wright, D.C., Geiger, P., Holloszy, J.O. & Han, D.-H. (2005) Contraction- and hypoxia-stimulated glucose transport is mediated by a Ca^{2+}-dependent mechanism in slow-twitch rat soleus muscle. *Am. J. Physiol. Endocrin. Metab.* **288**, E1062–E1066

10. Watt, M.J., Steinberg, G.R., Chan, S., Garnham, A., Kemp, B.E. & Febbraio, M.A. (2004) β-Adrenergic stimulation of skeletal muscle HSL can be overridden by AMPK signalling. *FASEB J.* **18**, 1445–1446

11. Ojuka, E.O., Jones, T.E., Han, D.-H., Chen, M. & Holloszy, J.O. (2003) Raising Ca^{2+} in L6 myotubes mimics effects of exercise on mitochondrial biogenesis in muscle. *FASEB J.* **17**, 675–681

12. Olson, E.N. & Williams, R.S. (2000) Remodeling muscles with calcineurin. *BioEssays* **22**, 510–519

13. Hardie, D.G. & Sakamoto, K. (2006) AMPK: a key sensor of fuel and energy status in skeletal muscle. *Physiology* **21**, 48–60

14. Fujii, N., Hayashi, T., Hirshman, M.F., Smith, J.T., Habinowski, S.A., Kaijser, L., Mu, J., Ljungqvist, O., Birnbaum, M.J., Witters, L.A. et al. (2000) Exercise induces isoform-specific increase in 5′ AMP-activated protein kinase activity in human skeletal muscle. *Biochem. Biophys. Res. Commun.* **273**, 1150–1155

15. Wojtaszewski, J.F.P., Nielsen, P., Hansen, B.F., Richter, E.A. & Kiens, B. (2000) Isoform-specific and exercise-intensity dependent activation of 5′-AMP-activated protein kinase in human skeletal muscle. *J. Physiol.* **528**, 221–226

16. Chen, Z.-P., McConell, G.K., Michell, B.J., Snow, R.J., Canny, B.J. & Kemp, B.E. (2000) AMPK signalling in contracting human skeletal muscle: acetyl-CoA carboxylase and NO synthase phosphorylation. *Am. J. Physiol. Endocrin. Metab.* **279**, E1202–E1206

17. Wojtaszewski, J.F., MacDonald, C., Nielsen, J.N., Hellsten, Y., Hardie, D.G., Kemp, B.E., Kiens, B., & Richter, E.A. (2003) Regulation of 5′AMP-activated protein kinase activity and substrate utilization in exercising human skeletal muscle. *Am. J. Physiol. Endocrinol. Metab.* **284**, E813–E822

18. Barnes B.B. & Zierath J.R. (2005) Role of AMP-activated protein kinase in the control of glucose homeostasis. *Curr. Mol. Medicine* **5**, 341–348

19. Rasmussen, B.B. & Winder, W.W. (1997) Effect of exercise intensity on skeletal muscle malonyl-CoA and acetyl-CoA carboxylase. *J. Appl. Physiol.* **83**, 1104–1109

20. Yu, M., Stepto, N.K., Chibalin, A.V., Fryer, L.G., Carling, D., Krook, A., Hawley, J.A. & Zierath, J.R. (2003) Metabolic and mitogenic signal transduction in human skeletal muscle after intense cycling exercise. *J. Physiol.* **546**, 327–335

21. Chen, Z.-P., Stephens, T.J., Murthy, S., Canny, B.J., Hargreaves, M., Witters, L.A., Kemp, B.E. & McConell, G.K. (2003) Effect of exercise intensity on skeletal muscle AMPK signalling in humans. *Diabetes* **52**, 2205–2212

22. McConell, G.K., Lee-Young, R.S., Chen, Z.-P., Stepto, N.K., Huynh, N.N., Stephens, T.J., Canny, B.J. & Kemp, B.E. (2005) Short-term exercise training in humans reduces AMPK signalling during prolonged exercise independent of muscle glycogen. *J. Physiol.* **568**, 665–676

23. Holmes, B.F., Kurth-Kraczek, E.J. & Winder, W.W. (1999) Chronic activation of 5′-AMP-activated protein kinase increases GLUT-4, hexokinase and glycogen in muscle. *J. Appl. Physiol.* **87**, 1990–1995

24. Winder, W.W., Holmes, B.F., Rubink, D.S., Jensen, E.B., Chen, M. & Holloszy, J.O. (2000)
     Activation of AMP-activated protein kinase increases mitochondrial enzymes in skeletal
     muscle. *J. Appl. Physiol.* **88**, 2219–2226

25. Jørgensen, S.B., Wojtaszewski, J.F.P., Viollet, B., Andreeli, F., Birk, J.B., Hellsten, Y., Schjerling,
     P., Vaulont, S., Neufer, P.D., Richter, E.A. & Pilegaard, H. (2005) Effects of α-AMPK knockout on
     exercise-induced gene activation in mouse skeletal muscle. *FASEB J.* **19**, 1146–1148

26. Long, Y.C., Widegren, U. & Zierath, J.R. (2004) Exercise-induced mitogen-activated protein kinase
     signalling in skeletal muscle. *Proc. Nutr. Soc.* **63**, 227–232

27. Widegren, U., Jiang, X.J., Krook, A., Chibalin, A.V., Bjornholm, M., Tally, M., Roth, R.A., Henriksson,
     J., Wallberg-Henriksson, H. & Zierath, J.R. (1998). Divergent effects of exercise on metabolic and
     mitogenic signalling pathways in human skeletal muscle. *FASEB J.* **12**, 1379–1389

28. Akimoto, T., Pohnert, S.C., Li, P., Zhang, M., Gumbs, C., Rosenberg, P.B., Williams, R.S. & Yan,
     Z. (2005). Exercise stimulates PGC-1α transcription in skeletal muscle through activation of the
     p38 MAPK pathway. *J. Biol. Chem.* **280**, 19587–19593

29. Whiteman, E.L., Cho, H. & Birnbaum, M.J. (2002) Role of Akt/protein kinase B in metabolism.
     Trends Endocrinol. Metab. **13**, 444–451

30. Bruss, M.D., Arias, E.B., Lienhard, G.E. & Cartee, G.D. (2005) Increased phosphorylation of Akt
     substrate of 160 kDa (AS160) in rat skeletal muscle in response to insulin or contractile activity.
     Diabetes **54**, 41–50

31. Deshmukh, A., Coffey, V.G., Zhong, Z., Chibalin, A.V., Hawley, J.A. & Zierath, J.R. (2006)
     Exercise-induced phosphorylation of the novel Akt substrates AS160 and filamin A in human skel-
     etal muscle. *Diabetes* **55**, 1776–1782

32. Watt, M.J., Howlett, K.F., Febbraio, M.A., Spriet, L.L. & Hargreaves, M. (2001) Adrenaline increases
     skeletal muscle glycogenolysis, pyruvate dehydrogenase activation and carbohydrate oxidation
     during moderate exercise in humans. *J. Physiol.* **534**, 269–278

33. Spriet, L.L. (2002) Regulation of skeletal muscle fat oxidation during exercise in humans. *Med. Sci.
     Sports Exerc.* **34**, 1477–1484

34. Brooks, G.A & Mercier, J. (1994) Balance of carbohydrate and lipid utilization during exercise: the
     'crossover concept'. *J. Appl. Physiol.* **76**, 2253–2261

35. Svedenhag, J., Henriksson, J. & Juhlin-Dannfelt, A. (1984) β-Adrenergic blockade and training in
     human subjects: effects on muscle metabolic capacity. *Am. J. Physiol.* **247**, E305–E311

36. Zierath, J.R. & Hawley, J.A. (2004) Skeletal muscle fiber type: influence on contractile and
     metabolic properties. *PLoS Biol.* **2**, e348

2

Control of gene expression and mitochondrial biogenesis in the muscular adaptation to endurance exercise

Anna-Maria Joseph*, Henriette Pilegaard†,
Anastassia Litvintsev‡, Lotte Leick† and
David A. Hood*‡[1]

*Department of Biology, York University, Toronto, Ontario,
Canada, M3J 1P3, †Copenhagen Muscle Research Centre, University
of Copenhagen, Copenhagen, Denmark, and ‡School of Kinesiology
and Health Science, York University, Toronto, Ontario, Canada,
M3J 1P3

Abstract

Every time a bout of exercise is performed, a change in gene expression occurs within the contracting muscle. Over the course of many repeated bouts of exercise (i.e. training), the cumulative effects of these alterations lead to a change in muscle phenotype. One of the most prominent of these adaptations is an increase in mitochondrial content, which confers a greater resistance to muscle fatigue. This essay reviews current knowledge on the regulation of exercise-induced mitochondrial biogenesis at the molecular level. The major steps involved include, (i) transcriptional regulation of nuclear-encoded genes encoding mitochondrial proteins by the coactivator peroxisome-proliferator-activated receptor γ coactivator-1, (ii) control of mitochondrial DNA gene

[1]To whom correspondence should be addressed (email dhood@yorku.ca).

expression by the transcription factor Tfam, (iii) mitochondrial fission and fusion mechanisms, and (iv) import of nuclear-derived gene products into the mitochondrion via the protein import machinery. It is now known that exercise can modify the rates of several of these steps, leading to mitochondrial biogenesis. An understanding of how exercise can produce this effect could help us decide whether exercise is beneficial for patients suffering from mitochondrial disorders, as well as a variety of metabolic diseases.

Introduction

Performing regular exercise has many health benefits. The consequences of exercise include improved cardiovascular function as well as a shift in substrate oxidation toward that of lipid, rather than carbohydrate. Endurance capacity for daily work tasks is enhanced, mainly as a result of a greater oxygen delivery and extraction by the exercising muscle. Oxygen extraction is a result of an improved capillary-to-fibre ratio, as well as a higher mitochondrial content within muscle. Although these adaptations have long been recognized, the molecular basis for these changes remain a matter of intense study. This is important because an understanding of the cellular processes involved could (i) help in the development of therapeutic applications other than exercise, and (ii) achieve a greater understanding of the pathology of mitochondrial diseases. The increase in mitochondrial content that occurs as a result of regular exercise is referred to as mitochondrial biogenesis. This process is complex because mitochondria are composed of proteins encoded by both nuclear and mtDNA (mitochondrial DNA). In addition, mitochondrial structure differs among cell types and even within different regions of a specific cell type. Recently, several breakthroughs in our understanding of this process have occurred, with the discovery of an important overall regulator of mitochondrial biogenesis, termed PGC-1α (peroxisome-proliferator-activated receptor γ coactivator-1α), as well as the recognition that mitochondria continually undergo fission and fusion events, processes that have an impact on mitochondrial morphology and function. In the present paper we will review our current understanding of mitochondrial regulatory proteins and organelle assembly patterns, as well as the response to exercise. Recent reviews on the topics discussed in this essay are also included [1–8].

PGC-1α

Transcriptional regulation by PGC-1α

PGC-1α has developed a reputation as a protein that is vital for mitochondrial biogenesis. It was discovered in the search for PPARγ (peroxisome-proliferator-activated receptor γ) interacting proteins from mouse BAT (brown adipose tissue) cells. PGC-1α binds many nuclear receptors that results in an increase in the transcriptional activity of their target genes [1,9]

Table 1. Examples of transcription factors and downstream target genes which are ultimately regulated by PGC-1α.

Transcription factor	Ultimate downstream target genes	Function
PPARγ, α, β	UCP 1	Lipid metabolism
Retinoid X receptor	UCP 2	Lipid metabolism
Thyroid hormone receptor β	CPT 1	Lipid metabolism
Oestrogen receptor and oestrogen related receptor α, γ	MCAD	Lipid metabolism
NRF-1 and NRF-2	CD36	Lipid metabolism
Myocyte enhancer factor (MEF) 2	Cytochrome c	Electron transport
Forkhead Box 01 (FOXO1)	NADH dehydrogenase	Electron transport
Farnesoid X receptor	COX subunit IV	Electron transport
	NRF-1	Transcriptional regulation
	NRF-2	Transcriptional regulation
	PGC 1α	Transcriptional regulation
	TFB1, TFB2	Transcriptional regulation
	Tfam	Transcriptional regulation
	Glut4	Carbohydrate metabolism
	PDK4	Carbohydrate metabolism

CD36, fatty acid translocase; CPT-1, carnitine palmitoyltransferase-1; Glut4, glucose transporter 4; MCAD, medium chain acetyl-coenzyme A dehydrogenase; PDK4, pyruvate dehydrogenase kinase 4.

(Table 1). Thus, PGC-1α is the transcriptional coactivator of a broad range of transcription factors regulating both nuclear and mitochondrial genes, with the potential to play an important coordinating role in regulating adaptive responses of the muscle cell. PGC-1α has the ability to increase the transcriptional activity of target genes by recruiting additional transcriptional regulators. These include proteins with histone acetyltransferase activity that are able to produce local alterations in chromatin structure, making the promoter region more accessible for the transcriptional machinery and thus more favourable for transcription.

Role of PGC-1α in BAT

The functional role of PGC-1α in BAT became evident from the findings that PGC-1α regulated the UCP1 (uncoupling protein 1) gene through activation of the transcription factors thyroid receptor and PPARγ, and that forced overexpression of PGC-1α in adipocytes elevated the mRNA content of the genes encoding UCP1 and many other mitochondrial proteins. Thus, WAT (white adipose tissue) with a low mitochondrial content obtained the characteristics of BAT with a higher mitochondrial concentration, when PGC-1α was induced. BAT is important in adaptive thermogenesis in which mitochondrial biogenesis and the increased expression of oxidative metabolism genes are important phenotypic characterisitics. Thus, PGC-1α is important in regulating adaptive thermogenesis. This interpretation is even further strengthened by the lower body temperature and marked cold-sensitivity of PGC-1α knockout mice [10]. In these animals, no change in BAT UCP1 expression is evident upon exposure to cold, whereas wild-type animals demonstrate a 3-fold increase of UCP1 mRNA in this tissue [10].

Role of PGC-1α in the heart

PGC-1α protein levels are very high in the heart, coincident with the extremely high mitochondrial content of this tissue [2]. The importance of PGC-1α in regulating cardiac mitochondrial number and metabolism first became clear from the increased expression of nuclear- and mitochondrial-encoded genes produced by the forced overexpression of PGC-1α in cardiac myocytes [11]. In contrast, the hearts of PGC-1α-deficient mice have reduced mRNA content of a broad range of genes encoding mitochondrial proteins, lower mitochondrial enzyme activities and poor cardiac contraction, with defects in the ability to increase cardiac work in response to physiological stimuli [12]. These data illustrate the importance of PGC-1α in the metabolism and function of the heart. However, extreme overexpression of PGC-1α also led to cardiomyopathy, presumably as a result of the uncoordinated up-regulation of key metabolic proteins.

Role of PGC-1α in skeletal muscle

A similar profound role of PGC-1α in regulating the expression of genes encoding mitochondrial proteins in skeletal muscle was convincingly shown by the changes induced by overexpressing PGC-1α both in myotubes [9] and in transgenic mice [13]. The overexpression of PGC-1α in myotubes induced mitochondrial biogenesis and increased the expression of genes involved in oxidative phosphorylation [9] (Figure 1). Interestingly, it was demonstrated that PGC-1α can coactivate the transcription factor NRF-1 (nuclear respiratory factor-1) to regulate Tfam (mitochondrial transcription factor A) levels, a nuclear-encoded protein which controls mtDNA replication and transcription (see below). This provides a mechanism through which PGC-1α can also control mitochondrially-encoded genes. In PGC-1α transgenic mice, normal 'white' muscles turned red. For example, the white vastus muscle, that normally has a low oxidative capacity, exhibited a dramatically elevated mRNA and protein content of myoglobin and COX (cytochrome c oxidase) subunits II and IV, proteins involved in oxidative metabolism. These changes occurred even when PGC-1α was expressed within the normal physiological range [13], emphasizing the physiological importance of PGC-1α. In contrast, in PGC-1α knockout mice, the lack of PGC-1α protein in skeletal muscles resulted in 30–60% reduced mRNA content of many genes encoding proteins involved in fatty acid metabolism, the tricarboxylic acid cycle and the respiratory chain [10], but surprisingly the mitochondrial volume was similar to that found

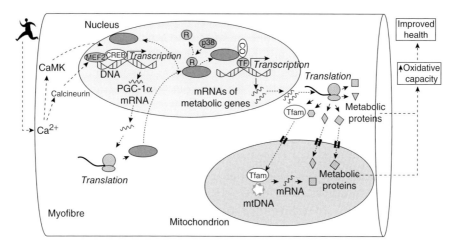

Figure 1. Exercise-induced up-regulation of PGC-1α expression and the concomitant effects of PGC-1α on the regulation of nuclear and mitochondrial encoded genes

Muscle contractions increase PGC-1α transcription, in part, through Ca^{2+}-mediated signalling via calcineurin and MEF2, as well as CaMK and CREB. PGC-1α transcripts translocate to the cytosol, where mRNA is translated. PGC-1α protein translocates back to the nucleus, where it regulates the transcription of many metabolic genes and transcription factors by binding to a broad range of transcription factors (TF) and recruiting other transcriptional regulators (coactivators; CO). PGC-1α also seems to regulate its own transcription. PGC-1α activity is inhibited when repressors (R) bind to PGC-1α, and this inhibition can be released by p38-induced phosphorylation of the repressor. One of the products of PGC-1α-mediated coactivation of the NRF-1 transcription factor is Tfam. Tfam and other metabolic proteins are imported into mitochondria. Tfam enhances the transcription of mitochondrially-encoded genes and the replication of mitochondrial DNA. Repeated bouts of exercise will thus increase mitochondrial biogenesis and skeletal muscle oxidative capacity leading to improved health and improved exercise performance.

in wild-type mice [12]. These data clearly support the view that PGC-1α is essential in maintaining normal metabolism in skeletal muscle. In agreement with intracellular metabolic disturbances due to changes in expression of mitochondrial proteins, skeletal muscles of PGC-1α knockout mice had an increased AMPK (AMP-activated protein kinase) activity [10]. Since this kinase is thought to be a sensor of intracellular energy charge, the increased AMPK activity is likely to be a compensatory mechanism in response to a lower intracellular ATP/ADP ratio in the PGC-1α knockout mice. PGC-1α is also suggested to contribute to the regulation of the redox status of the cell. This may be mediated by the PGC-1α-induced increase in the expression of uncoupling proteins [9], leading to reduced ROS (reactive oxygen species) production, along with a PGC-1α-regulated increased expression of scavenging enzymes [1].

Surprisingly, an influence of PGC-1α was also demonstrated on MHC (myosin heavy chain) fibre type changes, suggesting that it could act as a transcriptional coactivator that has a major influence in driving the formation of slow-twitch muscle fibres in transgenic mice. The observed change, however, was only 10 and 20% for type I and IIa fibres respectively [13]. Although this does suggest that PGC-1α plays a role in regulating MHC expression, it should be noted that the changes in metabolic gene expression were much more pronounced, emphasizing the major role of PGC-1α in regulating the expression of genes encoding proteins in oxidative metabolism. This view is supported by the findings that PGC-1α knockout mice had similar percentages of MHC type I and IIa fibres as in wild-type animals [12].

Intracellular signalling regulating PGC-1α expression

A likely role of calcium signalling in regulating PGC-1α expression became evident from the observed changes in transgenic mice expressing a constitutively active form of CaMK (calcium/calmodulin-dependent protein kinase) IV. In addition to an up-regulation of PGC-1α mRNA, the mRNA content of subunits of the NADH dehydrogenase (encoded by mtDNA), as well as nuclear gene products carnitine palmitoyl transferase I, cytochrome c and myoglobin were increased in the transgenic mice. Thus, CaMK overexpression appeared to induce a coordination of the nuclear and the mitochondrial genomes through PGC-1α [14]. In accordance with this, increasing cytosolic calcium in myotubes by caffeine incubation increased PGC-1α protein content. This induction was abolished by simultaneous treatment with dantrolene, an inhibitor of calcium release from the sarcoplasmic reticulum. In addition to the CaMK pathway, calcineurin signalling also appears to be involved in regulating PGC-1α expression in muscle cells. Co-transfection studies in C2C12 cells revealed that calcineurin seems to affect PGC-1α transcription through an effect on MEF2 (myocyte enhancer factor 2) at the PGC-1α promoter, whereas CAMKIV regulates the PGC-1α gene through phosphorylation of CREB (cAMP response element-binding protein), a binding protein that directly interacts with CRE (cAMP response element) and activates PGC-1α transcription. A cAMP signalling pathway is also likely to be involved in regulating PGC-1α expression. In hepatocytes, glucagon binding to the cell surface leads to increased cAMP, protein kinase A activation and the concomitant phosphorylation and activation of CREB. Similarly, insulin signalling through protein kinase B and FOXO1 (forkhead family transcriptional regulator) acting on insulin response sequences on the PGC-1α promoter has been demonstrated in hepatocytes [15]. In addition, AMPK has been suggested to be involved in regulating PGC-1α expression in skeletal muscle. This is because treatment of muscle cells with the AMPK activator AICAR (5-aminoimidazole-4-carboxamide-1-β-D-ribonucleoside) increases PGC-1α protein content. It should be noted, however, that the exercise-induced increases in PGC-1α transcription and mRNA content are not affected in mouse skeletal muscle by knocking out either the AMPKα1 or AMPKα2 isoforms [16]. Finally, PGC-1α seems to be able to activate its own transcription by coactivating MEF2 on the PGC-1α promoter, thereby exerting an autoregulatory influence on PGC-1α expression. This mechanism may help to ensure the stable transcription of PGC-1α during adaptive cellular responses [17].

In addition to regulation of PGC-1α via expression changes, the activity of PGC-1α is also controlled via changes in phosphorylation state. The p38 MAPK (mitogen-activated protein kinase)-induced phosphorylation of PGC-1α increases the stability of the protein, thus maintaining its activity for a longer period of time. In addition, changes in phosphorylation state also affect the activity of repressors that interfere with the interactions between PGC-1α and transcription factors [1,17,18]. It is suggested that the phosphorylation of a repressor by p38 MAPK promotes dissociation of the repressor from PGC-1α, which then becomes accessible for the transcription factors to allow transcriptional activation [18] (Figure 1).

Effect of exercise on PGC-1α gene expression

Regular physical activity is associated with a broad range of cellular adaptations in skeletal muscle including increased capillarization and mitochondrial enzyme content, leading to the improved oxidative capacity of skeletal muscles. The current understanding is that exercise-induced gene expression responses to each single acute exercise bout contributes to the ultimate cellular adaptations observed after exercise training. The final phenotypic adaptations stem from the cumulative effects of such transient gene expression responses. For this to be possible, only genes with a sufficiently prolonged expression response to acute exercise will have the potential to accumulate mRNA/protein when exercise is performed regularly. Genes encoding proteins such as citrate synthase, 3-hydroxy-acyl-dehydrogenase and cytochrome c seem to be among those possessing such responses [19]. The products of genes with more rapid turnover responses like UCP3, hexokinase II and PGC-1α [19] are less likely to accumulate when the activity is performed regularly. However, the responses of these genes are no doubt critical for the overall adaptation to physical activity. This may be due to their roles in re-establishing intracellular energy homoeostasis, or as transcriptional regulators of other metabolic genes important in this adaptive process. Acute exercise-induced increases in PGC-1α transcription, mRNA content and/or protein content have been demonstrated in rat [20] and human [19] skeletal muscle. Typical transcriptional and mRNA responses of PGC-1α in skeletal muscle occur within the initial 6 h of recovery from exercise. Increased PGC-1α protein expression was reported 18 h after the end of exercise in rats. This increased protein content was also observed after 5–7 days of repeated 3 h/day contractile activity bouts [2]. In addition, the acute transcriptional and mRNA responses of PGC-1α were enhanced by four weeks of exercise training in humans, although all other investigated genes had lower or similar responses to acute exercise after training [19] suggesting that the exercise-induced PGC-1α gene response is potentiated by regular exercise.

The functional role of the exercise-induced increase in PGC-1α gene expression lies in the ability of PGC-1α to coactivate a broad range of transcription factors, and thus a diverse set of target genes, leading to coordinated adaptive cellular responses to physical activity. In addition, the identification of specific phosphorylation sites in PGC-1α makes it possible that PGC-1α exerts its coordinating role through phosphorylation-mediated regulation of PGC-1α activity, without requiring an obligatory increase in PGC-1α protein levels. Whether such mechanisms are operative during exercise remains to be seen.

Potential role of PGC-1α in insulin resistance

The impact of PGC-1α on regulating the expression of metabolic genes has led to the search for potential roles of PGC-1α dysregulation in metabolically related diseases like T2D (type 2 diabetes). Insulin resistance and T2D were found to be associated with a lower mRNA expression of many NRF-1-regulated genes encoding proteins in oxidative metabolism. These changes coincided with reduced PGC-1α mRNA content in muscle obtained from individuals with T2D, as well as those who were non-diabetic but had a family history of diabetes [21]. PGC-1α is known to both regulate the expression of NRF-1 and to be a coactivator of NRF-1-mediated transcription. Therefore these findings suggest that lowered PGC-1α expression may be a factor leading to insulin resistance and T2D. Additionally, genetic variations in the PGC-1α gene seem to be implicated in the development of T2D. Thus, a frequent single nucleotide polymorphism (G482S) in the PGC-1α gene is associated with an increased risk of T2D in Danish Caucasians [22], and specific PGC-1α promoter polymorphisms seem to be associated with early onset T2D in a Korean population [23]. We speculate that such polymorphisms could influence the expression of PGC-1α or its rate of degradation, leading to reduced mRNA content in skeletal muscles of T2D patients, in addition to possible direct effects of a missense mutation on PGC-1α function. We propose that regular exercise may be beneficial in preventing the development of T2D because the exercise-induced increase in PGC-1α protein in skeletal muscle can lead to an increased oxidative capacity of skeletal muscle, including improved lipid oxidation.

mtDNA transcription factors

Mitochondria possess their own circular genome of about 16.5 kb termed mtDNA. mtDNA contains two ribosomal RNAs, 22 tRNAs and 13 mRNAs that encode proteins that function as subunits for respiratory complexes I, III and IV [3]. However, this represents only a small portion of the total number of genes that are necessary for the proper function of mitochondria. Indeed, the proteins that regulate the replication and transcription of mtDNA are nuclear-encoded, and need to be imported into the organelle (see below). One of the first identified, and most important of these regulatory proteins, is Tfam (Figure 2). Tfam plays a key role in maintaining the mitochondrial

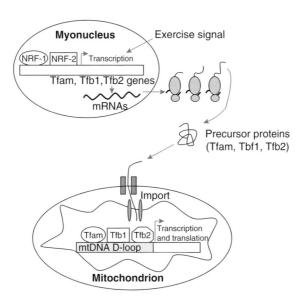

Figure 2. Mitochondrial DNA transcription and replication can be induced by physical activity through numerous signal transduction cascades
Exercise signals lead to the transcription of Tfam, Tfb1 and Tfb2 into mRNAs in the nucleus, which are then synthesized in the cytosol into precursor proteins and imported into mitochondria. Mature Tfam, Tfb1 and Tfb2 proteins activate mtDNA transcription and replication within the organelle. mtDNA gene products are then assembled into the electron transport chain.

copy number and transcriptional activity since the action of Tfam along with the mitochondrial RNA polymerase is necessary for the proper initiation of transcription of mammalian mtDNA from both heavy- and light-strand promoters [3]. The importance of Tfam is evident from the phenotype exhibited by Tfam knockout mice. Homozygous Tfam knockout leads to embryonic lethality. Embryos have delayed neural development, the absence of cardiac structures and either lack or have low levels of mtDNA. mtDNA copy number and respiratory chain complex activities are reduced in the heart of heterozygous Tfam knockout mice. Disruption of Tfam in cardiomyocytes results in dilated cardiomyopathy with atrioventricular conduction blocks, whereas inactivation of Tfam in β-cells results in the inability of the β-cell to release insulin in response to a glucose challenge. Massive neuronal degeneration has also been shown to result from a defect in the Tfam gene within cortical neurons. These studies demonstrate the critical role of Tfam in the maintenance of mtDNA and mitochondrial biogenesis in a variety of tissues.

It is now known that exercise increases the expression and function of Tfam in muscle. Gordon et al. [24] demonstrated that electrically stimulated-induced contractile activity of the rat tibialis anterior muscle leads to an increase in Tfam mRNA level after four days (Figure 2). Subsequent increases in Tfam import into mitochondria occurred by day five, leading to an accumulation of mitochondrial Tfam protein, an increase in Tfam–mtDNA binding and mtDNA transcript levels encoding COX subunit III, and a higher COX enzyme activity by day seven. A similar increase in Tfam expression has been found following endurance training in humans. Thus, the increase in Tfam expression during the progression of exercise training contributes substantially to mitochondrial biogenesis in skeletal muscle.

Although it was believed for some time that the proper initiation of transcription from heavy- and light-strand promoters was exclusively dependent upon mitochondrial RNA polymerase and Tfam [3], TFB1m and TFB2m, two human isoforms of mitochondrial specificity factor have recently been identified and shown to play an important role in transcription initiation [25]. TFB1m and TFB2m are localized to mitochondria in order to bind mtDNA and stimulate transcription from the L-strand promoter *in vitro*. However, TFB1m has about 10% of the transcriptional activity of TFB2m. It now appears that RNA polymerase, Tfam and the TFB isoforms are essential for proper mtDNA transcription, with Tfam playing a major role in this process since it regulates the activity of the TFB–RNA polymerase complex and transcriptional activity both *in vivo* and *in vitro*. Interestingly, TFB1m and TFB2m are transcriptionally regulated by NRF-1 and NRF-2, in a similar manner to Tfam (Figure 2). Since multiple nuclear genes encoding mitochondrial proteins also have recognition sequences for NRF-1 and -2, this indicates that common transcriptional regulators (NRF-1 and -2) link the expression of respiratory chain proteins to the mitochondrial transcriptional machinery [3]. This is likely to be important for coordinating the gene expression response to exercise, leading to an up-regulation of both nuclear and mitochondrial gene products and subsequent organelle biogenesis. More studies are necessary to reveal the expression and function of TFB1 and TFB2 in skeletal muscle during exercise.

Mitochondrial fusion and fission

Mitochondria are very dynamic structures. They have the ability to constantly fuse and divide and mitochondrial structure within the cell reflects a balance between mitochondrial fusion and division (i.e.fission). If fusion predominates, mitochondria become more interconnected and networked [26]. In contrast, excessive fission leads to mitochondrial network breakdown, the loss of mtDNA, an increase in ROS production and respiratory defects [4]. Despite the fact that the exact mechanisms responsible for mitochondrial fission and fusion events have not been identified, significant progress has been made in recognizing genes that play a critical role in these processes.

Several proteins within the outer and inner mitochondrial membrane are involved in the mitochondrial fusion process, including Mfn1 and Mfn2 (mitofusin 1 and 2) and OPA (a dynamin-related GTPase) [5]. The Mfn1 and Mfn2 isoforms are very similar in that they show a high degree of homology and

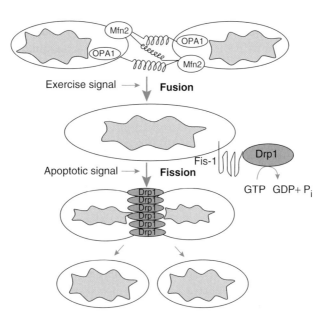

Figure 3. Schematic model of mitochondrial fusion and fission
GTPases are enzymes that have the ability to hydrolyse GTP. Mfn is an outer membrane mitochondrial protein. It has a cytosolic GTPase domain and two coiled-coil regions. Adjacent mitochondria start fusing by a process of oligomerization between Mfn molecules at the C-terminal coiled-coil region. Mfns coordinate fusion with the help of an OPA1 protein which is an intermembrane space GTPase. Mitochondrial fission is initiated by the cytosolic Drp1 protein that is recruited to the mitochondrial outer membrane by a presently unknown signal. It is proposed that Fis1 recruits Drp1 to the mitochondrial outer membrane, where activated Drp1 forms a ring-like complex and conveys signals to (or from) the inner membrane to coordinate mitochondrial membrane fission (modified from [23,25]).

topology. Both are GTPases located on the outer mitochondrial membrane with the N-terminal GTPase and their coiled-coil protruding into the cytosol [5]. Despite their similarity, Mfn1 can only promote functional elongation of mitochondria in the presence of OPA1, whereas Mfn2 does not require additional fusion proteins. Of interest is that OPA1 mutations have been shown to induce optic atrophy through mitochondrial impairment. In the absence of Mfn2, the degree of fusion events is low, leading to a discontinuous mitochondrial network. In contrast, overexpression of Mfn2 protein leads to the generation of a mitochondrial reticulum-like network. There is also evidence that Mfn2 has an effect on mitochondrial metabolism. Repression of Mfn2 expression in muscle myotubes reduced glucose oxidation as well as the mitochondrial membrane potential. The impairment of lipid and carbohydrate metabolism evident in obese Zucker rats may be related to the fact that Mfn2 is significantly reduced in the muscle of this animal model [27].

Mitochondrial fission is required during cell division when proper inheritance of mitochondria by daughter cells is of critical importance [6]. The mechanisms of mitochondrial fission are still poorly understood. Drp1 (dynamin-related protein 1) is a large GTPase protein and, along with Fis1 (mitochondrial fission protein), regulates fission in mammalian cells. The assembly of fission machinery occurs at scission points on the outer mito-chondrial membrane, where Fis1 recruits the Drp1 protein (Figure 3). The mitochondrial network becomes more fragmented when Fis1 expression is increased, whereas a decrease in Fis1 expression leads to more interconnected mitochondria.

Skeletal muscles have highly interconnected mitochondria, particularly in the intermyofibrillar region. In contrast, mitochondria within the subsarco-lemmal region of muscle cells appear more fragmented [7]. Endurance exercise training leads to an expansion of the mitochondrial reticulum during organelle biogenesis [8], yet little is known with regard to the specific mechanisms that control this process in muscle. A recent study has demonstrated an increase in Mfn1 and Mfn2 mRNA levels in human skeletal muscle 24 h post-exercise [28], but the regulation of the expression of these mitofusin isoforms, or the involvement of Fis1 or OPA have not yet been investigated. This remains an important area for future investigation in the study of mitochondrial structure and function in muscle.

Protein import

The biosynthesis of the mitochondrion is unique because it requires a high degree of intracellular communication between not one, but two distinct genomes. Given the limited capacity of the mitochondrion for gene transcription and translation, the nuclear genome is primarily responsible for encoding the majority of proteins essential for reticulum expansion and organelle biogenesis. In order for these polypeptides to transverse the mitochondrial membrane and be targeted to specific organelle compartments, they must first associate with, and utilize, a subset of proteins collectively referred to as the mitochondrial protein import machinery [8].

The protein import machinery is divided into two intricate sets of proteins (Figure 4). The first is the TOM (translocase of the outer membrane) complex, which in addition to several outer membrane receptor proteins, contains an approx. 400 kDa general import pore where precursor proteins traverse the outer membrane. The presence of specific targeting signals within the pri-mary structure of a newly synthesized protein dictates not only its localization within the mitochondria, but also the specific translocation pathway that it will take. The TIM (translocases of the inner membrane) complex comprise the sec-ond protein import machinery complex. These proteins rely on the mitochon-drial membrane potential ($\Delta\psi_\mathrm{m}$) for the translocation of precursor proteins across the inner membrane to the matrix.

To date, the regulation of the protein import pathways, and more specifi-cally the dynamics of assembly of these protein import complexes in response

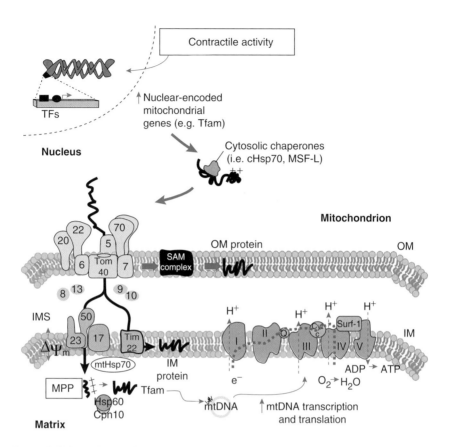

Figure 4. Effect of chronic contractile activity on mitochondrial protein import
Following an exercise stimulus, signalling pathways are activated which up-regulate the expression of several nuclear genes encoding mitochondrial proteins, including genes of the protein import machinery, as well as Tfam. Newly synthesized precursor proteins are subsequently targeted from the cytosol to the outer mitochondrial membrane (OM) via the cytosolic chaperones heat shock protein 70 (cHsp70) and mitochondrial import stimulating factor (MSF). The precursor protein associates with Tom20, Tom22 and Tom70 receptors and is transferred to the intermembrane space (IMS) via the TOM complex. Tim50 and the smaller TIM proteins direct the precursor protein either to the Tim22 channel to be inserted into the inner membrane, or to the Tim23 channel to be pulled into the matrix via the ATP-driven action of mtHsp70 and the membrane potential ($\Delta\Psi$m). Once inside the matrix, the presequence is cleaved by MPP (mitochondrial processing peptidase) and refolded by Hsp60 and Cpn10 into a mature protein. Mitochondrial proteins such as Tfam bind to mtDNA to induce the transcription and translation of proteins required for oxidative phosphorylation processes and ATP production.

to altered states of mitochondrial biogenesis, has remained elusive. However, there is evidence to suggest that the protein import machinery has the ability to respond to energy perturbations within the cell. For example, distinct mitochondrial subpopulations within skeletal muscle display different import capacities, which are believed to contribute to some of the biochemical and functional differences observed between these mitochondria. Furthermore, in response to an exercise stimulus, it has been shown that several components of the import machinery, including cytosolic molecular chaperones, outer membrane receptor proteins, and matrix chaperonins are increased [24,29]. These changes in the expression of the protein import apparatus are believed to contribute to the higher rate of precursor protein import that occurs following chronic contractile activity. As noted above, an increase in the import rate of Tfam observed with seven days of contractile activity may promote the transcription and replication of the mitochondrial genome, leading to increased mtDNA copy number and increased transcription of COX subunits.

The protein import machinery also adapts in response to pathological conditions of disease. In patients harbouring mtDNA mutations, a retrograde signalling pathway is activated, leading to a compensatory response within the nuclear genome. The result of this is an increased expression of specific protein import machinery components in an effort to maintain, or even increase protein import of nuclear-encoded mitochondrial proteins into the organelle [30,31]. The dynamic role of the protein import machinery has further been solidified with the finding that a mutation in DDP (the deafness dystonia protein), contributes to the human disease termed Mohr–Tranebjaerg syndrome, a rare neurodegenerative disorder characterized by hearing loss and dystonia. DDP is the human homologue of Tim8a which is located in the intermembrane space and is responsible for the proper insertion and assembly of the Tim23 protein. In addition, the recent finding that in response to an apoptotic stimulus, DDP is released from the mitochondria into the cytoplasm to promote Drp-1 mediated mitochondrial fission further implicates the importance of protein import in mitochondrial regulation [32].

Thus, given the above findings, it is now known that both changes in the expression, as well the assembly of the protein import machinery complexes into the mitochondrial membrane will affect the rate at which precursor proteins are imported into the mitochondria. Exercise stimulates import machinery expression, as well as import kinetics within the organelle. Whether this is also a result of an augmented assembly of protein import complexes remains to be determined. Theoretically, this improved capacity for import would allow for a lower requirement for rates of transcription and translation, implying a more efficient process of organelle assembly. Much work is still required to solidify the dynamic interactions of the assembly of these complexes in exercise-induced mitochondrial biogenesis.

Conclusions

Mitochondrial biogenesis is now recognized as a vital and exciting area of cell biology, the comprehension of which is relevant to an understanding of a large number of cellular pathological conditions. Exercise can play a significant role in accelerating the rate of mitochondrial biogenesis and likely serves to attenuate mitochondrial dysfunction present in a number of metabolic diseases. The study of the molecular basis of these exercise-induced effects remain relevant to exercise physiologists, clinicians dealing with mitochondrially based diseases, as well as molecular biologists seeking an understanding of the underlying mechanisms of organelle biogenesis.

Summary

- *Mitochondrial synthesis in muscle (biogenesis) is a consequence of endurance training and leads to fatigue resistance.*

- *Mitochondrial biogenesis is regulated at transcriptional and post-transcriptional levels of gene expression, as well as by fission and fusion processes.*

- *PGC-1α is an important transcriptional coactivator of nuclear genes encoding mitochondrial proteins, whilst Tfam regulates the expression of mitochondrial DNA.*

- *Exercise regulates the expression of PGC-1α, Tfam and protein import, but little is known about how exercise affects mitochondrial fission and fusion.*

- *Understanding the mechanisms by which exercise affects mitochondrial biogenesis can help us understand whether exercise is a viable treatment modality for metabolic diseases involving the organelle.*

Owing to space restrictions, references to certain works have not been included in the list below. A complete set of references is available from the corresponding author.

References

1. Lin, J., Handschin, C. & Spiegelman, B.M. (2005) Metabolic control through the PGC-1 family of transcription coactivators. *Cell Metab.* **1**, 361–370
2. Irrcher, I., Adhihetty, P.J., Joseph, A.M., Ljubicic, V. & Hood, D.A. (2003) Regulation of mitochondrial biogenesis in muscle by endurance exercise. *Sports Med.* **33**, 783–793
3. Shadel, G.S. & Clayton, D.A. (1993) Mitochondrial transcription initiation. Variation and conservation. *J. Biol. Chem.* **268**, 16083–16086
4. Yaffe, M.P. (1999) The machinery of mitochondrial inheritance and behavior. *Science* **283**, 1493–1497
5. Chen, H. & Chan, D.C. (2005) Emerging functions of mammalian mitochondrial fusion and fission. *Hum. Mol. Genet.* **14** (Spec No. 2), R283–R289
6. Bossy-Wetzel, E., Barsoum, M.J., Godzik, A., Schwarzenbacher, R. & Lipton, S.A. (2003) Mitochondrial fission in apoptosis, neurodegeneration and aging. *Curr. Opin. Cell Biol.* **15**, 706–716
7. Hood, D.A. & Irrcher, I. (2006) Mitochondrial biogenesis induced by endurance training. In ACSM's *Advanced Exercise Physiology*, (Tipton, C.M., Sawka, M.N., Tate, C.A., & Terjung, R.L. eds.), pp.437–452, Lippincott Williams & Wilkins, Baltimore
8. Hood, D.A. (2001) Invited Review: contractile activity-induced mitochondrial biogenesis in skeletal muscle. *J. Appl. Physiol.* **90**, 1137–1157
9. Wu, Z., Puigserver, P., Andersson, U., Zhang, C., Adelmant, G., Mootha, V., Troy, A., Cinti, S., Lowell, B., Scarpulla, R.C. & Spiegelman, B.M. (1999) Mechanisms controlling mitochondrial biogenesis and respiration through the thermogenic coactivator PGC-1. *Cell* **98**, 115–124

10. Lin, J., Wu, P.H., Tarr, P.T., Lindenberg, K.S., St-Pierre, J., Zhang, C.Y., Mootha, V.K., Jager, S., Vianna, C.R., Reznick, R.M. et al. (2004) Defects in adaptive energy metabolism with CNS-linked hyperactivity in PGC-1α null mice. *Cell* **119**, 121–135

11. Lehman, J.J., Barger, P.M., Kovacs, A., Saffitz, J.E., Medeiros, D.M. & Kelly, D.P. (2000) Peroxisome proliferator-activated receptor γ coactivator-1 promotes cardiac mitochondrial biogenesis. *J. Clin. Invest.* **106**, 847–856

12. Arany, Z., He, H., Lin, J., Hoyer, K., Handschin, C., Toka, O., Ahmad, F., Matsui, T., Chin, S., Wu, P.H. et al. (2005) Transcriptional coactivator PGC-1α controls the energy state and contractile function of cardiac muscle. *Cell Metab.* **1**, 259–271

13. Lin, J., Wu, H., Tarr, P.T., Zhang, C.Y., Wu, Z., Boss, O., Michael, L.F., Puigserver, P., Isotani, E., Olson, E.N. et al. (2002) Transcriptional co-activator PGC-1α drives the formation of slow-twitch muscle fibres. *Nature* **418**, 797–801

14. Wu, H., Kanatous, S.B., Thurmond, F.A., Gallardo, T., Isotani, E., Bassel-Duby, R. & Williams, R.S. (2002) Regulation of mitochondrial biogenesis in skeletal muscle by CaMK. *Science* **296**, 349–352

15. Daitoku, H., Yamagata, K., Matsuzaki, H., Hatta, M. & Fukamizu, A. (2003) Regulation of PGC-1 promoter activity by protein kinase B and the forkhead transcription factor FKHR. *Diabetes* **52**, 642–649

16. Jorgensen, S.B., Wojtaszewski, J.F., Viollet, B., Andreelli, F., Birk, J.B., Hellsten, Y., Schjerling, P., Vaulont, S., Neufer, P.D., Richter, E.A. & Pilegaard, H. (2005) Effects of α-AMPK knockout on exercise-induced gene activation in mouse skeletal muscle. *FASEB J.* **19**, 1146–1148

17. Handschin, C., Rhee, J., Lin, J., Tarr, P.T. & Spiegelman, B.M. (2003) An autoregulatory loop controls peroxisome proliferator-activated receptor gamma coactivator 1α expression in muscle. *Proc. Natl. Acad. Sci. U.S.A.* **100**, 7111–7116

18. Knutti, D., Kressler, D. & Kralli, A. (2001) Regulation of the transcriptional coactivator PGC-1 via MAPK-sensitive interaction with a repressor. *Proc. Natl. Acad. Sci. U.S.A.* **98**, 9713–9718

19. Pilegaard, H., Saltin, B. & Neufer, P.D. (2003) Exercise induces transient transcriptional activation of the PGC-1α gene in human skeletal muscle. *J. Physiol.* **546**, 851–858

20. Baar, K., Wende, A.R., Jones, T.E., Marison, M., Nolte, L.A., Chen, M., Kelly, D.P. & Holloszy, J.O. (2002) Adaptations of skeletal muscle to exercise: rapid increase in the transcriptional coactivator PGC-1. *FASEB J.* **16**, 1879–1886

21. Patti, M.E., Butte, A.J., Crunkhorn, S., Cusi, K., Berria, R., Kashyap, S., Miyazaki, Y., Kohane, I., Costello, M., Saccone, R. et al. (2003) Coordinated reduction of genes of oxidative metabolism in humans with insulin resistance and diabetes: Potential role of PGC1 and NRF1. *Proc. Natl. Acad. Sci. U.S.A.* **100**, 8466–8471

22. Ek, J., Andersen, G., Urhammer, S.A., Gaede, P.H., Drivsholm, T., Borch-Johnsen, K., Hansen, T. & Pedersen, O. (2001) Mutation analysis of peroxisome proliferator-activated receptor-γ coactivator-1 (PGC-1) and relationships of identified amino acid polymorphisms to Type II diabetes mellitus. *Diabetologia* **44**, 2220–2226

23. Kim, J.H., Shin, H.D., Park, B.L., Cho, Y.M., Kim, S.Y., Lee, H.K. & Park, K.S. (2005) Peroxisome proliferator-activated receptor γ coactivator 1 α promoter polymorphisms are associated with early-onset type 2 diabetes mellitus in the Korean population. *Diabetologia* **48**, 1323–1330

24. Gordon, J.W., Rungi, A.A., Inagaki, H. & Hood, D.A. (2001) Effects of contractile activity on mitochondrial transcription factor A expression in skeletal muscle. *J. Appl. Physiol.* **90**, 389–396

25. Falkenberg, M., Gaspari, M., Rantanen, A., Trifunovic, A., Larsson, N.G. & Gustafsson, C.M. (2002) Mitochondrial transcription factors B1 and B2 activate transcription of human mtDNA. *Nat. Genet.* **31**, 289–294

26. Rube, D.A. & van der Bliek, A.M. (2004) Mitochondrial morphology is dynamic and varied. *Mol. Cell Biochem.* **256–257**, 331–339

27. Bach, D., Pich, S., Soriano, F.X., Vega, N., Baumgartner, B., Oriola, J., Daugaard, J.R., Lloberas, J., Camps, M., Zierath, J.R. et al. (2003) Mitofusin-2 determines mitochondrial network architecture and mitochondrial metabolism. A novel regulatory mechanism altered in obesity. *J. Biol. Chem.* **278**, 17190–17197

28. Cartoni, R., Leger, B., Hock, M.B., Praz, M., Crettenand, A., Pich, S., Ziltener, J.L., Luthi, F., Deriaz, O., Zorzano, A. et al. (2005) Mitofusins 1/2 and ERRα expression are increased in human skeletal muscle after physical exercise *J. Physiol.* **567**, 349–358

29. Takahashi, M., Chesley, A., Freyssenet, D. & Hood, D.A. (1998) Contractile activity-induced adaptations in the mitochondrial protein import system. *Am. J. Physiol.* **274**, C1380–C1387

30. Joseph, A.M., Rungi, A.A., Robinson, B.H. & Hood, D.A. (2004) Compensatory responses of protein import and transcription factor expression in mitochondrial DNA defects. *Am. J. Physiol. Cell Physiol.* **286**, C867–C875

31. Rungi, A.A., Primeau, A., Nunes, C.L., Gordon, J.W., Robinson, B.H. & Hood, D.A. (2002) Events upstream of mitochondrial protein import limit the oxidative capacity of fibroblasts in multiple mitochondrial disease. *Biochim. Biophys. Acta* **1586**, 146–154

32. Arnoult, D., Rismanchi, N., Grodet, A., Roberts, R.G., Seeburg, D.P., Estaquier, J., Sheng, M. & Blackstone, C. (2005) Bax/Bak-dependent release of DDP/TIMM8a promotes Drp1-mediated mitochondrial fission and mitoptosis during programmed cell death. *Curr. Biol.* **15**, 2112–2118

3

Effects of acute exercise and training on insulin action and sensitivity: focus on molecular mechanisms in muscle

Jørgen F.P. Wojtaszewski and Erik A. Richter[1]

Copenhagen Muscle Research Centre, Institute of Exercise and Sport Sciences, University of Copenhagen, Denmark

Abstract

A single bout of exercise increases insulin sensitivity for several hours and the effect is mainly restricted to the muscles recruited during exercise. When exercise is repeated over time, adaptations to physical training occur that include more long-lasting increases in insulin sensitivity. The present review explores the molecular mechanisms involved in both the acute and chronic effects of exercise on insulin sensitivity in skeletal muscle.

Introduction

During dynamic exercise, the turnover of ATP in skeletal muscle increases greatly. This is mainly fuelled by the catabolism of carbohydrates (intramuscular glycogen and blood glucose) and fatty acids (intramuscular triglycerides and blood lipids) whereas protein oxidation does not increase significantly unless muscle glycogen stores are exhausted. During exercise in the postabsorptive state, the contribution of blood glucose to energy expenditure is initially relatively minor, but as exercise continues and muscle glycogen stores are depleted, the contribution of blood glucose becomes

[1]*To whom correspondence should be addressed (email erichter@ifi.ku.dk).*

more substantial, reaching about 35% of leg oxidative metabolism and close to 100% of muscle carbohydrate metabolism (for review see [1]). Following exercise, muscle glucose uptake decreases rapidly and, depending on the duration and intensity of the preceding exercise, glucose uptake reaches resting levels within a few hours if no food is ingested. However, the sensitivity of muscle towards insulin stimulation is enhanced for several hours (up to 48 h) after exercise [2]. This facilitates rapid glycogen resynthesis after exercise when food is ingested. In addition to the effect of a single bout of exercise, repeated exercise (physical training) leads to more long-lasting increases in insulin sensitivity [3]. The beneficial effect of both acute and chronic exercise on insulin sensitivity is the basis for recommending physical activity as an important tool in prevention and treatment of insulin resistance. In the present review we will discuss the possible mechanisms behind the increased metabolic effect of insulin in the period after a single bout of exercise, as well as after a period of regular training. This has been studied mainly from the perspective of insulin action on glucose transport, and to a somewhat lesser extent on GS (glycogen synthase) activity, whereas other potential metabolic roles of insulin, such as stimulation of amino acid transport and protein synthesis, have been studied remarkably little.

Insulin signalling: a complex web

The many biological effects of insulin are initiated by the binding of insulin to the α-subunits of the transmembrane heterotetrameric IR (insulin receptor), leading to autophosphorylation and activation of the kinase associated with β-subunits. A web of inter-related intracellular proteins then mediates the post-receptor signalling toward a diversity of both mitogenic and metabolic cellular bioeffects. Based on our limited knowledge, these signalling events are often depicted in a linear fashion but over recent years evidence has gathered to suggest a much more complex web-like arrangement, inhibiting and promoting cross talk within the web (Figure 1). For detailed information about the insulin signalling pathway the reader is referred to recent reviews [4,5].

The kinase of the IR phosphorylates other endogenous proteins on tyrosine residues. Such endogenous IR substrates (second messengers) are numerous, and include the IRS (insulin receptor substrate) family of proteins 1–4, CAP (c-Cbl associated protein) and APS (adapter proteins) associated with pleckstrin homology and SH2 (Src homology-2) domains [5]. Of these, the IRS family is by far the most studied group of substrates, and in fact the presence/function of the APS–Cbl–CAP complex in skeletal muscle is still unsolved. The IRS proteins do not themselves have catalytic activity. However, phosphorylation on tyrosine residues within specific motifs allow the IRS proteins to bind to other proteins containing the SH2 domain. In this fashion IRS proteins are thought to regulate and direct further signalling. The importance of IRS-1, and to a lesser extent IRS-2, to insulin-mediated glucose transport in muscle tissues/cells has

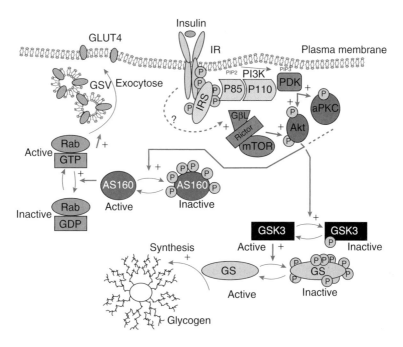

Figure 1. Insulin signalling
The figure depicts some of the events from insulin binding to its receptor to the activation of the effector proteins GLUT4 and glycogen synthase. aPKC, atypical protein kinase C; GSV, GLUT4 storage vesicles.

been underpinned by studies in which the protein has been eliminated by gene knockout or RNA silencing techniques [siRNA (small interfering RNA)] [6].

When tyrosine phosphorylated IRS interacts with the SH2 domain of the p85 regulatory subunit of the class IA PI3K (phosphatidylinositol 3-kinase), the p110 catalytic subunit of the enzyme is activated. This subsequently gives rise to an increased production of phosphatidylinositol-3-phosphate compounds [PI(3,4,5)P$_3$, PI(3,4)P$_2$, and PI(3)P] within the plasma membrane. The production of these compounds is also dependent on activation of additional lipid kinases acting on several of these sites as well. The essential role of class IA PI3K in glucose transport has been elucidated using many different techniques, including chemical poison and molecular inhibition [7]. Interestingly, increased levels of phosphatidylinositol-3-phosphate compounds seems to increase GLUT4 (glucose transporter 4) translocation to the plasma membrane, but does not increase glucose transport, raising the possibility that an additional signalling event is necessary for the full functionality of GLUT4 to be achieved at the plasma membrane. This could involve the newly identified protein AS160 (Akt substrate of 160 kDa) as discussed below.

Insulin stimulation leads to a PI3K-dependent dual phosphorylation and activation of the serine/threonine kinase, Akt, which exists in two isoforms in skeletal muscle, namely Akt 1 and Akt 2. Current evidence suggests that the insulin induced increase in PI(3,4,5)P$_3$ content initiates a recruitment of the PDK1 (phosphoinositol-dependent protein kinase 1) to the plasma membrane, as well as its activation. Apparently, Akt is recruited to the plasma membrane in association with PDK1 [4,5]. Akt is subsequently phosphorylated by PDK1 on its Thr[308] site. The full activation of Akt, however, requires additional phosphorylation by another kinase PDK2 (phosphoinositol-dependent protein kinase 2), on the Ser[473] site, which in fact may be the Rictor–mTOR kinase complex. An important role of Akt in insulin-stimulated glucose transport has been confirmed using transgenic approaches, as well as knockout and siRNA techniques. Through such studies, Akt 2 has been suggested to be more important in regulating glucose transport than Akt 1 [8].

PKCλ/ζ (protein kinase Cλ/ζ), atypical PKC isoforms, are also activated in response to insulin stimulation in a PI3K–PDK1-dependent manner. Phosphorylation by PDK1 induces autophosphorylation, and this is suggested to release auto-inhibition of these atypical PKCs. The role of PKCλ/ζ in insulin stimulated glucose transport has also been verified using overexpression of both kinase dead and active constructs, as well as siRNA [9].

Both Akt and PKCλ/ζ may regulate different aspects of the vesicular trafficking and membrane docking/fusion machinery enabling the GLUT4-containing vesicle translocation and fusion to the plasma membrane. Recently, a new substrate of Akt, AS160, was described. AS160 apparently links IR signalling and GLUT4 trafficking [10]. AS160 contains a GAP (GTPase-activating protein) homology domain, which has been shown to regulate the GTPase activity of certain Rab proteins *in vitro*. Phosphorylation of AS160 by Akt is likely to inhibit its GAP activity, such that as a consequence, the GTP form of this or these Rab protein(s) is/are formed, in turn increasing GLUT4 vesicle movement to, and/or fusion with, the plasma membrane. Insulin increases AS160 phosphorylation, likely in a PI3K-dependent manner, in 3T3-L1 adipocytes and skeletal muscle. Interestingly, AS160 is also phosphorylated (inactivated) during muscle contractions in an AMPK (AMP-activated protein kinase)-dependent manner [11].

Akt is at a crossroads at which insulin signals to regulate glycogen synthesis via regulation of GS activity. Upon insulin stimulation, Akt phosphorylates GSK3α/β (glycogen synthase kinase 3 α/β) in a PI3K-dependent manner leading to inactivation of GSK3 activity. Although GS action is regulated by multiple phosphorylations, the sites purported to affect its activity the most are the N-terminal site two and the C-terminal site three. Of these, GSK3 is only directly phosphorylating site three. The importance of GSK3 for insulin-induced GS activation has recently been firmly established using knockin experiments of mutated GSK3 in murine muscle resulting in failure of insulin to regulate GS activity [12]

An important route of regulation of the insulin signalling cascade is likely to be via negative feedback loops within the cascade. Over recent years it has become apparent that during insulin stimulation IRS-1 is heavily serine phosphorylated at the same time as it becomes tyrosine phosphorylated. Multiple serine residues have been described to undergo phosphorylation, and apparently these are induced by a variety of kinases [mTOR (mammalian target of rapamycin)/JNK (c-Jun N-terminal kinase), GSK3, Erk (extracellular signal-related kinase), Akt, S6K1 (ribosomal S6 protein kinase) and AMPK]. Although many aspects of these serine phosphorylations are unresolved, some seem to down-regulate whereas others appear to up-regulate the ability to signal through IRS-1. Another level of regulation occurs through the action of phosphatases acting on tyrosine residues, e.g. LAR (leukocyte antigen related phosphatase) and PTP1B (protein tyrosine phosphatase 1B) within the IR and IRS. In addition, insulin signalling may also be modified by the action of PP2A (serine/threonine phosphatases) acting on Akt, PKC, GSK3 and by the action of lipid phosphatases [PTEN (phosphatase and tensin homologue deleted on chromosome 10) and SHIP2 (SH2-containing inositol phosphatase 2)] down-regulating the levels of $PI(3,4,5)P_3$.

Exercise/contraction signalling in muscle: a web distinct from insulin's, but likely inter-woven

The factors thought to be involved in exercise-induced glucose transport have recently been reviewed [1]. In brief, glucose uptake during exercise increases due to a coordinated increase in (i) muscle glucose delivery due to greatly increased capillary perfusion; (ii) increased sarcolemmal and t-tubular transport of glucose from the interstitium to the muscle interior, aided by increased membrane content of the glucose transporter GLUT4; and (iii) increased metabolism of the transported glucose. Whereas each of these events is important, in this review we will focus on the molecular mechanisms activated by exercise/muscle contractions that lead to GLUT4 translocation. The importance of GLUT4 has been shown using muscle tissue from mice with systemic or muscle-specific knockout of GLUT4 [13], in which muscle glucose transport during contractions *in vitro* was abolished.

The molecular events leading to translocation of GLUT4 during muscle contractions are incompletely understood. It has been suggested that the regulation of glucose uptake during exercise can be divided in to a Ca^{2+}/calmodulin-dependent feed-forward mechanism, that is responsible for increasing muscle glucose uptake at the onset of contractions, and an AMPK-related feedback mechanism, responsible for adjusting glucose uptake to the energy needs of the muscle [1] (Figure 2).

Early evidence for a role of intracellular Ca^{2+} in increasing muscle glucose transport comes from older studies showing that pharmacologically induced increase in myoplasmic Ca^{2+}-concentration increases glucose transport in resting muscle [14]. More recently, Wright et al. in a series of studies based on inhibition of CaMK (Ca^{2+}/calmodulin dependent kinases) with the inhibitors KN62 and KN93 suggested that activation of CaMKII during muscle

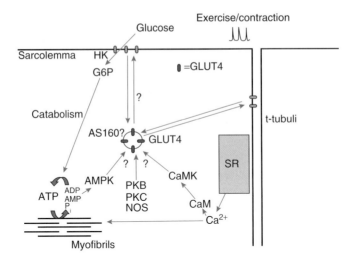

Figure 2. Contraction signalling in skeletal muscle during exercise/contractions
The higher glucose transport with exercise mainly occurs due to higher amounts of GLUT4 in
surface membranes, more specifically the sarcolemma and t-tubuli. The mechanisms behind this
may involve several kinases which sense and transduce signals relating to changes in the intracellular environment during contractions (i.e. higher Ca^{2+}, AMP concentrations) to other undefined
proteins involved in GLUT4 movement and insertion into membranes. CaM, calmodulin; G6P,
glucose-6-phosphate; HK, hexokinase; NOS, nitric oxide synthase; PKB, protein kinase B (also
known as Akt); SR, sarcoplasmic reticulum; t-tubuli, transverse tubuli.

contractions plays an essential role in activating glucose transport, especially
in slow-twitch fibres [15]. Notably, it was shown that the KN inhibitors did
not affect AMPK phosphorylation with exercise [16]. Other downstream
Ca^{2+}-dependent kinases of possible importance for translocation of GLUT4
include the conventional isoforms of PKC and the atypical isoforms of
PKC [17]. Since the atypical isoforms of PKC are involved in activating glucose transport during insulin stimulation, as discussed above, its activation
in muscle during exercise may suggest that it is also involved in stimulating
muscle glucose uptake during exercise.

The role of the AMPK in contraction-induced glucose uptake is at present
somewhat controversial. Pharmacological activation of AMPK with AICAR
(5-aminoimidazole-4-carboxamide-1-β-D-ribonucleoside) in resting muscle
results in activation of muscle glucose transport independently of insulin
(for review see [18]). Since AMPK is also activated in skeletal muscle during
contractions/exercise in both rodent and human skeletal muscle [18], it has
been speculated that AMPK may in fact be 'the' contraction activated kinase
responsible for increasing glucose transport. More definitive mechanistic
answers necessitate the use of genetically manipulated animals. Overexpression
of a dominant negative form of AMPK (a dead kinase) has in mice been
shown to inhibit electrically induced muscle glucose transport by 30–40%
in fast-twitch muscle of the kinase dead muscles compared with the wild
type [19]. This finding may suggest that contraction-induced glucose transport

is partly dependent upon AMPK via a feed-back pathway. Interestingly, however, knockout of either the α1 or the α2 catalytic subunit of AMPK, or the γ3 regulatory subunit, does not cause any inhibition of glucose transport in electrically stimulated incubated mouse muscle [20,21]. A recent study has added weight to the role of AMPK in contraction-induced glucose uptake. In LKB-1 knockout mice, in which the activation of AMPK during electrical stimulation is virtually abolished, uptake of glucose was also markedly inhibited [22]. Drawing conclusions from these experiments is difficult, but it would seem the sum of evidence supports a role for AMPK in contraction-induced glucose uptake. How significant this role is, and whether it varies in different kinds of contractions/exercise, awaits determination.

The regulation of GS activity during exercise has received less attention than glucose uptake. Nevertheless, GS is influenced by both stimulatory and inhibitory factors during exercise and the consequent effect of exercise on GS activity is a result of the relative strength of the various stimuli. Several human studies have shown that muscle GS activity is higher in a glycogen-depleted state compared with a glycogen-loaded state, and it has been suggested that exercise-induced GS activation is dependent on, and merely a result of, glycogen breakdown [23]. The mechanism behind this dependency is unknown, but at least in rodents seems to involve dephosphorylation of GS on site 3a and 3b and changes in the sub-cellular localization of GS [23]. Whether these two changes are linked is unknown, but cellular redistribution of GS induced by glycogen depletion could, for instance, make GS more susceptible to dephosphorylation. Conversely, the covalent modifications of GS, seen during conditions with high muscle glycogen content, are only partly reversible by phosphatase treatment, indicating the involvement of phosphorylation dependent regulatory mechanisms in addition to other unknown factors.

Effect of a single bout of exercise on insulin sensitivity

It has been shown that a single bout of cycle exercise, or stair climbing, improved insulin sensitivity of glucose clearance at the whole body level under hyperinsulinaemic euglycaemic clamp conditions (for review see [23,24]). These changes have been observed as long as two days after the bout of exercise. This effect is likely to be the result of increased insulin sensitivity localised to the muscles that performed the work, as shown in rats [25] and humans [2,26]. Increased insulin action seems to be mainly a result of a leftward shift in the dose–response curve for insulin action on glucose uptake (Figure 3). However, it should be noted that exercise does not always increase insulin action. For example, immediately after intense exercise, insulin action is impaired *in vivo* possibly due to elevated concentrations of catecholamines and non-esterified fatty acids. Likewise, eccentric exercise or physical activities with a dominant component of eccentric contractions elicit a prolonged decrease in insulin action, which may be caused by muscle damage and inflammation leading to

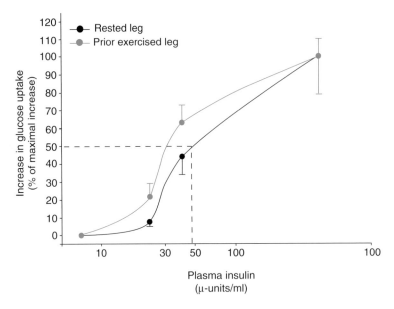

Figure 3. Exercise improves insulin sensitivity of glucose uptake in human muscle
Prior one-legged exercise enhances sensitivity of glucose uptake to insulin in the exercised compared with the rested leg in healthy human subjects as indicated by the decreased insulin concentration eliciting a half maximal glucose uptake response, when glucose uptake is given as a percentage of maximal increase. Data are extracted from Richter et al. [26].

altered protein expression and function [27,28]. Nevertheless, non-damaging dynamic exercise of a moderate intensity usually results in increased insulin sensitivity in the post-exercise period.

What are the mechanisms behind this effect of exercise on insulin sensitivity? A simple hypothesis is that exercise somehow potentiates the insulin signalling cascade. This could theoretically be via the exercise-induced muscle glycogen depletion, since a low glycogen concentration in rat skeletal muscle has been shown to enhance insulin signalling at the level of Akt [29]. However, when the proximal part of the insulin signalling cascade, from the IR through IRS-1 associated PI3K to Akt and GSK3, was analysed in human skeletal muscle, exercise-induced increased insulin action was not accompanied by enhanced signalling in this cascade [30]. On the contrary, IRS-1 associated PI3K activity was stimulated slightly less in the exercised muscle compared with the contralateral control muscle [2].

However, in human skeletal muscle two isoforms of IRS are expressed. Both IRS-1 and IRS-2 contribute to activation of PI3K during insulin stimulation [6], but the physiological role of IRS-2 associated PI3K activity in human skeletal muscle is not well described. Data from IRS knockout mice seem to indicate that IRS-1 is the major isoform mediating insulin-stimulated glucose uptake in skeletal muscle [31]. Still, knockout of IRS-2 results in the development of peripheral insulin resistance, but this could to some extent be a secondary consequence of prolonged exposure to hyperglycaemia due to hepatic insulin resistance and β-cell failure. Interestingly, immediately after *in vivo* exercise, activation of IRS-2 (but not IRS-1) associated PI3K activity in mouse skeletal muscle is markedly increased in response to a supraphysiological insulin stimulus compared with rested muscle [32]. Furthermore, we have recently shown that IRS-2 associated PI3K activity is increased for 60 min in human skeletal muscle 4 h after a single bout of knee-extensor exercise, but the effect of insulin on stimulation of IRS-2 associated PI3K activity is unchanged by prior exercise (unpublished observations by the authors). This results in a generally higher activity of IRS-2 associated PI3K activity in the exercised leg both at basal and during insulin stimulation. Theoretically, this should lead to a higher production of PIP_3 (phosphatidylinositol-3,4,5-trisphosphate). Downstream of PI3K, atypical PKC has emerged as an important signalling component stimulating GLUT4 translocation as discussed previously in this review. One way to activate atypical PKC is via PIP_3. Thus, increased IRS-2 associated PI3K activity in the exercised leg would be assumed to cause increased allosteric activation of atypical PKC. Interestingly, whilst the effect of insulin to activate atypical PKC is not enhanced by prior exercise, we have recently shown that exercise increases the ability of PIP_3 to activate atypical PKC (unpublished observations by the authors). Together, the increase in IRS-2 associated PI3K activity, and the increased ability of PIP_3 to activate atypical PKC in the exercised leg, may be the first indication of direct molecular interactions between exercise and insulin signalling.

Exercise leads to activation of AMPK in the contracting muscles as described above. It has been hypothesized that activation of AMPK is involved in increased sensitivity to insulin. Thus, in rats, pharmacological activation of AMPK by AICAR increased muscle insulin sensitivity in the absence of muscle contractions, suggesting that activation of AMPK increases subsequent insulin sensitivity [33]. However, proof of this concept requires studies utilizing genetic manipulation of muscles such as knockout of AMPK.

Exercise leads to expenditure of energy and decreased muscle glycogen levels. The duration of enhanced insulin sensitivity after a single bout of exercise has in some rodent studies been found to depend on the feeding status of the animals after exercise, such that the duration of enhanced insulin sensitivity is prolonged when carbohydrate intake is restricted after exercise. In humans, the amount of muscle glycogen degraded during exercise correlates significantly with insulin action determined 4 h after the cessation of exercise [24], suggesting that muscle glycogen plays a role in insulin sensitivity although the molecular mechanisms behind such an effect of glycogen remains to be established and may in fact not be directly causative.

Muscle contractions cause changes in gene expression. However, it is generally believed that the increase in insulin sensitivity after a single bout of exercise is not caused by exercise induced increases in the expression of signalling proteins or GLUT4 protein.

Effects of exercise training on insulin action

Whilst a single bout of exercise increases insulin action as discussed above, chronic changes in muscle use or disuse also causes more prolonged changes in insulin action. It should, however, be realised that by simply repeating a single bout of exercise regularly, the muscle will be maintained at a level of improved 'post-exercise' sensitivity. Still, exercise training also leads to changes in gene expression of key proteins involved in glucose handling which potentiates the action of insulin stimulation. Thus, discussing effects of exercise training cannot be done without taking into account that trained muscle is, more or less, chronically in a 'post-acute' exercise state.

Exercise training improves whole body insulin sensitivity in both healthy subjects and in people suffering insulin-resistant diseases. This effect is largely attributable to enhanced insulin induced glucose clearance in peripheral tissues, in particular in the trained skeletal muscle [34].

Skeletal muscle is a heterogeneous tissue composed of fibres with different metabolic and contractile characteristics. Use/disuse of skeletal muscle, i.e. contractile activity of the individual fibres affects these characteristics. For example, use/activity (endurance and strength training) induces changes in myosin heavy chain protein expression toward type IIa (from IIx), whereas disuse induces changes in the opposite direction. A shift in fibre type from IIx towards type IIa also means a shift to more oxidative fibres, generally thought to be more insulin sensitive than the mainly glycolytic fibres. Along the same lines, but not necessarily linked to changes in fibre types [35], use/disuse changes the expression profile of a range of other proteins. This includes the GLUT4 glucose transporter protein, known to be essential for insulin induced glucose uptake into skeletal muscle [13]. Thus, in rodents, exercise training increases GLUT4 protein and mRNA expression in skeletal muscle, an effect that seems to be rather early in onset. In human muscle similar plasticity is observed. Thus, both strength and endurance training increases, and physical inactivity decreases muscle GLUT4 mRNA and protein expression, and data suggest that those fibres recruited during the actual exercise performed are also those in which these adaptations are occurring [35]. In addition, endurance training induces increased capillarization of muscle leading to a generally lower mean diffusion distance from capillary to muscle, in this way facilitating delivery of insulin and glucose to the muscle. That this adaptation may be important is indirectly indicated by the fact that insulin sensitivity in a large sample of subjects has been shown to be related to capillary density [36].

In rodent muscle, insulin responsiveness to activate glucose transport is positively correlated with GLUT4 expression. Thus, a graded response of glucose uptake to insulin stimulation has been observed among rodent muscles expressing variable amounts of GLUT4, e.g. in genetically modified mice in which GLUT4 expression was manipulated (heterozygous and homozygous knockout of the GLUT4 gene), and in animals treated with streptozotocin in which muscle GLUT4 expression is decreased. In humans, a decrease in GLUT4 expression with age correlates with decreased whole body insulin sensitivity. Still, in type 2 diabetes, muscle insulin resistance is present in the face of normal muscle GLUT4 expression suggesting that other mechanisms may also be important for insulin action. In accordance, several studies have addressed the idea that exercise training not only increases the amount of GLUT4 in the muscle, but also leads to changes in insulin signalling capacity enabling the muscle cell to respond to insulin with an enhanced sensitivity.

In rodents, exercise training increases muscle mRNA encoding proteins within the signalling cascade (e.g. IR, IRS-1, P85/P110), as well as mRNA encoding 'effector proteins' (e.g. GLUT4 and GS). However, not all of these effects seem to be translated into changes in actual protein levels. Although increases in IR, p85 and IRS-2 protein levels have been reported [37], the vast majority of studies in rodents have reported no changes in insulin signalling protein expression (e.g. IR, IRS-1, IRS-2, Akt and PKC) despite increases in 'effector proteins' like GS and GLUT4, as well as insulin action. In human skeletal muscle available data is sparse. Short-term (a few weeks) exercise training studies have revealed no apparent changes in IR, IRS-1 or IRS-2 protein levels, whereas long-term training (endurance or strength) reveal increases in expression of IR and Akt protein levels, as well as the 'effector proteins' GLUT4 and GS, in addition to insulin action in muscle [38]. These responses to exercise training in muscle of both human and rodents are likely to be dependent on training mode (intensity and duration), animal species etc., yet the prevailing adaptive responses observed suggest that changes in the expression of the 'effector proteins' GLUT4 and GS are likely to be more important for the adaptive response in muscle (at the level of insulin action) than altered expression of the signalling proteins. Still, neither mRNA nor protein expression necessarily reflects adaptive responses in the signalling cascade upon activation. Thus, to address the question as to whether exercise training changes signalling sensitivity, a range of studies have also applied measurements at the signalling level, involving measurements of either activity or phosphorylation of different signalling elements.

Earlier studies investigating IR function *in vitro* using a wheat germ preparation have not reported any increases in IR tyrosine kinase activity after training in human skeletal muscle [39]. However, a recent study in humans [40] indicates that *in vitro* IR autophosphorylation capacity is increased after 7 days of training. In none of the studies did exercise training lead to changes in the amount of IR protein present. Similarly, some, but not all, studies in muscle of rodent models suggest improved receptor signalling after training [37]. Thus, from the available literature it can be concluded that exercise training under some conditions improves receptor function, and this may improve muscle sensitivity to insulin. In some of the rodent studies the improved IR function translates into increased activity at the post-receptor signalling level (IRS-1/IRS-2 PI3K activity), whereas in other studies this has not been found [41]. In human studies the picture is also not clear, as two studies have observed improved signalling at the level of PI3K and two have reported no improvement.

It is likely that this diversity of findings reflects the complexity of exercise training as a stimulus as well as our limited understanding of the intracellular signalling mechanism. A factor influenced by training is muscle glycogen content which is often increased by training. Glycogen has been shown to be a negative regulator of insulin signalling, at least at the level of Akt phosphorylation [29], and thus some of the variable signalling responses observed in different studies may relate to differences in glycogen modulation by the training regime used. Still, common to nearly all of these training studies is that besides improved muscle insulin action to glucose handling, the amount of 'effector proteins' like GLUT4 and GS is increased. One interpretation of this is that these adaptations are very important for the improved insulin action in trained muscle.

As discussed above, AMPK is activated during exercise, and may have important roles in regulating metabolic events both acutely and chronically. AMPK activation may also to some extent improve muscle insulin sensitivity [33]. Interestingly, we recently observed that AMPK activity in trained human muscle is increased at rest. Chemical activation of AMPK regulates a variety of genes involved in mitochondria biogenesis as well as GLUT4 in resting muscle. However, the obvious extension of these findings i.e. that AMPK is a regulator of insulin sensitivity by regulating the expression of the GLUT4 gene during training has not been verified in studies of genetic animal models. For example, both acute exercise- and training-induced GLUT4 gene transcription is AMPK independent [42,43]. Thus, the mechanisms behind the up-regulation of 'effector proteins' during exercise training are unclear at present.

Interestingly, a recent study in which subjects trained for 7 days showed that enhanced insulin sensitivity was only found if the subjects did not compensate for the training induced increase in energy expenditure [44]. In contrast, when the amount of calories expended during exercise training was carefully replaced by increased dietary intake mainly in the form of carbohydrates, no improvement in insulin sensitivity could be shown. Thus, decreased energy balance induced by exercise training may be important for development of increased insulin signalling, at least during short term training studies.

Conclusions

Insulin and exercise each stimulate muscle glucose uptake via distinct molecular mechanisms which eventually converge on GLUT4 translocation to the plasma membrane. A single bout of exercise increases insulin sensitivity for several hours maximally up to 48 h, and the effect is mainly found in the muscles recruited during exercise. The molecular mechanism behind this effect of exercise is presently largely unresolved, but is likely to be a complex phenomenon involving exercise induced changes in several signalling parameters as well as changes in muscle energy stores.

When exercise is repeated over time, adaptations to physical training occur, which include increased protein expression of GLUT4 and GS, muscle fibre type changes and increased capillarization. Changes in the expression or activation of signalling proteins are less consistently described. Because a single bout of exercise and regular physical training enhances insulin sensitivity, physical activity is considered a cornerstone in prevention and treatment of conditions of low insulin sensitivity such as the metabolic syndrome and type 2 diabetes.

Summary

- *Insulin and exercise each stimulate muscle glucose uptake via distinct molecular mechanisms.*
- *A single bout of exercise increases insulin sensitivity for several hours maximally up to 48 h.*
- *Adaptations to physical training include increased protein expression of GLUT4 and GS, muscle fibre type changes and increased capillarization.*
- *Changes in the expression or activation of signalling proteins are less consistently described.*
- *Physical activity is considered a cornerstone in prevention and treatment of conditions of low insulin sensitivity such as the metabolic syndrome and type 2 diabetes.*

The study was supported by grants from the Danish Medical Research Council, The Danish Natural Science Research Council, the Novo Nordisk Foundation, the Danish Diabetes Association, the Copenhagen Muscle Research Centre, an Integrated Project Funded by the European Union (#LSHM-CT-2004-005272) and the Lundbeck Foundation. J.F.P.W. was supported by a Hallas Møller fellowship from the Novo Nordisk Foundation.

References

1. Rose, A.J. & Richter, E.A. (2005) Skeletal muscle glucose uptake during exercise: how is it regulated? *Physiology (Bethesda)* **20**, 260–270
2. Wojtaszewski, J.F., Hansen, B.F., Kiens, B. & Richter, E.A. (1997) Insulin signaling in human skeletal muscle: time course and effect of exercise. *Diabetes* **46**, 1775–1781
3. Mikines, K., Sonne, B., Farrell, P., Tronier, B. & Galbo, H. (1989) Effect of training on the dose-response relationship for insulin action in men. *J. Appl. Physiol.* **66**, 695–703
4. Thong, F.S., Dugani, C.B. & Klip, A. (2005) Turning signals on and off: GLUT4 traffic in the insulin-signaling highway. *Physiology (Bethesda)* **20**, 271–284

5. Chang, L., Chiang, S.H. & Saltiel, A.R. (2004) Insulin signaling and the regulation of glucose
    transport. *Mol. Med.* **10**, 65–71
6. White, M.F. (2002) IRS proteins and the common path to diabetes. *Am. J. Physiol. Endocrinol.
    Metab.* **283**, E413–E422
7. Shepherd, P.R. (2005) Mechanisms regulating phosphoinositide 3-kinase signalling in
    insulin-sensitive tissues. *Acta Physiol. Scand.* **183**, 3–12
8. Whiteman, E.L., Cho, H. & Birnbaum, M.J. (2002) Role of Akt/protein kinase B in metabolism.
    Trends Endocrinol. Metab. **13**, 444–451
9. Sajan, M.P., Rivas, J., Li, P., Standaert, M.L. & Farese, R.V. (2006) Repletion of atypical protein
    kinase C following RNA interference-mediated depletion restores insulin-stimulated glucose
    transport. *J. Biol. Chem.* **281**, 17466–17473
10. Watson, R.T. and Pessin, J.E. (2006) Bridging the GAP between insulin signaling and GLUT4
    translocation. *Trends Biochem. Sci.* **31**, 215–222
11. Treebak, J.T., Glund, S., Deshmukh, A., Klein, D.K., Long, Y.C., Jensen, T.E., Jorgensen, S.B.,
    Viollet, B., Andersson, L., Neumann, D. et al. (2006) AMPK-mediated AS160 phosphorylation in
    skeletal muscle is dependent on AMPK catalytic and regulatory subunits. *Diabetes* **55**, 2051–2058
12. McManus, E.J., Sakamoto, K., Armit, L.J., Ronaldson, L., Shpiro, N., Marquez, R. & Alessi, D.R.
    (2005) Role that phosphorylation of GSK3 plays in insulin and Wnt signalling defined by knockin
    analysis. *EMBO J.* **24**, 1571–1583
13. Zisman, A., Peroni, O.D., Abel, E.D., Michael, M.D., Mauvais-Jarvis, F., Lowell, B.B., Wojtaszewski,
    J.F., Hirshman, M.F., Virkamaki, A., Goodyear, L.J., Kahn, C.R. & Kahn, B.B. (2000) Targeted
    disruption of the glucose transporter 4 selectively in muscle causes insulin resistance and glucose
    intolerance. *Nat. Med.* **6**, 924–928
14. Holloszy, J. & Narahara, H. (1967) Enhanced permeability to sugar associated with muscle
    contraction. *J. Gen. Physiol.* **50**, 551–562
15. Wright, D.C., Geiger, P.C., Holloszy, J.O. & Han, D.H. (2005) Contraction- and
    hypoxia-stimulated glucose transport is mediated by a Ca^{2+}-dependent mechanism in
    slow-twitch rat soleus muscle. *Am. J. Physiol. Endocrinol. Metab.* **288**, E1062–E1066
16. Wright, D.C., Hucker, K.A., Holloszy, J.O. & Han,D.H. (2004) Ca^{2+} and AMPK both mediate
    stimulation of glucose transport by muscle contractions. *Diabetes.* **53**, 330–335
17. Richter, E.A., Vistisen, B., Maarbjerg, S.J., Sajan, M., Farese, R.V. & Kiens, B. (2004) Differential
    effect of bicycling exercise intensity on activity and phosphorylation of atypical protein kinase C
    and extracellular signal-regulated protein kinase in skeletal muscle. *J. Physiol.* **560**, 909–918
18. Jorgensen, S.B., Richter, E.A. & Wojtaszewski, J.F. (2006) Role of AMPK in skeletal muscle
    metabolic regulation and adaptation in relation to exercise. *J. Physiol.* **574**, 17–31
19. Mu, J., Brozinick, Jr, J.T., Valladares, O., Bucan, M. & Birnbaum, M.J. (2001) A role for
    AMP-activated protein kinase in contraction- and hypoxia-regulated glucose transport in skeletal
    muscle. *Mol. Cell* **7**, 1085–1094
20. Jorgensen, S.B., Viollet, B., Andreelli, F., Frosig, C., Birk, J.B., Schjerling, P., Vaulont, S., Richter,
    E.A. & Wojtaszewski, J.F. (2004) Knockout of the α2 but not α1 5′-AMP-activated protein
    kinase isoform abolishes 5-aminoimidazole-4-carboxamide-1-β-4-ribofuranosidebut not
    contraction-induced glucose uptake in skeletal muscle. *J. Biol. Chem.* **279**, 1070–1079
21. Barnes, B.R., Marklund, S., Steiler, T.L., Walter, M., Hjalm, G., Amarger, V., Mahlapuu, M., Leng,
    Y., Johansson, C., Galuska, D. et al. (2004) The 5′-AMP-activated protein kinase γ3 isoform has
    a key role in carbohydrate and lipid metabolism in glycolytic skeletal muscle. *J. Biol. Chem.* **279**,
    38441–38447
22. Sakamoto, K., Goransson, O., Hardie, D.G. & Alessi, D.R. (2004) Activity of LKB1 and
    AMPK-related kinases in skeletal muscle: effects of contraction, phenformin, and AICAR. *Am. J.
    Physiol. Endocrinol. Metab.* **287**, E310–E317
23. Nielsen, J.N., Derave, W., Kristiansen, S., Ralston, E., Ploug, T. & Richter, E.A. (2001) Glycogen
    synthase localization and activity in rat skeletal muscle is strongly dependent on glycogen content.
    J. Physiol. **531**, 757–769

24. Wojtaszewski, J.F., Nielsen, J.N. & Richter, E.A. (2002) Invited Review: Effect of acute exercise on insulin signaling and action in humans. *J. Appl. Physiol.* **93**, 384–392

25. Richter, E.A., Garetto, L.P., Goodman, M.N. & Ruderman, N.B. (1984) Enhanced muscle glucose metabolism after exercise: modulation by local factors. *Am. J. Physiol.* **246**, E476–E482

26. Richter, E.A., Mikines, K.J., Galbo, H. & Kiens, B. (1989) Effect of exercise on insulin action in human skeletal muscle. *J. Appl. Physiol.* **66**, 876–885

27. Kristiansen, S., Jones, J., Handberg, A., Dohm, G.L. & Richter, E.A. (1997) Eccentric contractions decrease glucose transporter transcription rate, mRNA, and protein in skeletal muscle. *Am. J. Physiol.* **272**, C1734–C1738

28. Del Aguila, L.F., Krishnan, R.K., Ulbrecht, J.S., Farrell, P.A., Correll, P.H., Lang, C.H., Zierath, J.R. & Kirwan, J.P. (2000) Muscle damage impairs insulin stimulation of IRS-1, PI 3-kinase, and Akt-kinase in human skeletal muscle. *Am. J. Physiol. Endocrinol. Metab.* **279**, E206–E212

29. Derave, W., Hansen, B.F., Lund, S., Kristiansen, S. & Richter, E.A. (2000) Muscle glycogen content affects insulin-stimulated glucose transport and protein kinase B activity. *Am. J. Physiol. Endocrinol. Metab.* **279**, E947–E955

30. Wojtaszewski, J.F.P., Hansen, B.F., Gade, J., Kiens, B., Markuns, J.F., Goodyear, L.J. & Richter, E.A. (2000) Insulin signaling and insulin sensitivity after exercise in human skeletal muscle. *Diabetes* **49**, 325–331

31. Previs, S.F., Withers, D.J., Ren, J.M., White, M.F. & Shulman, G.I. (2000) Contrasting effects of IRS-1 versus IRS-2 gene disruption on carbohydrate and lipid metabolism *in vivo*. *J. Biol. Chem.* **275**, 38990–38994

32. Howlett, K.F., Sakamoto, K., Hirshman, M.F., Aschenbach, W.G., Dow, M., White, M.F. & Goodyear, L.J. (2002) Insulin signaling after exercise in insulin receptor substrate-2-deficient mice. *Diabetes* **51**, 479–483

33. Fisher, J.S., Gao, J., Han, D.H., Holloszy, J.O. & Nolte, L.A. (2002) Activation of AMP kinase enhances sensitivity of muscle glucose transport to insulin. *Am. J. Physiol. Endocrinol. Metab.* **282**, E18–E23

34. Dela, F., Larsen, J.J., Mikines, K.J., Ploug, T., Petersen, L.N. & Galbo, H. (1995) Insulin-stimulated muscle glucose clearance in patients with NIDDM. Effects of one-legged physical training. *Diabetes* **44**, 1010–1020

35. Daugaard, J.R. & Richter, E.A. (2001) Relationship between muscle fibre composition, glucose transporter protein 4 and exercise training: possible consequences in non-insulin-dependent diabetes mellitus. *Acta Physiol. Scand.* **171**, 267–276

36. Lillioja, S., Young, A., Culter, C., Ivy, J., Abbott, W.G., Zawadzki, J.K., Yki-Järvinen, H., Christin, L., Secomb, T.W. & Bogardus, C. (1987) Skeletal muscle capillary density and fiber type are possible determinants of *in vivo* insulin resistance in man. *J. Clin. Invest.* **80**, 415–424

37. Chibalin, A.V., Yu, M., Ryder, J.W., Song, X.M., Galuska, D., Krook, A., Wallberg-Henriksson, H. & Zierath, J.R. (2000) Exercise-induced changes in expression and activity of proteins involved in insulin signal transduction in skeletal muscle: differential effects on insulin-receptor substrates 1 and 2. *Proc. Natl. Acad. Sci. U.S.A.* **97**, 38–43

38. Holten, M.K., Zacho, M., Gaster, M., Juel, C., Wojtaszewski, J.F. & Dela, F. (2004) Strength training increases insulin-mediated glucose uptake, GLUT4 content, and insulin signaling in skeletal muscle in patients with type 2 diabetes. *Diabetes* **53**, 294–305

39. Dela, F., Handberg, Aa., Mikines, K.J., Vinten, J. & Galbo, H. (1993) GLUT4 and insulin receptor binding and kinase activity in trained human muscle. *J. Physiol.* **469**, 615–624

40. Youngren, J.F., Keen, S., Kulp, J.L., Tanner, C.J., Houmard, J.A. and Goldfine, I.D. (2001) Enhanced muscle insulin receptor autophosphorylation with short-term aerobic exercise training. *Am. J. Physiol. Endocrinol. Metab.* **280**, E528–E533

41. Zierath, J.R. (2002) Invited review: Exercise training-induced changes in insulin signaling in skeletal muscle. *J. Appl. Physiol.* **93**, 773–781

42. Holmes, B.F., Lang, D.B., Birnbaum, M.J., Mu, J. & Dohm, G.L. (2004) AMP kinase is not required
     for the GLUT4 response to exercise and denervation in skeletal muscle. *Am. J. Physiol. Endocrinol.
     Metab.* **287**, E739–E743
43. Jorgensen, S.B., Treebak, J.T., Viollet, B., Schjerling, P., Vaulont, S., Wojtaszewski, J.F. & Richter
     E.A. (2006) Role of α2-AMPK in basal, training- and AICAR-induced GLUT4, hexokinase II and
     mitochondrial protein expression in mouse muscle. *Am. J. Physiol. Endocrinol. Metab.*, doi: 10.1152/
     ajpendo.00243.2006
44. Black, S.E., Mitchell, E., Freedson, P.S., Chipkin, S.R. & Braun, B. (2005) Improved insulin action
     following short-term exercise training: role of energy and carbohydrate balance. *J. Appl. Physiol.*
     99, 2285–2293

4

Lipid metabolism, exercise and insulin action

Arend Bonen[*][1], G. Lynis Dohm[†] and Luc J.C. van Loon[‡]

Department of Human Health and Nutritional Sciences, University of Guelph, Guelph, Ontario, Canada N1G 2W1, †Department of Physiology, East Carolina University, Greenville, NC, 27858-4353 U.S.A., and ‡Department of Movement Sciences, Maastricht University, Maastricht, The Netherlands, 6200 MD

Abstract

Skeletal muscle constitutes 40% of body mass and takes up 80% of a glucose load. Therefore, impaired glucose removal from the circulation, such as that which occurs in obesity and type 2 diabetes, is attributable in large part to the insulin resistance in muscle. Recent research has shown that fatty acids, derived from adipose tissue, can interfere with insulin signalling in muscle. Hence, insulin-stimulated GLUT4 translocation to the cell surface is impaired, and therefore, the rate of glucose removal from the circulation into muscle is delayed. The mechanisms provoking lipid-mediated insulin resistance are not completely understood. In sedentary individuals, excess intramyocellular accumulation of triacylglycerols is only modestly associated with insulin resistance. In contrast, endurance athletes, despite accumulating large amounts of intramyocellular triacylglycerols, are highly insulin sensitive. Thus it appears that lipid metabolites, other than triacylglycerols, interfere with insulin signalling. These metabolites, however, are not expected to accumulate

[1]*To whom correspondence should be addressed (abonen@uoguelph.ca).*

in athletic muscles, as endurance training increases the capacity for fatty acid oxidation by muscle. These observations, and others in severely obese individuals and type 2 diabetes patients, suggest that impaired rates of fatty acid oxidation are associated with insulin resistance. In addition, in obesity and type 2 diabetes, the rates of fatty acid transport into muscle are also increased. Thus, excess intracellular lipid metabolite accumulation, which interferes with insulin signalling, can occur as a result of impaired rates of fatty acid oxidation and/or increased rates of fatty acid transport into muscle. Accumulation of excess intramyocellular lipid can be avoided by exercise, which improves the capacity for fatty acid oxidation.

Introduction

The prevalence of obesity and type 2 diabetes has increased dramatically in recent years. There is good reason to believe that changes in lifestyle (reduced physical activity and increased energy intake) have contributed to this problem in the latter half of the twentieth century. Indeed, a landmark study has shown that a modest change in lifestyle over 2.8 years [i.e. brisk walking 150 min/week and a restricted energy intake to induce a 7% or approx. 5.6 kg (12.3 lb) weight loss] is twice as effective, and far more economic, than daily drug (metformin) treatment in preventing the onset of type 2 diabetes [1]. However, the molecular mechanisms that are at the root of lifestyle-induced type 2 diabetes remain elusive.

Causes of insulin resistance in skeletal muscle

Glucose uptake into muscle occurs via a well-known facilitated diffusion process involving the glucose transporter GLUT4. Under basal conditions most of the GLUT4 protein is present within intramyocellular depot(s). When glucose levels in the circulation are increased, as is normally the case after a meal, insulin levels also rise. At the plasma membrane of the muscle cell, insulin binds to its receptor, which then initiates a signalling cascade that serves to induce the translocation of GLUT4 from its intracellular depot(s) to the cell surface, thereby increasing the rate of glucose transport into the muscle cell (for a review see [2]) (Figure 1). Muscle contraction can also recruit GLUT4 to the cell surface by activating a signalling system that is independent of the insulin signalling system. Insulin resistance occurs when inadequate quantities of GLUT4 are recruited to the cell surface by insulin, due to impairments in the insulin signalling cascade.

   Type 2 diabetes patients, as well as a high proportion of obese individuals, exhibit insulin resistance. It is now widely recognized that skeletal muscle is one of the key sites in which insulin resistance is present. Under normal circumstances, about 80% of a glucose load is taken up by the skeletal muscles of the human body. Because skeletal muscle comprises about 40% of body weight, insulin resistance in this tissue accounts for a major proportion of

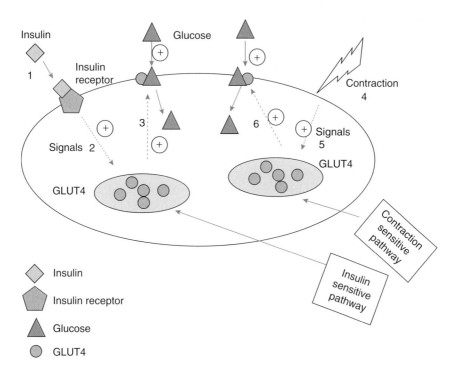

Figure 1. Schematic view of insulin-stimulated and muscle contraction-stimulated glucose transport into muscle

Insulin binds to its receptor at the cell surface. This begins an insulin signalling cascade as detailed elsewhere (see Chapter 3). GLUT4 proteins are then recruited to and inserted into the plasma membrane allowing glucose to be transported into the cell. Contraction also stimulates GLUT4 translocation. The contraction signalling system differs from the insulin signalling system. AMPK activation is one of the signals involved in recruiting GLUT4 to the cell surface. Others signals are also likely to be needed but these have proved elusive. Once the proper contraction signal is received, GLUT4 is then recruited to and inserted into the plasma membrane allowing glucose to be transported into the cell.

the whole body insulin resistance (i.e. delayed clearance of glucose from the circulation in response to insulin).

The decreased ability of insulin to stimulate glucose transport in muscle of individuals with insulin resistance could be caused by a block in insulin signal transduction or an inability to move the GLUT4 transporter to the membrane. To differentiate between these alternatives, several studies have investigated whether signals other than insulin could stimulate glucose transport in insulin resistant muscle; if so, then the insulin resistance must be caused by inadequate insulin signal transduction. Most such studies (for a review see [3]) demonstrate that glucose transport is stimulated normally by muscle contraction and hypoxia. There are also a number of studies that directly demonstrate that insulin signalling is depressed in insulin resistant muscle of obese and diabetic animals and humans. It has been demonstrated that insulin receptor autophosphorylation, IRS-1 (insulin receptor substrate 1) tyrosine phosphorylation, as well as insulin activation of phosphatidylinositol 3-kinase and PKB/Akt (protein kinase B) were depressed in muscle of morbidly obese patients (for a review see [3]). These changes were accompanied by serine phosphorylation of the insulin receptor and IRS-1, both of which have been shown to depress the tyrosine kinase activity of the insulin receptor.

These changes in insulin signal transduction raise the question of which kinase phosphorylates the insulin receptor/IRS-1 and what activates that kinase in insulin resistant muscle. Several lines of evidence support the hypothesis that lipid accumulation in muscles of obese and diabetic individuals activates PKC (protein kinase C) which leads to serine phosphorylation and inactivation of IRS-1 and the insulin receptor. The β-isoform of PKC is elevated in insulin resistant muscle of morbidly obese patients and lipid-treated human subjects. In obese animal models and in rats infused with lipid, the θ-isoform of PKC is activated. These studies demonstrate an association between insulin resistance and PKC but do not demonstrate a cause and effect relationship. However, when human muscle is incubated with a PKC activator the muscle becomes less responsive to insulin and when insulin resistant human muscle is treated with a PKC inhibitor insulin sensitivity is restored. These studies support the role of PKC as an agent of insulin resistance. However, other factors, such as oxidative stress (accumulation of reactive oxygen species) and reduced fat oxidation may also play a role in causing insulin resistance.

Fatty acids and skeletal muscle insulin resistance in obesity and type 2 diabetes

It is now known that fatty acids contribute to insulin resistance in skeletal muscle. Whilst insulin resistance can be induced rapidly within about 4–5 h in humans, when fatty acids are infused [4], the mechanisms involved in this process are not fully understood. Traditionally, the well-known Randle (glucose–fatty acid) cycle has been widely used to explain the mechanism behind fatty acid-induced insulin resistance in skeletal muscle. However, this explanation has been questioned.

Recently, research has begun to identify other mechanisms by which fatty acids or their metabolites induce insulin resistance. These studies have begun to suggest that an increase in intramyocellular lipid accumulation and/or a reduction in fatty oxidation induce defects in the insulin signalling cascade that impairs the recruitment of GLUT4 to the cell surface (i.e. skeletal muscle insulin resistance). However, the mechanisms promoting the intramyocellular accumulation of triacylglycerols and fatty metabolites (fatty acyl-CoA, ceramides and diacylglycerol) are not clear. Such increases can be attributed to an increase in circulating fatty acid concentrations, increased rates of fatty acid transport into muscle and/or reductions in the rates of fatty acid oxidation. Below we examine how some of these processes are associated with insulin resistance in skeletal muscle. Understanding these processes provide direction for therapeutic strategies, especially exercise intervention. This is a healthy, economic and non-pharmacological approach by which to combat insulin resistance in obesity and type 2 diabetes in modern industrialized societies.

Fatty acids and intramyocellular lipids

Fatty acids are stored primarily as triacylglycerols in subcutaneous and deep visceral adipose tissue. These depots are large (in a 70 kg male there is 9–15 kg adipose tissue, or 350–586 MJ) and represent approx. 95% of the total energy stores in humans. Physiologic signals (e.g. catecholamines, cortisol and reduced insulin concentrations) lead to the hydrolysis of triacylglycerol thereby releasing fatty acids into the circulation that are delivered to a number of tissues, including skeletal muscle. These blood-borne fatty acids are a primary source for skeletal muscle fatty acid oxidation, and precursors for the formation of intramyocellular fatty acyl-CoAs, diacylglycerols, ceramides and triacylglycerols.

When calculated across the entire muscle mass of the human body, the total quantity of intramuscular triacylglycerol is very small constituting only 1–2% of the triacylglycerol depot that is present in the adipose tissue mass in the human body (e.g. in a 70 kg male with 28 kg muscle the total intramyocellular triacylglycerol pool is estimated to be approx. 0.2 kg or 7.8 MJ). Within muscle, triacylglycerols are present as small lipid droplets, located adjacent to the muscle mitochondria (Figure 2), and may therefore function as a readily available fuel for oxidative metabolism, particularly during exercise. Indeed, despite earlier work to the contrary, recent research using stable isotope methodology,

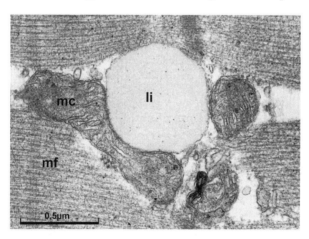

Figure 2. Electron photomicrograph of a longitudinal section of skeletal muscle tissue
In the centre, on the level of the Z-line, are intermyofibrillar mitochondria with a lipid droplet immediately adjacent. Li, lipid droplet; mc, central mitochondria; mf, myofilaments; marker indicates 0.5 μm (reproduced from [24]). Reproduced by permission from Macmillan Publishers Ltd: *International Journal of Obesity* (1999) vol. 23, pages s7–s10. Copyright (1999); www.nature.com/ijo.

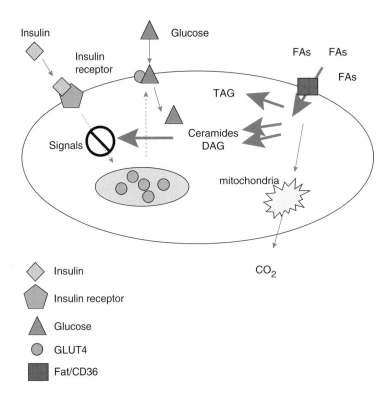

Figure 3. Schematic view of insulin-stimulated glucose transport into muscle and intramyocellular lipid interference with insulin signalling.
In sedentary individuals fatty acid products (diacylglycerol and ceramides) accumulate in the muscle cell, possibly because of insufficient exercise during the day. These fatty acid metabolites (diacylglycerol and ceramides) interfere with some steps in the insulin signalling cascade, resulting in impaired GLUT4 translocation to the plasma membrane, and therefore glucose entry into the muscle cell is impaired.

[1]H-magnetic resonance spectroscopy and electron and/or immunofluorescence microscopy, have all shown that a substantial amount of energy is liberated from the hydrolysis and subsequent oxidation of intramyocellular triacylglycerol depots in type 1 muscle fibres with endurance exercise (for a review see [5]).

Intramyocellular triacylglycerols and insulin resistance

Despite their low concentrations within the muscle cell, intramyocellular lipids, when present in excess, appear to be very significant in causing interference with insulin signalling in the muscle cell. In this manner intramyocellular lipids interfere with the recruitment of the glucose transporter, GLUT4, to the cell surface, that then results in a lowered rate of insulin-stimulated glucose transport into the muscle cell (i.e. insulin resistance) (Figure 3).

The first suggestion that intramyocellular lipids were associated with insulin resistance in muscle resulted from work showing that increases in intramyocellular triacylglycerol were positively, but modestly, associated with the severity of insulin resistance [6]. An association between intramyocellular triacylglycerol accumulation and insulin resistance has now been confirmed in many other studies, particular those in which high fat feeding trials have been used to induce skeletal muscle insulin resistance.

There are, however, exceptions to this intramyocellular triacylglycerol-insulin resistance linkage, which seemingly produces a paradox. First, type 1 (oxidative) skeletal muscle fibres have a 3-fold higher content of intramyocellular triacylglycerols than type 2 (glycolytic) muscle fibres; yet, type 1 muscle fibres are more insulin sensitive than type 2 muscle fibres. Secondly, endurance trained athletes have higher concentrations of intramyocellular triacylglycerols than sedentary and/or diabetic individuals; yet, because of their training, these athletes are far more insulin sensitive than sedentary individuals.

However, these examples may be much less paradoxical than it appears. The greater intramuscular triacylglycerol storage in type 1 fibres or in the trained athlete allows a greater contribution of the intramuscular triacylglycerol pool as a substrate source during exercise [5], as rates of fatty acid oxidation are high in type 1 fibres or in muscles of athletes because of endurance training. In contrast, in the obese and/or type 2 diabetes patient, elevated intramuscular triacylglycerol stores seem to be secondary to increased plasma fatty acid concentrations and increased skeletal muscle fatty acid uptake. In these individuals, in whom fatty acid oxidation may be impaired, this leads to accumulation of intramuscular triacylglycerol and fatty acid intermediates (fatty acyl-CoAs, diacylglycerols and ceramides). These intermediates, rather than intramuscular triacylglycerol themselves, impair insulin signalling [7–9]. Therefore, intramyocellular triacylglycerol content is probably only a surrogate marker for dysregulated fatty acid metabolism in muscle of obese individuals and type 2 diabetes patients, whilst in trained athletes intramyocellular triacylglycerol content is not related to impaired fatty acid metabolism.

Fatty acid oxidation and insulin resistance

Intramyocellular triacylglycerol concentrations are not always a good marker of insulin resistance. Therefore it has been suggested that skeletal muscle oxidative capacity may provide a better relationship to insulin sensitivity. This conclusion would be consistent with the observation that (i) in type 2 diabetes patients, skeletal muscle oxidative capacity is a better predictor of insulin sensitivity than either intramyocellular triacylglycerol concentration or long-chain fatty acyl-CoA content [10], and (ii) the increase in the muscles' oxidative capacity and the increase in insulin sensitivity are highly correlated when individuals undergo a rigorous exercise training program (reviewed in [11]).

Consistent with the suggestion that the capacity for fatty acid oxidation may be related to insulin sensitivity, several groups have demonstrated that mitochondrial content and oxidative capacity are reduced in insulin resistant obese and diabetes patients (for a review see [3]). The recent report that mito-chondrial density is lower in insulin-resistant offspring of type 2 diabetic patients suggests that reduced oxidative capacity may represent an early factor in the development of insulin resistance and type 2 diabetes [12].

Further support for the key role of impaired fatty acid oxidation in insulin resistance has come from studies in L6 muscle cells and studies using isolated muscles. In both systems palmitate induced insulin resistance by inhibiting the activation of the key insulin signalling kinase, Akt/PKB. This how-ever was reversed when rates of fatty acid oxidation were increased either by transfecting L6 cells with CPT 1 (carnitine palmitoyltransferase 1) [13], or by stimulating fatty acid oxidation in isolated muscle by stimulating AMPK (AMP-activated protein kinase) with the exercise-mimetic agent AICAR (5-aminoimidazole-4-carboxamide-1-β-D-ribonucleoside) [14]. The rescue of insulin resistance was not accompanied by the reduction of intramuscular lipid metabolites, either in L6 cells or in isolated muscles. However, in isolated mus-cle the degree of insulin resistance and its rescue were highly correlated with the improved capacity for fatty acid oxidation [14].

In humans, skeletal muscle fatty acid oxidation is reduced in severely obese individuals (BMI = 54 kg/m^2), but not in less severe obese individuals (BMI = 30–35 kg/m^2) (for a review see [3]). In addition, morbidly obese patients have depressed fat oxidation measured at the whole body level, in muscle homoge-nates, and in muscle cells in culture, and these changes correlate with insulin resistance. However, when these patients lose weight after gastric bypass sur-gery, insulin sensitivity is restored but fatty acid oxidation remains depressed (for a review see [3]). Thus, alterations in fatty acid oxidation in the latter individuals are not obviously associated with impairment in insulin sensitivity. Therefore, other mechanisms may also be involved in fatty acid-induced insu-lin resistance in skeletal muscle.

Increased fatty acid uptake and insulin resistance

Intramuscular triacylglycerol and fatty acid intermediate accumulation may also be associated with an increase in circulating concentrations of fatty acids and mechanisms regulating their uptake. Insulin resistance and type 2 diabetes are often associated with increased fat intake and obesity. A greater fat mass increases the basal, whole-body lipolytic rate, as in the insulin resistant state adipose tissue lipolysis is less inhibited. This can result in higher circulating concentrations of fatty acids, which would result in a greater accumulation of intramuscular triacylglycerol and fatty acid intermediates. Lowering the circulating concentrations of fatty acids by inhibition of adipose tissue lipolysis, increases the oxidation of intramuscular triacylglycerol, and presumably also reduces intramuscular fatty acid intermediates, at rest

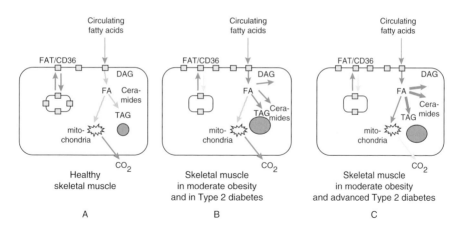

Figure 4. Possible model of how FAT/CD36 mediated fatty acid influx contributes to the accumulation of intramyocellular lipids
(A) Under normal circumstances fatty acids enter the cell, a process assisted by the protein FAT/CD36, which cycles between an intracellular depot and the plasma membrane. **(B)** In moderately obese individuals and patients with type 2 diabetes more FAT/CD36 is present at the plasma membrane, allowing a more rapid entry of fatty acids into the cell. In these individuals fatty acid oxidation is not impaired. **(C)** In more severely obese individuals and severely diabetic individuals, oxidation of fatty acids is also reduced leading to an even greater fatty acid accumulation. Note also that in situations where circulating fatty acids are also increased, the same process would still be occurring but even more triacylglycerol, diacyglycerol and ceramides would accumulate. TAG, triacylglycerol; DAG, diacylglycerol; FA, fatty acids. (Figure based on data presented in [18]).

and during exercise, in overweight type 2 diabetes patients [5,15]. Reducing circulating fatty acids is an effective strategy to improve insulin sensitivity in type 2 diabetes patients [5,15,16].

Increased fatty acid transport and insulin resistance

Recently, it has been found that fatty acid uptake into the muscle cell occurs via a highly regulated protein mediated mechanism, involving a number of fatty acid transporters (for review see [17]). A key fatty acid transporter is FAT/CD36 (fatty acid translocase), the homologue of human CD36. Thus, an increased rate of entry of fatty acids into muscle could be yet another mechanism whereby excess fatty acids accumulate within the muscle cell.

In insulin resistant skeletal muscle in humans and animals, rates of fatty acid transport into muscle are markedly increased [18–20]. Such increased rates of fatty acid transport are already evident at an early age before type 2 diabetes is evident in diabetic fatty Zucker rats [20]. In obese humans, the increased rates of fatty acid transport into muscle are highly correlated with an increase in triacylglycerol accumulation, whereas rates of fatty acid oxidation are not increased [18]. In these studies, a permanent relocation of FAT/CD36 to the plasma membrane, but not an increase in FAT/CD36 expression, facilitates the increased rate of fatty acid transport into the insulin resistant skeletal muscles of obese and type 2 diabetic individuals [18]. This means that for a given level of circulating fatty acids, more will be taken up into the muscle when the plasma membrane FAT/CD36 content has been increased. This has led to a model which suggests that intramyocellular lipids accumulate in response to a greater rate of FAT/CD36-mediated fatty acid influx into the muscle cell, in the absence of any changes in fatty acid oxidation (Figure 4B). This is further supported by the inverse correlation between the plasma membrane content of the fatty acid transporter FAT/CD36 and the glucose transporter GLUT4 ($r = -0.91$) [20], during the transition from insulin resistance to severe type 2 diabetes in diabetic fatty Zucker rats. Thus in insulin resistant muscles, the subcellular locations of FAT/CD36 and GLUT4 are juxtaposed, with GLUT4 being retained in its intracellular depots whilst FAT/CD36 is permanently relocated to the plasma membrane. Clearly, the increased rate of fatty acid transport into the muscle cell is yet another mechanism that is associated with insulin resistance in this tissue.

It is also possible that changes in fatty acid transport across the plasma membrane are associated with changes in fatty acid oxidation, as unexpectedly FAT/CD36 is also present in the mitochondrion in rat [21] and human muscle [22,23], where it appears to interact with CPT 1. Blocking FAT/CD36 at the mitochondrion reduced fatty acid oxidation by 90%. During exercise in rats [21] and humans [23] muscle mitochondrial FAT/CD36 is increased via its translocation from an unknown intracellular depot. However, the significance of mitochondrial FAT/CD36 in insulin resistance and type 2 diabetes is not yet understood.

Conclusion

There is little doubt that lipids contribute to the onset of insulin resistance in muscle. Research is needed at several levels. In particular, we need to develop an understanding of the molecular mechanisms that contribute to the intramyocellular accumulation of lipid metabolites and their interference with insulin signalling. In addition, there is already sufficient knowledge to pursue important research at the applied level. Specifically, without knowing the molecular basis of action of lipid metabolites, effective exercise and dietary regimens need to be investigated, i.e. ones that limit intramyocellular lipid accumulation, either by limiting the availability of fatty acids in the diet and/or by effectively oxidizing them in muscle, as occurs when an exercise programme is maintained. These healthy, low cost, non-pharmacological strategies can provide an opportunity to prevent or even reverse insulin resistance.

Summary

- *Intramyocellular triacylglycerol depots are modestly correlated with insulin resistance, but are unlikely to be the direct cause of insulin resistance.*
- *Accumulation of lipid metabolites (fatty acyl-CoAs, diacylglycerols and ceramides) within the muscle contribute to insulin resistance by interfering with the insulin activation of the signalling pathway involved in recruiting GLUT4 to the cell surface.*
- *It has been hypothesized that the fatty acid metabolites (fatty acyl-CoAs, diacylglycerols and ceramides) activate protein kinase C, which then leads to serine phosphorylation and inactivation of IRS-1. The latter is regarded as a molecular key event leading to insulin resistance as it prevents tyrosine phosphorylation and activation of IRS-1.*
- *Reduced rates of fatty acid oxidation by muscle may be a better indicator of insulin resistance than intramyocellular lipid accumulation.*
- *Reduced rates of fatty acid oxidation have been related to insulin resistance in severely obese individuals (BMI > 35 kg/m²), since this probably leads to the accumulation of intramyocellular lipid metabolites.*
- *Increased rates of fatty acid transport into muscle, due to the increased presence of a fatty acid transport protein (FAT/CD36) at the cell surface, is another mechanism whereby muscle can accumulate excess intramyocellular lipids.*
- *The imbalance between plasma fatty acids, skeletal muscle fatty acid uptake, storage and oxidation collectively contribute to the development of skeletal muscle insulin resistance. Therefore, limiting fatty acid accumulation in muscle, as occurs with regular exercise, is an effective strategy to maintain insulin sensitivity.*

References

1. Knowler, W.C., Barrett-Connor, E., Fowler, S.E., Hamman, R.F., Lachin, J.M., Walker, E.A. & Nathan, D.M. (2002) Reduction in the incidence of type 2 diabetes with lifestyle intervention or metformin. *N. Engl. J. Med.* **346**, 393–403
2. Saltiel, A.R. & Kahn, C.R. (2001) Insulin signalling and the regulation of glucose and lipid metabolism. *Nature* **414**, 799–806
3. Thyfault, J.P. & Dohm, G.L. (2006) Metabolic alterations in muscle associated with obesity. In. *Nutrition and Diabetes. Pathophysiology and Management.* (E. Opara ed.) pp 79–98 Taylor & Frances Group, Boca Raton
4. Boden, G. (1996) Role of fatty acids in the pathogenesis of insulin resistance and NIDDM. *Diabetes* **45**, 3–10
5. van Loon, L.J. (2004) Use of intramuscular triacylglycerol as a substrate source during exercise in humans. *J. Appl. Physiol.* **97**, 1170–1187
6. Pan, D.A., Lillioja, S., Kriketos, A.D., Milner, M.R., Baur, L.A., Jenkins, A.B. & Storlien, L.H. (1997) Skeletal muscle triglyceride levels are inversely related to insulin action. *Diabetes* **46**, 983–988

7.   Ellis, B.A., Poynten, A., Lowy, A.J., Furler, S.M., Chisholm, D.J., Kraegen, E.W. & Cooney, G.J.
     (2000) Long chain acyl-CoA esters as indicators of lipid availability and insulin sensitivity in rat and
     human muscle. *Am. J. Physiol. Endocrinol. Metab.* **279**, E554–E560

8.   Chavez, J.A., Holland, W.L., Bar, J., Sandhoff, K. & Summers, S.A. (2005) Acid ceramidase overex-
     pression prevents the inhibitory effects of saturated fatty acids on insulin signaling. *J. Biol. Chem.*
     280, 20148–20153

9.   Yu, C., Chen, Y., Cline, G.W., Zhang, D., Zong, H., Wang, Y., Bergeron, R., Kim, J.K., Cushman,
     S.W., Cooney, G.W. et al. (2002) Mechanism by which fatty acids inhibit insulin activation of insu-
     lin receptor substrate-1 (IRS-1)-associated phosphatidylinositol 3-kinase activity in muscle. *J. Biol.
     Chem.* **277**, 50230–50236

10. Bruce, C.R., Anderson, M.J., Carey, A.L., Newman, D.G., Bonen, A., Kriketos, A.D., Cooney, G.J.
     & Hawley, J.A. (2003) Muscle oxidative capacity is a better predictor of insulin sensitivity than
     lipid status. *J. Clin. Endocrinol. Metab.* **88**, 5444–5451

11. Goodpaster, B.H. & Brown, N.F. (2005) Skeletal muscle lipid and its association with insulin
     resistance: what is the role for exercise? *Exerc. Sport Sci. Rev.* **33**, 150–154

12. Morino, K., Petersen, K.F., Dufour, S., Befroy, D., Frattini, J., Shatzkes, N., Neschen, S., White,
     M.F., Bilz, S., Sono, S., et al. (2005) Reduced mitochondrial density and increased IRS-1 serine
     phosphorylation in muscle of insulin-resistant offspring of type 2 diabetic parents. *J. Clin. Invest.*
     115, 3587–3593

13. Perdomo, G., Commerford, S.R., Richard, A.M., Adams, S.H., Corkey, B.E., O'Doherty, R.M. &
     Brown, N.F. (2004) Increased β-oxidation in muscle cells enhances insulin-stimulated glucose
     metabolism and protects against fatty acid-induced insulin resistance despite intramyocellular
     lipid accumulation. *J. Biol. Chem.* **279**, 27177–27186

14. Alkhateeb, H. & Bonen, A. (2005) Fatty acid induced insulin resistance and its amelioration in
     isolated soleus muscle. *2nd Northern Lights Conference. Canadian Federation of Biological Societies,*
     (Abstract F25).

15. Boden, G., Lebed, B., Schatz, M., Homko, C. & Lemieux, S. (2001) Effects of acute changes of
     plasma free fatty acids on intramyocellular fat content and insulin resistance in healthy subjects.
     Diabetes **50**, 1612–1617

16. van Loon, L.J.C., Manders, R.J.F., Koopman, R., Kaastra, B., Stegen, J.H.C.H., Gijsen, A.P., Saris,
     W.H.M. & Keizer, H.A. (2005) Inhibition of adipose tissue lipolysis increases intramuscular lipid
     use in type 2 diabetic patients. *Diabetologia* **48**, 2097–2107

17. Koonen, D.P., Glatz, J.F., Bonen, A. & Luiken, J.J. (2005) Long-chain fatty acid uptake and FAT/
     CD36 translocation in heart and skeletal muscle. *Biochim. Biophys. Acta* **1736**, 163–180

18. Bonen, A., Parolin, M.L., Steinberg, G.R., Calles-Escandon, J., Tandon, N.N., Glatz, J.F.C., Luiken,
     J.J.F.P., Heigenhauser, G.J.F. & Dyck, D.J. (2004) Triacylglycerol accumulation in human obesity
     and type 2 diabetes is associated with increased rates of skeletal muscle fatty acid transport and
     increased sarcolemmal FAT/CD36. *FASEB J.* **18**, 1144–1146

19. Luiken, J.J.F.P., Arumugam, Y., Dyck, D.J., Bell, R.C., Pelsers, M.L., Turcotte, L.P., Tandon, N.N.,
     Glatz, J.F.C. & Bonen, A. (2001) Increased rates of fatty acid uptake and plasmalemmal fatty acid
     transporters in obese Zucker rats. *J. Biol. Chem.* **276**, 40567–40573

20. Chabowski, A., Chatham, J.C., Tandon, N.N., Calles-Escandon, J., Glatz, J.F.C., Luiken, J.J.F.P. &
     Bonen, A. (2006) Fatty acid transport and FAT/CD36 are increased in red but not in white muscle
     skeletal muscle of Zucker diabetic fatty (ZDF) rats. *Am. J. Physiol. Endocrinol. Metab.* **29**, E675–E682

21. Campbell, S.E., Tandon, N.N., Woldegiorgis, G., Luiken, J.J.F.P., Glatz, J.F.C. & Bonen, A. (2004) A
     novel function for FAT/CD36: involvement in long chain fatty acid transfer into the mitochondria.
     J. Biol. Chem. **279**, 36325–36341

22. Bezaire, V., Bruce, C.R., Heigenhauser, G.J., Tandon, N.N., Glatz, J.F., Luiken, J.J., Bonen, A. &
     Spriet, L.L. (2006) Identification of fatty acid translocase on human skeletal muscle mitochondrial
     membranes: essential role in fatty acid oxidation. *Am. J. Physiol. Endocrinol. Metab.* **290**, E509–E515

23. Holloway, G.P., Bezaire, V., Heigenhauser, G.J., Tandon, N.N., Glatz, J.F., Luiken, J.J., Bonen, A. & Spriet, L.L. (2006) Mitochondrial long chain fatty acid oxidation, fatty acid translocase/CD36 content and carnitine palmitoyltransferase I activity in human skeletal muscle during aerobic exercise. *J. Physiol.* **571**, 201–210

24. Hoppeler, H. (1999) Skeletal muscle substrate metabolism. *Int. J. Obes. Relat. Metab. Disord.* **23** (suppl 3), S7–S10

5

Resistance exercise, muscle loading/unloading and the control of muscle mass

Keith Baar[*][1], Gustavo Nader[†] and Sue Bodine[‡]

Division of Molecular Physiology, University of Dundee, Dundee U.K., †Research Center for Genetic Medicine, Children's National Medical Center, Washington D.C., U.S.A. and, ‡College of Biological Sciences, University of California, Davis, CA, U.S.A.

Abstract

Muscle mass is determined by the difference between the rate of protein synthesis and degradation. If synthesis is greater than degradation, muscle mass will increase (hypertrophy) and when the reverse is true muscle mass will decrease (atrophy). Following resistance exercise/increased loading there is a transient increase in protein synthesis within muscle. This change in protein synthesis correlates with an increase in the activity of protein kinase B/Akt and mTOR (mammalian target of rapamycin). mTOR increases protein synthesis by increasing translation initiation and by inducing ribosomal biogenesis. By contrast, unloading or inactivity results in a decrease in protein synthesis and a significant increase in muscle protein breakdown. The decrease in synthesis is due in part to the inactivation of mTOR and therefore a decrease in translation initiation, but also to a decrease in the rate of translation elongation. The increase in degradation is the result of a co-ordinated response of the calpains, lysosomal proteases and the ATP-dependent ubiquitin-proteosome. Caspase 3 and the calpains act upstream of the ubiquitin–proteosome system to assist in the complete breakdown of the myofibrillar proteins. Two muscle specific E3 ubiquitin ligases, MuRF1 and MAFbx/atrogen-1, have been identified as

[1]*To whom correspondence should be addressed (email k.baar@dundee.ac.uk).*

key regulators of muscle atrophy. In this chapter, these pathways and how the balance between anabolism and catabolism is affected by loading and unloading will be discussed.

Introduction

Skeletal muscle produces the forces that allow us to move, is the primary storehouse for both amino acids and glucose and, because of its high metabolic rate, is also the primary determinant of our basal metabolic rate [1]. Our overall amount of muscle tissue is therefore not only essential for maintaining an active lifestyle, but is also an important determinant of our longevity [2], adiposity [3] and insulin sensitivity [1]. Muscle mass is determined by the balance between protein synthesis and protein degradation. Following resistance exercise/increased loading in the fed state, the rate of protein synthesis exceeds breakdown, whilst unloading has the reverse effect. The result is that increasing loading results in skeletal muscle hypertrophy (increased muscle mass) and increased force production whereas unloading results in skeletal muscle atrophy (decreased muscle mass) and frailty. Over the last ten years a number of important discoveries have shed light on how loading determines muscle mass and much of this work will be briefly reviewed below. For a more extensive description, we suggest a number of very good reviews for both hypertrophy [4] and atrophy [5,6].

Muscle hypertrophy

Skeletal muscle hypertrophy occurs following repeated bouts of high resistance exercise. Whilst each individual bout of high resistance exercise is necessary, it is not sufficient to produce hypertrophy. This indicates that, following acute exercise, there is a transient alteration within the muscle that, when repeated, produces skeletal muscle hypertrophy. Therefore, in order to understand what drives the increase in muscle mass we must understand what happens immediately following a single bout of resistance exercise. The most important acute response to resistance exercise is an increase in the rate of protein synthesis.

Control of protein synthesis by hypertrophic stimuli

In humans, a bout of high resistance exercise increases the fractional rate of protein synthesis 50% after 4 h, and 115% by 24 h [7]. In some studies the increase in protein synthesis is maintained out to 48 h before returning to control levels [8]. Theoretically, this increase could be due to an increase in RNA levels leading to an increase in protein synthesis through a mass action effect. However, needle biopsies taken from the subjects showed that there was no change in the RNA content of the muscle at either 4 h or 24 h following a single bout of resistance exercise [7], suggesting that the immediate changes in protein synthesis are the result of an increase in the amount of protein synthesized per molecule of RNA, not an increase in total RNA, thus it is the efficiency of translation or mRNA activity, that is increased following loading. An immediate increase in the rate of protein synthesis following an acute bout of resistance exercise has also been shown in a number of animal models. The most well-controlled studies addressing the initial response of skeletal muscle to a hypertrophic stimulus are those of Wong and Booth [9,10]. In these studies the initial response to an acute bout of shortening and lengthening contractions was a 25–50% increase in protein synthesis. This increase in protein synthesis was observed 12–17 h after the exercise bout at a time when the accumulation of RNA and DNA was unchanged. The authors concluded that increases in RNA do not have a primary role in increased protein synthesis after a single bout of resistance exercise [10]. Hamosch et al. [11] conclusively demonstrated that an increase in protein synthesis occurs during hypertrophy using cell free extracts taken from hypertrophied muscle. This study demonstrated that following the addition of equal amounts of mRNA, the rate of amino acid incorporation was 120% higher in extracts from hypertrophied muscle than in extracts from normal muscle, indicating that the RNA activity of muscle is increased following high resistance exercise.

Control of protein synthesis by phosphorylation

Protein synthesis is the process by which the genetic code, carried by mRNA, is translated into the amino acids that form proteins. The polymerization of the amino acids is catalysed by a large molecule know as the ribosome that binds to the mRNA and scans to find the translation start site (initiation), translates the mRNA by sequentially inserting one amino acid for every codon as it travels the length of the mRNA (elongation), and is released from the mRNA when it completes the protein and reaches a stop codon (termination). To determine what step of protein synthesis was affected by resistance exercise, Baar and Esser used polysome profiles to show that there was an increase in the association of mRNA with ribosomes (Figure 1) suggesting that the rate of initiation of protein synthesis had increased more than the rate of elongation and termination [12].

Initiation can largely be separated into two regulated steps. The binding of the initiator tRNA to the 40S ribosomal subunit to make the 43S preinitiation complex which is regulated by eIF2 (eukaryotic initiation factor 2), and the cap-dependent binding of mRNA to the 43S preinitiation complex which is regulated by eIF4E (eukaryotic initiation factor 4E) and its repressor 4E-BP (eIF4E binding protein) (for a review see [13]). Both of these processes can be controlled following loading by the mTOR (mammalian target of rapamycin) and PDK1 (phosphoinositol-dependent protein kinase 1) pathway (Figure 2). mTOR exists in two important complexes within cells. The first is with its binding partners raptor and GβL in TORC1 (TOR complex 1) and the second is a complex with rictor and GβL termed TORC2 (TOR complex 2). TORC1 has been widely studied for its role in controlling protein synthesis through

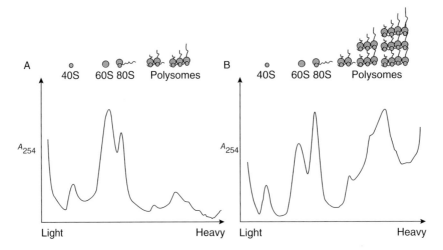

Figure 1. Resistance exercise increases polysomal RNA
Polysome traces from the tibialis anterior muscle of rats (**A**) without resistance exercise and
(**B**) 6 h after a single bout of resistance exercise. As denoted above the figures, the peaks on
the curve (from left-to-right) are: the 40S ribosomal subunit, the 60S ribosomal subunit, the
80S ribosome, two ribosomes on a single mRNA, three ribosomes on an mRNA etc. Note the
increase in heavy RNA molecules indicative of an increase in the number of ribosomes associated with RNA. Adapted from Barr and Esser (1999) *American Journal of Physiology*, vol. 276, pages
C120–C127, with permission from The American Physiological Society.

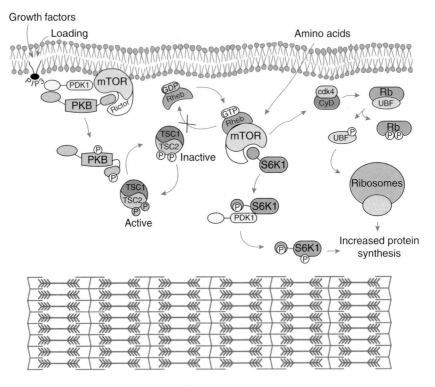

**Figure 2. Schematic diagram of molecular signals leading to an increase in the rate
of protein synthesis via the activation of PKB and mTOR**
For details, see text.

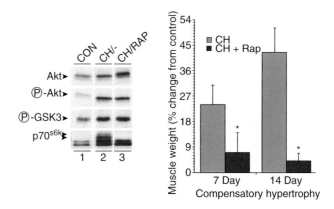

Figure 3. Rapamycin prevents overload-induced phosphorylation of S6K1 (p70^S6k)
and muscle hypertrophy without affecting PKB/Akt and GSK3
Compensatory hypertrophy (CH) increases phosphorylation of PKB, GSK3, and S6K1 and only
the activation of S6K1 is blocked by rapamycin (CH/RAP). Even without blocking PKB activity,
rapamycin inhibits 67% of hypertrophy at 7 days and 90% of hypertrophy at 14 days. Reproduced
by permission from Macmillan Publishers Ltd: *Nature Cell Biology* vol. 3, pages 1014–1019,
Copyright (2001); www.nature.com/ncb.

phosphorylation of its downstream targets the translational inhibitor 4E–BP
and the 70 kDa S6K1 (ribosomal S6 kinase). TORC2 is the recently identified
kinase upstream of PKB (protein kinase B)/Akt. Phosphorylation of S6K1
by TORC1 and PKB by TORC2 changes the conformation of the proteins
making them substrates for the constitutively active PDK1. Following PDK1
phosphorylation, the proteins are fully active and function to increase the rate
of protein synthesis. The importance of PDK1 in determining cell size has
been demonstrated in mice with significantly decreased PDK1 protein levels.
These mice are 40% smaller than their wild type littermates due to a decrease
in cell size and no change in cell number [14].

Resistance exercise is known to induce a transient increase in the phosphorylation of mTOR [15], PKB [16], 4E-BP [17] and S6K1 [12], as well as
the activity of eIF2 [18]. The increase in S6K1 phosphorylation 6 h after a
single bout of resistance exercise correlates with the increase in muscle mass
following 6 weeks of training, suggesting that mTOR may play an important
role in regulating muscle mass [12]. In support of this hypothesis, blocking
mTOR activity, with the bacterial macrolide antibiotic rapamycin, blocks the
activation of S6K1, the increase in eIF2 activity and the increase in muscle
mass following overload (Figure 3) [18,19] and muscle mass is decreased in
S6K1 knockout mice [20].

Control of protein synthesis by increasing protein synthetic machinery
Along with increasing the rate of initiation, another way to promote increases
in protein synthesis rates is to increase the number of ribosomes within
muscle following increased loading. The number of ribosomes in a cell plays a
fundamental role in growth regulation because it affects the amount of protein

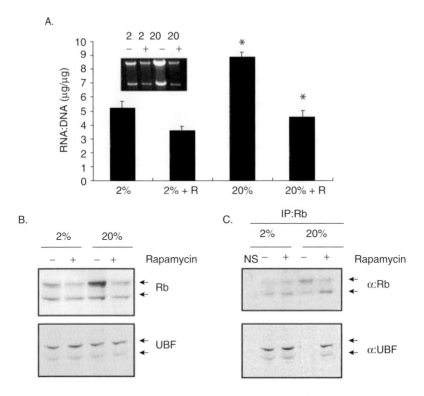

Figure 4. Serum increases ribosomal RNA and Rb phosphorylation in a rapamycin-dependent manner

The (**A**) increased ribosomal RNA, (**B**) Rb phosphorylation, and (**C**) decrease in the amount of UBF bound to Rb in response to serum treatment (20%) of L6 cells is reversed by rapamycin treatment. Adapted from Nader, McLoughlin and Esser (2005) *American Journal of Physiology Cell Physiology*, vol. 289, pages C1457–C1465 with permission from The American Physiological Society.

being synthesized per mRNA molecule. The cellular content of ribosomes is mainly regulated by an increase in their biosynthesis, which requires the co-ordinated synthesis of approx. 80 ribosomal proteins and four RNA species in addition to several hundred accessory enzymes [21].

Expression of the genes encoding ribosomal proteins can be regulated at both transcriptional and translational levels. Ribosomal protein gene transcription is regulated by the RNA polymerase II holoenzyme, and although transcriptional regulation is possible, ribosomal protein expression is controlled mainly by translational mechanisms. The typical ribosomal protein mRNA is characterized by a motif of 5–20 pyrimidines followed by a GC-rich sequence of approximately 40 nucleotides in its 5′ UTR (terminal oligopyrimidine tract or 5′ TOP). The 5′ TOP confers selectivity for translational regulation of the ribosomal proteins during specific cellular demands, e.g. growth [22].

The expression of the ribosomal RNA subunits requires RNA polymerase I, UBF (upstream binding factor), and a series of associated factors. The ability of UBF to control rRNA expression is regulated by its own level of expression, phosphorylation on its C-terminus (that enhances UBF activity), as well as sequestration by retinoblastoma (that decreases UBF activity) [21]. Retinoblastoma can in turn be regulated by phosphorylation by the cyclins and cdks (cyclin-dependent kinases) [23]. Nader et al. [24] have recently reported that ribosome biogenesis during skeletal muscle hypertrophy is regulated, in part, by a cell cycle mechanism that is dependent on mTOR signalling. Serum stimulation of differentiated L6 rat myotubes resulted in an increase in ribosomal RNA content, cyclin D1-dependent phosphorylation of retinoblastoma, and release of the Rb binding partner UBF (Figure 4). All of these effects could be blocked by treatment with rapamycin, suggesting that mTOR controls ribosome synthesis via cyclin D1-dependent phosphorylation of retinoblastoma and an increase in UBF availability (Figure 2). Whether or not UBF phosphorylation plays a role in ribosome biosynthesis during muscle hypertrophy remains to be determined. However, in proliferating NIH 3T3 cells, mTOR regulates rRNA synthesis via release and phosphorylation of UBF [25] suggesting that increasing the amount of phosphorylated UBF within muscle may increase ribosome biogenesis in an mTOR dependent fashion.

Control of protein breakdown by increased loading

As well as increasing protein synthesis, resistance exercise increases the rate of protein degradation. The importance of the increase in degradation can be seen in the correlation between the fractional synthesis rate and the fractional breakdown rate in muscle following loading [8]. As the rate of protein breakdown increases there is a concomitant rise in protein synthesis suggesting that there might be a molecular link between the two processes. However, the association is not always seen. Eating a meal rich in essential amino acids can decrease the effects of resistance exercise on protein degradation whilst at the same time increasing the rate of protein synthesis [26]. Taking in a carbohydrate or mixed amino acids meal decreases the rate of degradation, possibly by decreasing circulating corticosteroids, without affecting the rate of synthesis. Therefore, it is only in the fed state that the net protein balance (protein synthesis minus degradation) becomes positive allowing the muscle to grow [26].

Muscle atrophy

Muscle atrophy can result from a decrease in the recruitment of a muscle, a decrease in the loading of a muscle, ageing and metabolic diseases. Whilst all of these processes have the same global effect, a decrease in muscle mass, the underlying molecular mechanisms are different. What appears to be consistent across all forms of atrophy is that there is an overall shift in the balance between synthesis and degradation towards degradation leading to the loss of muscle mass. Under unloading conditions, the decrease in protein synthesis appears to acutely drive the decrease in muscle mass, whilst the rate of protein degradation remains fairly constant [27].

Control of protein synthesis by atrophic stimuli

As with muscle hypertrophy, the early changes in the rate of muscle protein synthesis correlate with alterations in the phosphorylation of translation factors. As opposed to resistance loading, unloading of muscle leads to a decrease in the phosphorylation of PKB and S6K1, an increase in the association of 4E-BP with eIF4E [19], and a likely decrease in the rate of translation initiation. However, initiation may not be the only site of translational regulation. Indeed, the *wasted* mouse shows a progressive muscle wasting as the result of a mutation in an elongation factor known as eEF1α2 [28]. Further, muscle loss due to unloading has been associated with a decrease in translation elongation [29] and an increase in the phosphorylation of the elongation repressor eEF2 [30]. These data suggest that multiple levels of translation are repressed under atrophic conditions resulting in a reduction of protein synthesis.

Control of protein breakdown by atrophic stimuli

Whilst protein synthesis is inhibited by atrophic stimuli, maintaining the rate of protein degradation is equally important in the development of muscle atrophy. Support for this hypothesis comes from transgenic mouse studies showing that inhibiting protein degradation can decrease muscle wasting in response to atrophic stimuli [30]. A number of proteolytic systems are involved in muscle wasting and blocking one or more of these systems can attenuate muscle loss. The primary proteolytic systems: the calcium-dependent calpain system, the lysosomal proteases (i.e. cathepsins) and the ATP-dependent ubiquitin–proteosome system will be described below.

Calpains are a family of calcium-dependent cysteine proteases that localize to the Z-line of the sarcomere. These proteins are activated in response to elevated levels of calcium and phosphatidylinositides and are inactivated by the calpain-specific inhibitor calpistatin. The calpains can target structural proteins within the myofibrillar lattice such as titin, C-protein and nebulin [31] and may aid in the disassembly of the myofilaments and degradation by other proteases. Blocking calpain activity with either a dominant negative form of m-calpain or calpistatin overexpression reduced the rate of protein degradation, in muscle cells *in vitro* stimulated to atrophy by nutrient withdrawal, 30% and 60% respectively. Interestingly, blocking calpain activation *in vivo* blocks unloading induced muscle atrophy, but has no effect on inactivity-induced muscle loss [32]. This suggests that calpains might play a specific role in controlling protein degradation in response to decreased loading.

Lysosomal proteases are primarily involved in the breakdown of proteins in the sarcolemma such as growth factor receptors, channels and transporters. Since growth factors like insulin and insulin-like growth factor 1 play an important role in the maintenance of muscle cell size, increasing the degradation of these receptors could lead to a progressive loss of muscle mass. Blocking lysosomal protease activity decreases the amount of muscle loss

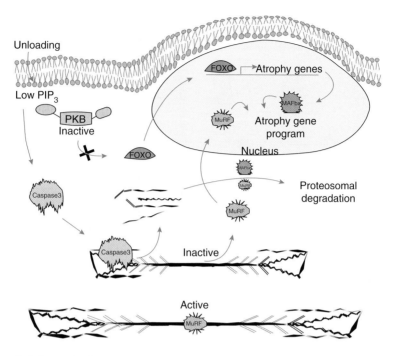

Figure 5. Schematic diagram of the molecular signals leading to muscle atrophy following unloading

In active muscle, MuRF is bound to the m-line of muscle through its interaction with titin. In inactive muscle, MuRF is released and shuttles to the nucleus whilst the decrease in PIP_3 levels at the membrane lead to caspase 3 proteolysis of the myofibrillar proteins and inactivation of PKB. When PKB is inactive, FOXO is unphosphorylated and can move to the nucleus resulting in an increase in the expression of catabolic genes.

following denervation, but has no effect on atrophy due to unloading [32]. Since denervation normally leads to greater atrophy than unloading, and inhibiting lysosomal proteases eliminates this difference, this suggests that denervation induces a lysosomal-dependent loss of growth factor signalling that results in greater muscle atrophy.

Another way that muscle protein can be degraded is through the caspase-3/ATP-dependent ubiquitination pathway (Figure 5). This system uses caspase-3 to breakdown intact sarcomeres and liberate fragments of actin and myosin that can later be degraded in the proteosome [33]. In order for proteins to be degraded in the proteosome they have to be targeted by the addition of a polyubiquitin chain. Ubiquitin is added to proteins that are targeted for degradation in the proteosome by a process involving at least three classes of proteins called E1 (ubiquitin-activating enzyme), E2 (ubiquitin-conjugating enzyme) and E3 (ubiquitin ligase). In skeletal muscle, two novel E3 ubiquitin ligases have been clearly linked to muscle atrophy. The MAFbx (muscle atrophy F-box)/atrogin 1 and the MuRF1 (muscle ring finger protein -1) proteins are E3 ubiquitin ligases that are selectively expressed

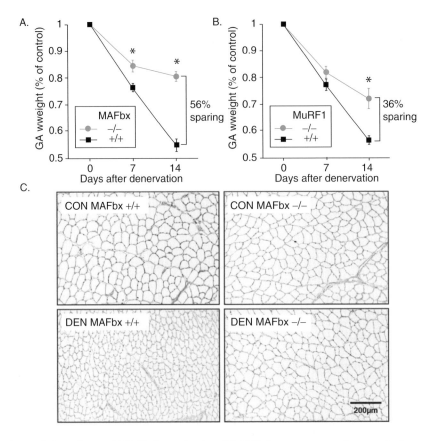

Figure 6. Knockout of MAFbx/atrogin -1 or MuRF1 decreases muscle atrophy in response to denervation
(**A**) and (**B**) Quantification and (**C**) cross-sections of muscle atrophy following 7 and 14 days denervation (den) in MAFbx and MuRF1 knockout mice. Adapted with permission from Bodine, S.C. et al. (2001) Identification of ubiquilin ligases required for skeletal muscle atrophy. *Science* vol. 294, pages 1704–1708. Copyright (2001) the American Association for the Advancement of Science.

in skeletal, cardiac and smooth muscle. MAFbx is characteristic of F-box proteins that are components of Skp/Cullin/F-box ubiquitin–ligase complexes [34], and both MuRF1 and MAFbx exhibit E3 ligase activity *in vitro* when incubated with appropriate E1 and E2 ligases. Both MuRF1 and MAFbx are up-regulated in almost all atrophy models tested to date and this up-regulation appears to be the result of an increase in the amount of FOXO (forkhead transcription factor) in the nucleus [35,36]. One current theory is that a decrease in activity/loading in muscle decreases growth factor signalling, resulting in decreased phosphorylation of FOXO by its upstream kinase PKB. In the hypophosphorylated form, FOXO translocates to the nucleus and increases atrogene expression. Knocking out either MAFbx/atrogin-1 or MuRF1 spares muscle loss following denervation by 56% and 36% respectively (Figure 6). To date there is little information regarding the physiological function or target substrates of these genes; however, it is assumed that they function in some manner to regulate protein degradation since they are expressed early in the atrophy process and their peak expression occurs during the peak of protein degradation and muscle loss. MuRF1 is a member of a gene family that consists of MuRF1, MuRF2 and MuRF3, all of which are expressed in skeletal and cardiac muscle. Of the three family members, MuRF1 is the only one that is significantly up-regulated under atrophy inducing conditions. Using yeast two-hybrid methods, MuRF1 and MuRF2 have been shown to associate with each other, and both have been detected in the nucleus, indicating that they may play a role in the regulation of transcription via ubiquitination of specific transcription factors. MuRF proteins have been shown to interact with the kinase domain of titin, the 3 MDa muscle protein that extends from the Z-line to the M-line and provides passive tension within a muscle. When MuRF binding to titin is disrupted, either through expression of MuRF mutants or through inactivity, the different MuRF family members can move to the nucleus where they interact with the SRF (serum response factor) and GMEB-1 (glucocorticoid modulatory element binding protein 1) [37,38]. MuRF-1 appears to specifically bind and localize to the same nuclei as GMEB-1 whereas when MuRF-2 moves to the nucleus it specifically binds to SRF and induces the cytosolic translocation of SRF [37,38]. Through GMEB-1, nuclear MuRF-1 could increase the expression of degradation genes, whereas in excluding SRF from the nucleus, MuRF-2 would decrease the synthesis of muscle genes thus again increasing degradation and inhibiting synthesis. The transcriptional regulation of MuRF1 and MAFbx is intriguing since both genes are co-regulated under most atrophy-inducing conditions. Interestingly, the promoters of both MAFbx and MuRF1 contain FOXO binding sites, and the expression of MAFbx/atrogin 1 has been shown to be controlled by PKB–FOXO signalling, connecting growth factors to the regulation of protein degradation.

Conclusion

Muscle wasting is a major feature of ageing, and pathologies such as cancer, diabetes and neuromuscular diseases. Preventing the loss of muscle mass has been shown to increase lifespan [2]. Further, having greater muscle mass decreases frailty and increases independence in the elderly, therefore maintaining muscle mass is essential to a long happy life. The primary determinant of muscle size is the interaction of molecular signalling pathways that affect the rates of protein synthesis and degradation. Increasing synthesis more than degradation leads to greater muscle mass whilst the opposite leads to decreased muscle mass. We are beginning to understand how a change in loading/recruitment is sensed by the muscle and converted into a chemical signal that increases or decreases muscle size. However, there are still a number of questions that remain unanswered. First, what is the sensor of the strain on a muscle? Titin seems to be involved in transducing a signal that controls degradation, but is this same signal important in activating synthesis? What other signals are important: integrin signals such as muselin, autophagy signals through Vps34, inactivation of phosphoinositide phosphatases such as SHIP (SH2-containing inositol phosphatase) and PTEN (phosphatase and tensin homologue) or could it be a new as yet undiscovered mechanism? Secondly, the activation of PKB following resistance exercise seems to be quite central to increasing muscle mass and yet its activation is quite transient, returning to baseline levels within 30 min whilst S6K1 activity remains high for 3–6 h. If PKB is required for the increase in S6K1 activity why are the kinetics of inactivation so different? Thirdly, what role does protein degradation play in the development of muscle hypertrophy? Is the increase in protein degradation after resistance exercise required for muscle hypertrophy? If so, why? Why doesn't decreasing degradation increase muscle cell size in either transgenic animals or tissue culture? What are the physiological targets and functions of the E3 ligases, MuRF1 and MAFbx? With the growing rise in muscle wasting conditions and the resulting metabolic syndrome, we must be able to answer these and other questions concerning the control of muscle size so that the increase in lifespan is associated with an increased quality of life.

Summary

- *Muscle mass is determined by the sum of protein synthesis and protein degradation.*
- *Following resistance exercise there is an mTOR-dependent increase in translation initiation and ribosome biogenesis.*
- *The increase in protein degradation following resistance exercise correlates with the increase in the rate of protein synthesis suggesting that the two processes may be linked.*
- *Unloading results in attenuation of translation initiation and elongation leading to a decrease in protein synthesis.*
- *Calpains, lysosomal proteases and the ATP-dependent ubiquitin–proteosome system all play a role in muscle protein breakdown.*
- *MuRF1 and MAFbx contain FOXO binding sites and are co-regulated in response to atrophy-inducing conditions.*

References

1. Karakelides, H. & Sreekumaran Nair, K. (2005) Sarcopenia of aging and its metabolic impact. *Curr. Top. Dev. Biol.* **68**, 123–148
2. Cai, D., Frantz, J.D., Tawa, Jr, N.E., Melendez, P.A., Oh, B.C., Lidov, H.G., Hasselgren, P.O., Frontera, W.R., Lee, J., Glass, D.J. & Shoelson, S.E. (2004) IKKβ/NF-κB activation causes severe muscle wasting in mice. *Cell* **119**, 285–298
3. Petersen, K.F., Befroy, D., Dufour, S., Dziura, J., Ariyan, C., Rothman, D.L., DiPietro, L., Cline, G.W. & Shulman, G.I. (2003) Mitochondrial dysfunction in the elderly: possible role in insulin resistance. *Science* **300**, 1140–1142

4.   Nader, G.A. (2005) Molecular determinants of skeletal muscle mass: getting the 'AKT' together. *Int. J. Biochem. Cell Biol.* **37**, 1985–1996

5.   Kandarian, S.C. & Jackman, R.W. (2006) Intracellular signaling during skeletal muscle atrophy. *Muscle Nerve* **33**, 155–165

6.   Jackman, R.W. & Kandarian, S.C. (2004) The molecular basis of skeletal muscle atrophy. *Am. J. Physiol. Cell. Physiol.* **287**, C834–C843

7.   Chesley, A., MacDougall, J.D., Tarnopolsky, M.A., Atkinson, S.A. & Smith, K. (1992) Changes in human muscle protein synthesis after resistance exercise. *J. Appl. Physiol.* **73**, 1383–1388

8.   Phillips, S.M., Tipton, K.D., Aarsland, A., Wolf, S.E. & Wolfe, R.R. (1997) Mixed muscle protein synthesis and breakdown after resistance exercise in humans. *Am. J. Physiol.* **273**, E99–E107

9.   Wong, T.S. & Booth, F.W. (1990) Protein metabolism in rat gastrocnemius muscle after stimulated chronic concentric exercise. *J. Appl. Physiol.* **69**, 1709–1717

10.   Wong, T.S. & Booth, F.W. (1990) Protein metabolism in rat tibialis anterior muscle after stimulated chronic eccentric exercise. *J. Appl. Physiol.* **69**, 1718–1724

11.   Hamosch, M., Lesch, M., Baron, J. & Kaufman, S. (1967) Enhanced protein synthesis in a cell free system from hypertrophied skeletal muscle. *Science* **157**, 935–937

12.   Baar, K. & Esser, K. (1999) Phosphorylation of p70(S6k) correlates with increased skeletal muscle mass following resistance exercise. *Am. J. Physiol.* **276**, C120–C127

13.   Sonenberg, N. & Dever, T.E. (2003) Eukaryotic translation initiation factors and regulators. *Curr. Opin. Struct. Biol.* **13**, 56–63

14.   Lawlor, M.A., Mora, A., Ashby, P.R., Williams, M.R., Murray Tait, V., Malone, L., Prescott, A.R., Lucocq, J.M. & Alessi, D.R. (2002) Essential role of PDK1 in regulating cell size and development in mice. *EMBO J* **21**, 3728–3738

15.   Parkington, J.D., Siebert, A.P., LeBrasseur, N.K. & Fielding, R.A. (2003) Differential activation of mTOR signaling by contractile activity in skeletal muscle. *Am. J. Physiol. Regul. Integr. Comp. Physiol.* **285**, R1086–R1090

16.   Nader, G.A. & Esser, K.A. (2001) Intracellular signaling specificity in skeletal muscle in response to different modes of exercise. *J. Appl. Physiol.* **90**, 1936–1942

17.   Bolster, D.R., Kubica, N., Crozier, S.J., Williamson, D.L., Farrell, P.A., Kimball, S.R. & Jefferson, L.S. (2003) Immediate response of mammalian target of rapamycin (mTOR) mediated signalling following acute resistance exercise in rat skeletal muscle. *J. Physiol.* **553**, 213–220

18.   Kubica, N., Bolster, D.R., Farrell, P.A., Kimball, S.R. & Jefferson, L.S. (2005) Resistance exercise increases muscle protein synthesis and translation of eukaryotic initiation factor 2Bε mRNA in a mammalian target of rapamycin dependent manner. *J. Biol. Chem.* **280**, 7570–7580

19.   Bodine, S.C., Stitt, T.N., Gonzalez, M., Kline, W.O., Stover, G.L., Bauerlein, R., Zlotchenko, E., Scrimgeour, A., Lawrence, J.C., Glass, D.J. & Yancopoulos, G.D. (2001) Akt/mTOR pathway is a crucial regulator of skeletal muscle hypertrophy and can prevent muscle atrophy *in vivo. Nat. Cell Biol.* **3**, 1014–1019

20.   Ohanna, M., Sobering, A.K., Lapointe, T., Lorenzo, L., Praud, C., Petroulakis, E., Sonenberg, N., Kelly, P.A., Sotiropoulos, A. & Pende, M. (2005) Atrophy of S6K1(−/−) skeletal muscle cells reveals distinct mTOR effectors for cell cycle and size control. *Nat. Cell Biol.* **7**, 286–294

21.   Hannan, R., Taylor, L., Cavanaugh, A.H., Hannan, K.M. & Rothblum, L. (1998) UBF and the regulation of ribosomal DNA transcription. Springer Verlag, Berlin

22.   Jefferies, H.B., Thomas, G. & Thomas, G. (1994) Elongation factor 1 α mRNA is selectively translated following mitogenic stimulation. *J. Biol. Chem.* **269**, 4367–4372

23.   Goodrich, D.W., Wang, N.P., Qian, Y.W., Lee, E.Y. & Lee, W.H. (1991) The retinoblastoma gene product regulates progression through the G1 phase of the cell cycle. *Cell* **67**, 293–302

24.   Nader, G.A., McLoughlin, T.J. & Esser, K.A. (2005) mTOR function in skeletal muscle hypertrophy: increased ribosomal RNA via cell cycle regulators. *Am. J. Physiol. Cell Physiol.* **289**, C1457–C1465

25.   Hannan, K.M., Brandenburger, Y., Jenkins, A., Sharkey, K., Cavanaugh, A., Rothblum, L., Moss, T., Poortinga, G., McArthur, G.A., Pearson, R.B. & Hannan, R.D. (2003) mTOR dependent

regulation of ribosomal gene transcription requires S6K1 and is mediated by phosphorylation of the carboxy terminal activation domain of the nucleolar transcription factor UBF. *Mol. Cell Biol.* **23**, 8862–8877

26. Tipton, K.D., Ferrando, A.A., Phillips, S.M., Doyle, Jr, D. & Wolfe, R.R. (1999) Postexercise net protein synthesis in human muscle from orally administered amino acids. *Am. J. Physiol.* **276**, E628–E634

27. Ferrando, A.A., Lane, H.W., Stuart, C.A., Davis Street, J. & Wolfe, R.R. (1996) Prolonged bed rest decreases skeletal muscle and whole body protein synthesis. *Am. J. Physiol.* **270**, E627–E633

28. Hafezparast, M. & Fisher, E. (1998) Wasted by an elongation factor. *Trends Genet.* **14**, 215–217

29. Ku, Z., Yang, J., Menon, V. & Thomason, D.B. (1995) Decreased polysomal HSP 70 may slow polypeptide elongation during skeletal muscle atrophy. *Am. J. Physiol.* **268**, C1369–C1374

30. Hornberger, T.A., Hunter, R.B., Kandarian, S.C. & Esser, K.A. (2001) Regulation of translation factors during hindlimb unloading and denervation of skeletal muscle in rats. *Am. J. Physiol. Cell Physiol.* **281**, C179–C187

31. Huang, J. & Forsberg, N.E. (1998) Role of calpain in skeletal muscle protein degradation. *Proc. Natl. Acad. Sci. U.S.A.* **95**, 12100–12105

32. Tischler, M.E., Rosenberg, S., Satarug, S., Henriksen, E.J., Kirby, C.R., Tome, M. & Chase, P. (1990) Different mechanisms of increased proteolysis in atrophy induced by denervation or unweighting of rat soleus muscle. *Metabolism* **39**, 756–763

33. Du, J., Wang, X., Miereles, C., Bailey, J.L., Debigare, R., Zheng, B., Price, S.R. & Mitch, W.E. (2004) Activation of caspase-3 is an initial step triggering accelerated muscle proteolysis in catabolic conditions. *J. Clin. Invest.* **113**, 115–123

34. Bodine, S.C., Latres, E., Baumhueter, S., Lai, V.K., Nunez, L., Clarke, B.A., Poueymirou, W.T., Panaro, F.J., Na, E., Dharmarajan, K. et al. (2001) Identification of ubiquitin ligases required for skeletal muscle atrophy. *Science* **294**, 1704–1708

35. Sandri, M., Sandri, C., Gilbert, A., Skurk, C., Calabria, E., Picard, A., Walsh, K., Schiaffino, S., Lecker, S.H. & Goldberg, A.L. (2004) FOXO transcription factors induce the atrophy related ubiquitin ligase atrogin-1 and cause skeletal muscle atrophy. *Cell* **117**, 399–412

36. Stitt, T.N., Drujan, D., Clarke, B.A., Panaro, F., Timofeyva, Y., Kline, W.O., Gonzalez, M., Yancopoulos, G.D. & Glass, D.J. (2004) The IGF 1/PI3K/Akt pathway prevents expression of muscle atrophy induced ubiquitin ligases by inhibiting FOXO transcription factors. *Mol. Cell* **14**, 395–403

37. McElhinny, A.S., Kakinuma, K., Sorimachi, H., Labeit, S. & Gregorio, C.C. (2002) Muscle-specific RING finger-1 interacts with titin to regulate sarcomeric M-line and thick filament structure and may have nuclear functions via its interaction with glucocorticoid modulatory element binding protein-1. *J. Cell Biol.* **157**, 125–136

38. Lange, S., Xiang, F., Yakovenko, A., Vihola, A., Hackman, P., Rostkova, E., Kristensen, J., Brandmeier, B., Franzen, G., Hedberg, B. et al. (2005) The kinase domain of titin controls muscle gene expression and protein turnover. *Science* **308**, 1599–1603

6

Resistance training, insulin sensitivity and muscle function in the elderly

Flemming Dela* and Michael Kjaer†[1]

*Institute for Biomedical Sciences, University of Copenhagen, Denmark, and †Institute of Sports Medicine, Copenhagen University Hospital at Bispebjerg, Denmark.

Abstract

Ageing is associated with a loss in both muscle mass and in the metabolic quality of skeletal muscle. This leads to sarcopenia and reduced daily function, as well as to an increased risk for development of insulin resistance and type 2 diabetes. A major part, but not all, of these changes are associated with an age-related decrease in the physical activity level and can be counteracted by increased physical activity of a resistive nature. Strength training has been shown to improve insulin-stimulated glucose uptake in both healthy elderly individuals and patients with manifest diabetes, and likewise to improve muscle strength in both elderly healthy individuals and in elderly individuals with chronic disease. The increased strength is coupled to improved function and a decreased risk for fall injuries and fractures. Elderly individuals have preserved the capacity to improve muscle strength and mass with training, but seem to display a reduced sensitivity towards stimulating protein synthesis from nutritional intake, rather than by any reduced response in protein turnover to exercise.

[1] To whom correspondence should be addressed (email m.kjaer@mfi.ku.dk)

Introduction

Getting older and ageing is associated with an increase in life-style related metabolic diseases as well as with a loss in overall function. Intimately linked to these events is on one side a reduction in insulin sensitivity that plays a major role in the development of the metabolic syndrome and diabetes, and on the other side a reduction in the skeletal muscle mass that plays a major role for the decrease in functional performance (Figure 1). For both metabolic and functional impairment with ageing it is not clear to what extent this can solely be explained by the age-associated reduction in activity levels. It is clear that ageing has an influence upon skeletal muscle loss, but it is also clear that metabolic impairment and functional losses can be largely counteracted by physical training especially of a resistive nature. With increasing age the amount of skeletal muscle is decreasing due both to a reduction in the number of muscle fibres and due to a reduction in the protein content and thus cross-sectional area of individual muscle fibres. Interestingly, the loss of muscle fibres and area is more pronounced in fast contracting type II fibres compared with the slower oxidative type I fibres, and therefore decreased ability to generate fast movements (maximal muscle power output or force over the first 100–200 ms) is more pronounced (around 3%/year after the age of 60) than the loss in maximal force (peak force generation independent of time; around 1%/year). In addition to loss of muscle fibres, a loss in spinal motor neurons, a reduced axon conduction speed in the remaining neurons and a reduced excitability of the remaining motor neurons contributes to the loss of force and power.

The loss of muscle protein with ageing is not fully explained, but can result in sarcopenia which is defined as: muscle mass/height^2 that is more than two standard deviations below the standard value for young individuals. Using this definition, it is found that approximately 20% of people over 70 years

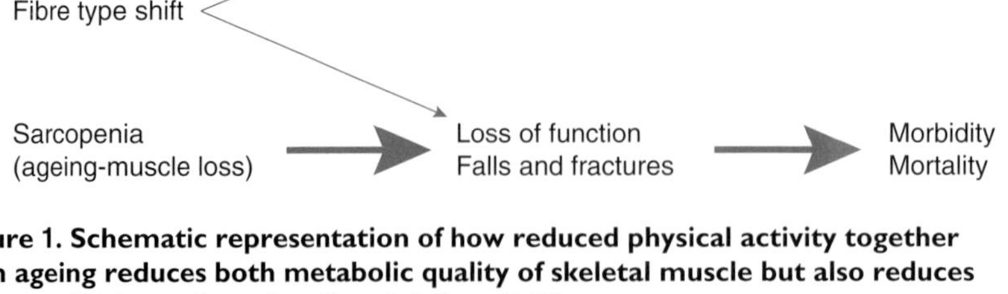

Skeletal muscle

Figure 1. Schematic representation of how reduced physical activity together with ageing reduces both metabolic quality of skeletal muscle but also reduces the capacity to perform functional daily activities
Both these effects will lead to increased morbidity and mortality.

and 50% of all over 80 years are classified as sarcopenic. The implications of being sarcopenic is that the muscle mass drops below the critical value needed to perform everyday activities, which causes elderly people to become less independent, and rely on help from others in their daily life. With increasing adiposity in ageing, and thus increase in body weight due to fat, the function in sarcopenic elderly subjects will worsen. In addition to these functional implications associated with loss of muscle mass, both reduced activity and shift in muscle fibre characteristics from II to I will contribute to a reduced insulin-mediated glucose uptake in skeletal muscle of elderly subjects.

Resistance training has the overall aim to improve muscle strength and power for use either in relation to competitive performance, recreational sports or in a more clinical setting where increased muscle strength results in increased functional capacity as a part of rehabilitation after disease or injury. Especially in elderly subjects, resistance exercise has become increasingly important in order to avoid functional decline and disability. Resistance exercise results in both a net increase in muscle protein synthesis and thus a rise in muscle fibre cross-sectional area, as well as in an increased ability to activate motor units in a more synchronized way. Together these changes contribute to increased force output after training.

Resistance training and insulin sensitivity in the elderly

The headline may imply that insulin resistance is a natural development that inevitably follows ageing. This is not the case. With 'healthy' ageing, i.e. maintenance of a physically active lifestyle and avoidance of obesity, insulin-mediated glucose uptake rates in skeletal muscle does not necessarily decrease with age. When insulin resistance is so often associated with ageing, it is mostly due to a marked decrease in daily physical activity, decreased muscle mass, increased intramyocellular lipid deposits and accumulation of adipose tissue. For obvious reasons no longitudinal, randomized studies of this have been carried out, but studies of glucose tolerance and skeletal muscle biochemistry in master athletes [1–3] as well as measurements of muscle glucose uptake rates in elderly and young healthy subjects [4] support this notion.

Nevertheless, it is a fact, that with advancing age the prevalence of glucose intolerance and insulin resistance (type 2 diabetes) is increased, and for these patients non-pharmacological treatment should be the first 'drug of choice'. Life-style modifications, focusing on changing dietary habits and energy restriction, have proved to be difficult and are often perceived as a limitation (i.e. disallowing a behaviour). In contrast, when prescribing exercise as a tool to prevent glucose intolerance developing into overt type 2 diabetes or even to treat established insulin resistance, this is perceived as adding an element, not taking something away or prohibiting a behaviour. However, as with any other treatment a successful intervention requires that the individual is motivated and quickly experiences a solid effect of the personal efforts. Thus an important task for the health care professional is to visualize and explain such effects, e.g. by simple measurements of blood glucose, strength or aerobic capacity [5].

Apart from the positive effect on insulin resistance, exercise training also has wholesome effects on all of the other conditions associated with the metabolic syndrome (e.g. hypertension, dyslipidaemia, obesity and athero-sclerosis), which is also seen more frequently with advanced age. In patients with diagnosed type 2 diabetes, and in pre-diabetic states such as impaired glucose tolerance, an increase in daily physical activity has been shown to prevent type 2 diabetes, improve insulin-mediated glucose uptake rates, glu-cose tolerance and the insulin response to glucose. The majority of interven-tion studies have used endurance/aerobic training programs and the effects of such programs on insulin sensitivity are undisputed. However, aerobic training may be difficult for many of the patients, due to the existence of co-morbidities or simply because the majority of the patients are overweight if not severely obese. For these patients, resistance exercise represents an attractive alternative.

The number of studies on the effects of resistance training on glycaemic control and insulin sensitivity in middle aged to elderly healthy subjects and patients with insulin resistance has increased substantially in the past 15 years. We have identified 25 such studies, but the limitations of the present chapter do not allow for a detailed review of these studies. However, in a review from 2003 [6] several of them are described. In general, the interpretation and indi-vidual comparison of intervention studies using resistance training is to some extent difficult, because there is no uniform agreement in how the exercise intervention is described in terms of intensity and/or number of repetitions. Some studies merely report that the used workload was e.g. 8RM, whereas others report the number of repetitions at a given percentage of max. workload. Furthermore, some studies describe in detail the use of progressive resist-ance training, while others do not give this kind of information. Therefore, a clear dose–response relationship between the training intensity and the effect on strength is difficult to obtain in these studies. Furthermore, a clear dose–response relationship as regards insulin sensitivity cannot be deduced from the published studies, but from a biological point of view it is difficult to imagine that such a relationship should not exist, at least up to a yet undefined maxi-mum. In those studies where insulin sensitivity has been measured, the major-ity have shown a significant effect. With some uncertainty the percentage of maximal workload can be calculated from given data on RM, and by doing so it appears that resistance training at an intensity range of 45–80% of maximal load results in approx. 30% (range 10–75%) increase in strength and approx. 28% (range 15–48%) increase in insulin sensitivity. The duration of the inter-vention is in most studies more than three months, but as little as six weeks of training have shown marked improvements in insulin sensitivity [7].

The mechanism by which resistance training improves insulin action is not merely a function of increased muscle mass [8]. Several proteins increase

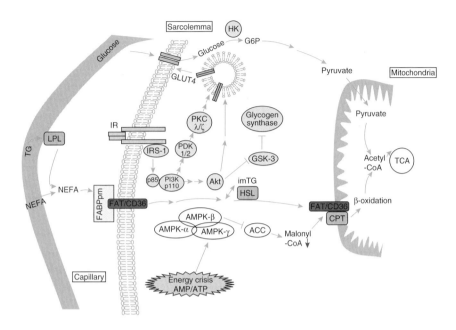

Figure 2. Key players in strength and/or endurance training induced improvements in fat- and carbohydrate metabolism in skeletal muscle
The depicted signals and pathways are not representing the complete picture. Rather the most important proteins and enzymes in relation to physical training are shown. See text for details. ACC, acetyl-CoA carboxylase; FABPpm, fatty acid binding protein in the plasma membrane; GSK-3, glycogen synthase kinase-3; HK, hexokinase; HSL, hormone sensitive lipase; IRS-1, insulin receptor substrate-1; LPL, lipoprotein lipase; PDK 1/2, phosphoinositide-dependent kinase 1/2; PI3K, phosphatidylinositol 3-kinase; PKC, protein kinase C; NEFA, non-esterified fatty acid; TG, triacylglycerol.

in abundance and/or activity, and below is given a short overview of the key players. Minor discrepancies may exist between effects of strength and endurance training, but in general the effects are similar and therefore a discrimination between the two training regimens is not made (Figure 2).

Insulin binding to the IR (insulin receptor) is not affected by training in rats [9] or humans [10]. The number of IRs has been shown to increase with training in rats [11] and in humans [7], to decrease in humans [12] and in rats [13] or remain unchanged in humans [14]. Insulin receptor kinase activity seems unchanged with training in humans [10,14]. Insulin receptor substrate-1 protein has been shown to decrease [13] in rats whilst remaining unchanged in humans [7].

The protein levels of the regulatory subunit, p85, of the phosphatidyl-inositol 3-kinase (PI3K), is not changed with training [7], whereas activity of the catalytic subunit, p110, has been shown to increase with training in rats [13,15]. Further along the pathway leading to GLUT4 (glucose transporter 4) translocation, protein kinase C λ/ζ activity increases with training [15]. One of the most robust findings is the training induced increase in GLUT4 protein and mRNA levels in humans [10,16]. Akt (protein kinase B) protein levels also increase with training in rats [13] and in humans [7] as does Akt activity in rats [15]. Akt inhibits glycogen synthase kinase-3, which in turn, has an inhibitory effect on the GS (glycogen synthase) enzyme. Thus, an increase in Akt may ultimately lead to a stimulation of GS and glycogen formation. Another robust finding is the training induced increase in GS activity [7].

As glucose enters the cytoplasm of the muscle cell, it is rapidly phosphorylated into glucose 6-phosphate by the enzyme, hexokinase. The third robust finding in training studies, is an increase in the activity of hexokinase [17].

In addition to the above-mentioned training effects on carbohydrate metabolism in skeletal muscle, it is well-known that physical training (in particular endurance training) increases the β-oxidative capacity (e.g. by enhancing the activity of hydroxy-acyl-CoA-dehydrogenase). More recently, it has been found that the maximal activity of CPT 1 (carnitine palmitoyltransferase 1), which is the rate-limiting step for mitochondrial oxidation of long-chain fatty acids, is increased with training [18]. In addition, these authors also found that training diminished the sensitivity of CPT 1 to inhibiton by malonyl-CoA [18]. The fatty acid translocase, FAT/CD36, has now been found to be present in mitochondria [19], and furthermore, it co-immunoprecipitates with CPT 1 and this association increases with training [20]. Further up-stream of this pathway (Figure 2), the contents of FAT/CD36 and the fatty acid binding protein in the plasma membrane has been shown to increase with training [21–23]. All of these effects on proteins involved in the transport of fatty acids to the mitochondria form the basis for the increased capacity for fatty acid oxidation. One might expect that also the activity of the hormone sensitive lipase is increased with training, but so far this has not been shown [24]. In contrast, lipoprotein lipase activity increases with training [23,25,26], again improving the overall capacity for trained muscle to metabolize fatty acids at the expense of carbohydrates.

AMPK (AMP-activated protein kinase) plays a key role in regulating fuel combustion in skeletal muscle, and the amount of this protein is also highly influenced by the training status of the individual. Thus, AMPKα1 and AMPKβ2 protein expression increases, whilst AMPKγ3 protein and gene expression decreases with training [27,28]. Activation of AMPK by e.g. exercise, will cause a drop in malonyl CoA, which in turn will facilitate fatty acid transport into mitochondria and stimulate fatty acid oxidation. The effect is mediated via inhibition of acetyl-CoA carboxylase, which also increases in expression with training [27].

Recently, a study compared the mechanisms behind comparable increases in insulin-mediated glucose disposal after aerobic and resistance training in older men [29]. The authors reported a significant increase in skeletal muscle glycogen synthase activity only in the aerobically trained men, but a significant increase in muscle mass, muscle glycogen content or citrate synthase activity could not be demonstrated in any of the groups [29], which normally is a characteristic finding after training programs. With aerobic training for months, an increase in capillary density is a common finding in both healthy and insulin resistant humans. This increase facilitates diffusion of glucose from the capillaries into the muscle cells, and is therefore also a part of the mechanism behind the increase in insulin action seen after aerobic training. Capillary density is normally not increased by resistance training, so the mechanisms behind the enhancement of insulin action with the two different training regimens are not completely identical, but most likely the mechanisms differ only in minor details. Further studies may clarify this issue.

Resistance training, muscle hypertrophy and function in the elderly

Cross-sectional data on elite master athletes demonstrate that regular strength training throughout life can preserve a last part of the muscle mass from a young age. Intervention studies on a variety of groups of elderly individuals from around 60 and up to 100 years of age has shown that improvements in both muscle strength and muscle volume can be achieved by resistance training. This beneficial effect of training is seen not only in healthy elderly individuals, but also in frail elderly, and older individuals with co-morbidities [30]. The main question is, to what extent elderly individuals can counteract their skeletal muscle loss, and what role training and nutrition plays. Trained elderly individuals often have the strength of young untrained individuals, and intervention with strength training often show a 'strength-rejuvenation' of 20–30 years. Strength training studies demonstrate an improvement in everyday functional abilities like chair rising and stair climbing.

The regulation of muscle growth in the elderly is not completely understood. Synthesis of myofibrillar protein in relation to exercise has been shown to be either lower or identical to young individuals, and similarly degradation of muscle protein has been found to be similar to or somewhat higher than in younger counter parts [31,32]. If the findings of reduced synthesis and increased breakdown should be true the muscle loss in the elderly would be larger than is actually seen. It is clear that the mTOR pathway involving p70 S6 kinase phosphorylation in elderly individuals is active, and interestingly this pathway can also interact synergistically with high amino acid concentrations [33]. Interestingly, it is known that elderly individuals when compared with younger counterparts do not respond as efficiently in using nutritional supplementation like amino acids [34]. This implies that the elderly possess anabolic insensitivity and that the ability to benefit sufficiently from their food intake is reduced. Ingestion of food will be associated with an increase in circulating insulin levels, which activates the insulin signalling cascade all the way down to p70 S6 kinase and 4EBP1. After resistance training this stimulating effect of insulin is enhanced by a mechanism that is not fully understood. The lower anabolic response to nutritional intake in the elderly can be shown both with ingestion of relatively small amounts of protein/amino acids and with

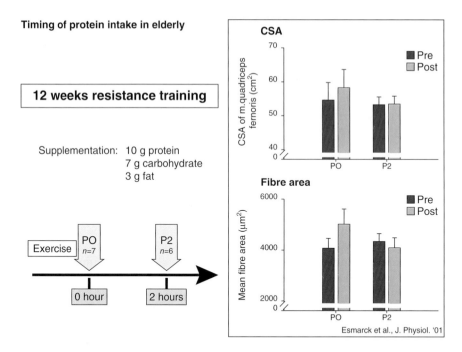

Figure 3. The effect of early administration of protein (mixed with carbohydrate and fat) to elderly subjects on muscle hypertrophy associated with resistance training
Determinations of whole muscle cross-sectional area (CSA) from magnetic resonance imaging of the thigh and CSA of individual muscle fibres (fibre area) from individual biopsies of the human thigh muscle. Reproduced from B. Esmarck, J.L. Andersen, S. Olsen, E.A. Richtér, M. Mizuno and M. Kjaer (2001) Timing of postexercise protein intake is important for muscle hypertrophy with resistance training in elderly humans. The Journal of Physiology **535**, 301–311 with permission from Blackwell Publishers.

the combination of carbohydrate and protein administration. The latter finding is at least suggestive for the idea that elderly individuals have a reduced anabolic action of insulin. This could be due to an impaired capacity of insulin to stimulate the protein signalling pathway, but could also be due to a reduced capacity of insulin to stimulate muscle perfusion and thus amino acid availability to the skeletal muscle. Resistance training is known to cause an increased expression and protein synthesis of GH (growth hormone), IGF-1 (insulin-like growth factor-1) and the IGF-1 isoform entitled MGF (mechano growth factor), which has been suggested to be specific for skeletal muscle [35], but recently has been shown also to be up-regulated by exercise in connective tissue such as tendon [36]. The influence of IGF-1/MGF may result in a post exercise activation either via the insulin signalling pathway or via activation of satellite cells. Suggestions have also been made that the calcium/calmodulin dependent protein kinase plays a role in the acute effect of resistance exercise and the long-term adaptation and fibre type shift with resistance exercise. Amino acids can stimulate mTOR independently from insulin but also activate p70 S6 kinase and 4EBP1 independently from insulin. Whether these pathways have a reduced capacity in elderly individuals compared with young counterparts is not known. Administration of GH to elderly individuals in amounts that double the circulating levels of IGF-1 did not enhance the muscle hypertrophy that was achieved by strength training alone [37]. In accordance with a reduced ability to benefit from nutritional supplementation in the elderly, administration of protein together with carbohydrate and fat in healthy elderly individuals after strength training resulted in an improvement in strength and muscle volume, only if supplementation was given immediately after training [38]. If given 2 h after training, the hypertrophy effect of strength training was abolished (Figure 3). Earlier classical studies have found varying results as to the effect of protein supplementation [30]. Although these reports all described the given dose, they did not report the timing for the administration, and this may be important. The exact mechanism behind the interaction between nutrition and strength training induced muscle hypertrophy is not elucidated, but it can be shown that in elderly individuals the protein balance is only positive if protein is taken, and that it is superior to carbohydrate intake.

Hormones like testosterone in elderly men and oestrogen in middle aged and elderly women have been shown to positively stimulate muscle growth [39]. In contrast, counteracting the age-related reduction in GH secretion (somatopenia) seen with ageing, does not improve muscle growth either alone nor in addition to strength training. A further factor that has been discussed in relation to ageing and skeletal muscle is the number and activity of satellite cells. In younger individuals its appreciated that satellite cells not only are active in the case of tissue injury and repair but also play a physiological role in providing new myonuclei as the muscle fibre grows in relation to strength training. Recently it has been shown that elderly individuals, independent of gender, increase their number of satellite cells in response to physiological strength training. This indicates that this pathway for forming new myonuclei is maintained in elderly individuals. What role nutrition may have in relation to satellite cells in the elderly is unknown.

Therefore, more studies are beginning to look at the response to training in individuals 'at risk' who typically have sub-optimal function and co-morbidities [40,41]. In such a study, elderly women who had experienced a fall injury (contusions but without fracture) were enrolled to either a training group or a non-training control group. After 6 months of strength training, women who trained improved their muscle strength significantly as well as their muscle power, evaluated as the ability to perform quick knee extensions in specialized and validated equipment. This increase in muscle power could indicate that training increased type II muscle fibre volume more than type I, but not all studies have been able to find a relative increase in type II to I fibre content as a result of training. An additional explanation for the increased muscle power could lie in the connective tissue. Although tendons of elderly individuals are thicker compared with younger individuals, they are also weaker, and interestingly it has been shown that strength training makes the ageing human tendon stiffer. This would cause less extensibility in the tendon during muscle contraction and thus result in a more rapid force transmission. The better muscle force and power in the frail elderly women after fall injury following training also resulted in improved everyday function. Interestingly, the maximal walking speed of these individuals was identical to the required speed which you need to have in order to be able to cross a street with traffic lights, and after resistance training the relative load to perform this task was lowered to 80–85% of maximal walking speed.

Low muscle mass is correlated with not only lower functional capacity, but is associated with a higher risk of falls, fractures and mortality. Low grip strength is associated with higher mortality, and low knee extension strength is related to incidence of early mortality after hip fracture. It was shown that those individuals with the highest knee extension strength had an almost 10-fold reduction in the mortality in association with a hip fracture compared with those individuals who had the weakest knee extension strength. Such a study is too small to detect whether strength training can not only influence factors of importance for falls but can also prevent *de facto* falls and injuries. Large scale studies comparing exercise training with vision control and managing of home hazards showed that exercise was the only intervention that had a significant effect upon fall frequency. Furthermore, looking at the larger studies within this area has shown that strength training in the elderly at risk from falls can reduce both frequency of falls as well as frequency of injuries with fractures by about a third. Thus there is good evidence that strength training, both supervised in a hospital setting as well as home-based exercises, is effective in counteracting falls and fractures.

In several groups with chronic diseases it has been shown that strength training can improve function (Figure 4). In patients with severe chronic obstructive lung disease increases in both muscle strength and in muscle volume after strength training was accompanied by a marked improvement in walking speed, stair climbing and activity of daily living. Furthermore, both in heart disease, osteoporosis and arthrosis it has been demonstrated that strength training will improve symptoms and function. Finally, in regards to depression, sleep pattern and mental well-being, strength training has been shown to be beneficial in elderly individuals. Training studies in patients vary often, but seem to be closely related to the compliance of the participants, rather than to detailed differences in the training pattern.

Strength training has been shown to play a positive role following surgery. With severe hip osteoarthritis, post-operative treatment with strength training was superior to electrical stimulation and standard mobilization regimens [42]. The increase in muscle strength that was obtained with strength training resulted in a neutralization of the side-to-side difference in strength that was observed prior to surgery, which is important considering that a difference in leg strength is a major risk factor for falls in the elderly. In addition to these improvements, with strength training, the functional performances improved

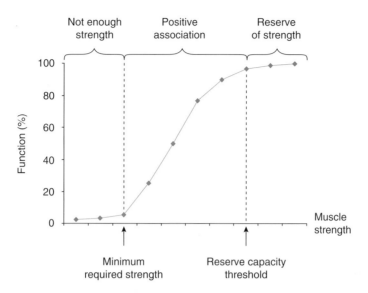

Figure 4. A schematic correlation demonstrates the relationship between the skeletal muscle strength and daily function
A well functioning elderly person will be placed far to the right, whereas a bedridden very weak sick elderly individual will be to the far left.

and correlated with the rate of force development of the thigh muscle. In addition the period of rehabilitation before the patients were discharged was reduced. Although these findings cannot be generalized to all surgical interventions it does show that training, in association with surgery is beneficial, and helps with restoring both muscle strength and functional performance [42].

Conclusions

Despite the fact that ageing is associated with a decreased muscle oxidative capacity and a reduced muscle function, a major part of this decline can be counteracted by physical activity, especially by resistance training. It is interesting that resistance training improves insulin sensitivity beyond the effect of just adding muscle mass, and this raises the question of whether heavy loading of muscle in the elderly causes similar effects on muscle that endurance activities would also create. The studies on protein turnover in skeletal muscle in the elderly are still not comprehensive enough to explain the mechanisms, and especially methods for the study of muscle protein degradation are not sufficiently accurate to draw major conclusions. Thus, adequate and timely nutrition support should accompany physical resistance training in elderly, and this advice should be followed whilst the mechanism behind the effect of exercise and nutrition is further investigated.

Summary

- *Muscle mass and strength is lost with ageing both due to muscle fibre atrophy and loss of motor units.*
- *Resistance training can improve insulin sensitivity not only due to development of more muscle but also due to improved muscle quality.*
- *Improvement of strength and especially of power through resistance training prevents falls and injury in elderly people.*
- *Patients with chronic disease or who are post-operative can benefit from strength training and improve muscle strength as well as daily function.*
- *Elderly and young people respond to resistance training with a similar increase in muscle protein synthesis, but elderly people have a reduced nutrition-induced increase in protein synthesis.*

References

1. Rogers, M.A., King, D.S., Hagberg, J.M., Ehsani, A.A. & Holloszy, J.O. (1990) Effect of 10 days of physical inactivity on glucose tolerance in master athletes. *J. Appl. Physiol.* **68**, 1833–1837
2. Coggan, A.R., Spina, R.J., Rogers, M.A., King, D.S., Brown, M., Nemeth, P.M. & Holloszy, J.O. (1990) Histochemical and enzymatic characteristics of skeletal muscle in master athletes. *J. Appl. Physiol.* **68**, 1896–1901
3. Heath, G.W., Hagberg, J.M., Ehsani, A.A. & Holloszy, J.O. (1981) A physiological comparison of young and older endurance athletes. *J. Appl. Physiol.* **51**, 634–640
4. Dela, F., Mikines, K.J., Larsen, J.J. & Galbo, H. (1996) Training-induced enhancement of insulin action in human skeletal muscle: The influence of aging. *J. Gerontol.* **51A**, B247–B252
5. Fritz, T. & Rosenqvist, U. (2001) Walking for exercise: immediate effect on blood glucose levels in type 2 diabetes. *Scand. J. Prim. Health Care* **19**, 31–33
6. Willey, K.A. & Singh, M.A. (2003) Battling insulin resistance in elderly obese people with type 2 diabetes: bring on the heavy weights. *Diabetes Care* **26**, 1580–1588
7. Holten, M.K., Zacho, M., Gaster, M., Juel, C., Wojtaszewski, J.F.P. & Dela, F. (2004) Strength training increases insulin-mediated glucose uptake, GLUT4 content and insulin signaling in skeletal muscle in patients with Type 2 diabetes. *Diabetes* **53**, 294–305
8. Andersen, J.L., Schjerling, P., Andersen, L.L. & Dela, F. (2003) Resistance training and insulin action in humans: effects of de-training. *J. Physiol.* **551**, 1049–1058
9. Grimditch, G.K., Barnard, J., Kaplan, S.A. & Sternlicht, E. (1986) Effect of training on insulin binding to rat skeletal muscle sarcolemmal vesicles. *Am. J. Physiol.* **250**, E570–E575
10. Dela, F., Handberg, A., Mikines, K.J., Vinten, J. & Galbo, H. (1993) GLUT 4 and insulin receptor binding and kinase activity in trained human muscle. *J. Physiol.* **469**, 615–624
11. Dohm, G.L., Sinha, M.K. & Caro, J.F. (1987) Insulin receptor binding and protein kinase activity in muscles of trained rats. *Am. J. Physiol.* **252**, E170–E175
12. Yu, M., Blomstrand, E., Chibalin, A.V., Wallberg-Henriksson, H., Zierath, J.R. & Krook, A. (2001) Exercise-associated differences in an array of proteins involved in signal transduction and glucose transport. *J. Appl. Physiol.* **90**, 29–34
13. Chibalin, A.V., Yu, M., Ryder, J.W., Song, X.M., Galuska, D., Krook, A., Wallberg-Henriksson, H. & Zierath, J.R. (2000) Exercise-induced changes in expression and activity of proteins involved in insulin signal transduction in skeletal muscle: differential effects on insulin-receptor substrates 1 and 2. *Proc. Natl. Acad. Sci. U.S.A.* **97**, 38–43

14. Bak, J.F., Jacobsen, U.K., Jørgensen, F.S. & Pedersen, O. (1989) Insulin receptor function and glycogen synthase activity in skeletal muscle biopsies from patients with insulin-dependent diabetes mellitus: Effects of physical training. *J. Clin. Endocrinol. Metab.* **69**, 158–164

15. Yaspelkis, III, B.B. (2006) Resistance training improves insulin signaling and action in skeletal muscle. *Exerc. Sport Sci. Rev.* **34**, 42–46

16. Dela, F., Ploug, T., Handberg, A., Petersen, L.N., Larsen, J.J., Mikines, K.J. & Galbo, H. (1994) Physical training increases muscle GLUT-4 protein and mRNA in patients with NIDDM. *Diabetes* **43**, 862–865

17. Saltin, B. & Gollnick, P.D. (1983) Skeletal muscle adaptability: significance for metabolism and performance. In *Handbook of Physiology. Section 10: Skeletal muscle*, Peachey, L.D., Adrian, R.H., & Geiger, S.R., pp. 555–631. American Physiological Society, Bethesda, MD.

18. Bruce, C.R., Thrush, A.B., Mertz, V.A., Bezaire, V., Chabowski, A., Heigenhauser, G.J. & Dyck, D.J. (2006) Endurance training in obese humans improves glucose tolerance, mitochondrial fatty acid oxidation and alters muscle lipid content. *Am. J. Physiol. Endocrinol. Metab.* **291**, E99–E109

19. Bezaire, V., Bruce, C.R., Heigenhauser, G.J., Tandon, N.N., Glatz, J.F., Luiken, J.J., Bonen, A. & Spriet, L.L. (2006) Identification of fatty acid translocase on human skeletal muscle mitochondrial membranes: essential role in fatty acid oxidation. *Am. J. Physiol. Endocrinol. Metab.* **290**, E509–E515

20. Schenk, S. & Horowitz, J.F. (2006) Coimmunoprecipitation of FAT/CD36 and CPT I in skeletal muscle increases proportionally with fat oxidation after endurance exercise training. *Am. J. Physiol. Endocrinol. Metab.* **291**, E254–E260

21. Tunstall, R.J., Mehan, K.A., Wadley, G.D., Collier, G.R., Bonen, A., Hargreaves, M. & Cameron-Smith, D. (2002) Exercise training increases lipid metabolism gene expression in human skeletal muscle. *Am. J. Physiol. Endocrinol. Metab.* **283**, E66–E72

22. Kiens, B., Kristiansen, S., Jensen, P., Richter, E.A. & Turcotte, L.P. (1997) Membrane associated fatty acid binding protein (FABPpm) in human skeletal muscle is increased by endurance training. *Biochem. Biophys. Res. Commun.* **231**, 463–465

23. Kiens, B., Roepstorff, C., Glatz, J.F., Bonen, A., Schjerling, P., Knudsen, J. & Nielsen, J.N. (2004) Lipid-binding proteins and lipoprotein lipase activity in human skeletal muscle: influence of physical activity and gender. *J. Appl. Physiol.* **97**, 1209–1218

24. Helge, J.W., Biba, T.O., Galbo, H., Gaster, M. & Donsmark, M. (2006) Muscle triacylglycerol and hormone-sensitive lipase activity in untrained and trained human muscles. *Eur. J. Appl. Physiol.* **97**, 566–572

25. Kiens, B. & Lithell, H. (1989) Lipoprotein metabolism influenced by training-induced changes in human skeletal muscle. *J. Clin. Invest.* **83**, 558–564

26. Nikkila, E.A., Taskinen, M.R., Rehunen, S. & Harkonen, M. (1978) Lipoprotein lipase activity in adipose tissue and skeletal muscle of runners: relation to serum lipoproteins. *Metabolism* **27**, 1661–1667

27. Wojtaszewski, J.F., Birk, J.B., Frosig, C., Holten, M., Pilegaard, H. & Dela, F. (2005) 5 AMP activated protein kinase expression in human skeletal muscle: effects of strength training and type 2 diabetes. *J. Physiol.* **564**, 563–573

28. Langfort, J., Viese, M., Ploug, T. & Dela, F. (2003) Time course of GLUT4 and AMPK protein expression in human skeletal muscle during one month of physical training. *Scand. J. Med. Sci. Sports* **13**, 169–174

29. Ferrara, C.M., Goldberg, A.P., Ortmeyer, H.K. & Ryan, A.S. (2006) Effects of aerobic and resistive exercise training on glucose disposal and skeletal muscle metabolism in older men. *J. Gerontol. Ser. A* **61**, 480–487

30. Fiatarone, M.A., O'Neill, E.F., Ryan, N.D. & Evans, W.J. (1994) Exercise training and nutritional supplementation for physical frailty in very elderly people. *N. Engl. J. Med.* **330**, 1769–1775

31. Welle, S., Thornton, C., Jozefowicz, R. & Statt, M. (1993) Myofibrillar protein synthesis in young and old men. *Am J. Physiol.* **264**, E693–E698

32. Trappe, T., Williams, R., Carrithers, J., Raue, U., Esmarck, B., Kjaer, M. & Hickner, R. (2004) Influence of age and resistance exercise on human skeletal muscle proteolysis: a microdialysis approach. *J. Physiol.* **554**, 803–813

33. Guillet, C., Prod'homme, M., Balage, M., Gachon, P., Giraudet, C. & Boirie, Y. (2004) Impaired anabolic response of muscle protein synthesis is associated with S6K1 dysregulation in elderly individuals. *FASEB J.* **18**, 1586–1587

34. Cuthbertson, D., Smith, K., Babraj, J., Leese, G., Waddell, T., Atherton, P., Wackerhage, H., Taylor, P.M. & Rennie, M.J. (2005) Anabolic signaling deficits underlie amino acid resistance of wasting, ageing muscle. *FASEB J.* **19**, 422–424

35. Hameed, M., Lange, K.H.W., Andersen, J.L., Scherling, P., Kjær, M., Harridge, S.D.R. & Goldspink, G. (2004) The effect of recombinant human growth hormne and resistance training on IGF-I mRNA expression in the muscles of elderly men. *J. Physiol.* **555**, 231–240

36. Olesen, J.L., Heinemeier, K.M., Haddad, F., Langberg, H., Flyvbjerg, A., Kjaer, M. & Baldwin, K.M. (2006) Expression of insulin-like growth factor I, insulin-like growth factor binding proteins, and collagen mRNA in mechanically loaded plantaris tendon. *J. Appl. Physiol.* **101**, 183–188

37. Lange, K.H., Andersen, J.L., Beyer, N., Isaksson, F., Larsson, B., Rasmussen, M.H., Juul, A., Bülow, J. & Kjær, M. (2002) GH administration changes myosin heavy chain isoforms in skeletal muscle but does not augment muscle strength or hypertrophy, either alone or combined with resistance exercise training in healthy elderly men. *J. Clin. Endocrinol. Metab.* **87**, 513–523

38. Esmarck, B., Andersen, J.L., Olsen, S., Richter, E.A., Mizuno, M. & Kjaer, M.(2001) Timing of postexercise protein intake is important for muscle hypertrophy with resistance training in elderly humans. *J. Physiol.* **535**, 301–311

39. Urban, R.J., Bodenberg, Y.H., Gilkison, C., Foxworth, J., Coggan, A.R., Wolfe, R.R. & Ferrando, A. (1995) Testosterone administration to elderly men increases muscle strength and protein synthesis. *Am. J. Physiol.* **268**, E268–E276

40. Lexell, J., Taylor, C.C. & Sjöström, M. (1988) What is the cause of the ageing atrophy? Total number, size and proportions of different fiber types studied in whole vastus lateralis muscle from 15- to 83-year old men. *J. Neurol. Sci.* **84**, 275–294

41. Skelton, D.A., Greig, C.A., Davies, J.M. & Young, A. (1994) Strength, power and related functional ability of healthy people aged 65–89 years. *Age Ageing* **23**, 371–377

42. Suetta, C., Magnusson, S.P., Rosted, A., Aagaard, P., Jacobsen, A.K., Duus, B. & Kjær, M. (2004) Resistance training in the early post-operative phase reduces hospitalization and leads to muscle hypertrophy in elderly hip surgery patients - a controlled randomized study. *J. Am. Ger. Soc.* **52**, 2016–2022

7

Fatty acid metabolism in adipose tissue, muscle and liver in health and disease

Keith N. Frayn*[1], Peter Arner† and Hannele Yki-Järvinen‡

*Oxford Centre for Diabetes, Endocrinology and Metabolism, University of Oxford, Churchill Hospital, Oxford OX3 7LJ, U.K., †Department of Medicine, Karolinska Institute, Huddinge University Hospital, S 141 86 Huddinge, Sweden, and ‡Department of Medicine, Division of Diabetes, University of Helsinki, PO Box 340, 00029 Helsinki, Finland

Abstract

Fat is the largest energy reserve in mammals. Most tissues are involved in fatty acid metabolism, but three are quantitatively more important than others: adipose tissue, skeletal muscle and liver. Each of these tissues has a store of triacylglycerol that can be hydrolysed (mobilized) in a regulated way to release fatty acids. In the case of adipose tissue, these fatty acids may be released into the circulation for delivery to other tissues, whereas in muscle they are a substrate for oxidation and in liver they are a substrate for re-esterification within the endoplasmic reticulum to make triacylglycerol that will be secreted as very-low-density lipoprotein. These pathways are regulated, most clearly in the case of adipose tissue. Adipose tissue fat storage is stimulated, and fat mobilization suppressed, by insulin, leading to a drive to store energy in the fed state. Muscle fatty acid metabolism is more sensitive to physical activity, during which fatty acid utilization from extracellular and

[1]To whom correspondence should be addressed (email keith.frayn@oxlip.ox.ac.uk).

intracellular sources may increase enormously. The uptake of fat by the liver seems to depend mainly upon delivery in the plasma, but the secretion of very-low-density lipoprotein triacylglycerol is suppressed by insulin. There is clearly cooperation amongst the tissues, so that, for instance, adipose tissue fat mobilization increases to meet the demands of skeletal muscle during exercise. When triacylglycerol accumulates excessively in skeletal muscle and liver, sometimes called ectopic fat deposition, then the condition of insulin resistance arises. This may reflect a lack of exercise and an excess of fat intake.

Introduction

Triacylglycerol (or triglyceride) is a concentrated form in which to store energy. Triacylglycerol circulates in the plasma in lipoproteins and is also present as lipid droplets within cells. The 'energy density' of lipid stored in cells in this way is approx. 37 kJ/g. The energy density of whole adipose tissue (with cytoplasm, connective tissues etc.) is approx. 30 kJ/g. In contrast, glycogen in pure form has an energy density of approx. 17 kJ/g, but when stored in hydrated form with about three times its own weight of water (as it is in cells), this reduces to approx. 4 kJ/g. There are three main organs that store triacylglycerol in a regulated way and hydrolyse it to release fatty acids, either for export or for internal consumption. These are, in order of amount of triacylglycerol typically stored, adipose tissue, skeletal muscle and the liver. Recent years have seen an enormous increase in our understanding of

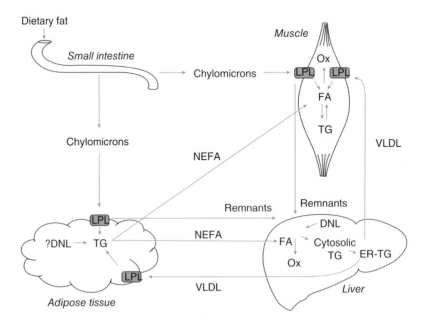

Figure 1. Lipid exchanges between gut, adipose tissue, skeletal muscle and liver
Note that adipose tissue LPL also releases NEFA into the plasma, making further fatty acids available for uptake by muscle and liver. ER, endoplasmic reticulum; FA, fatty acids; Ox, β-oxidation.

Table 1. Characteristics of fatty acid and TG metabolism compared in adipose tissue, skeletal muscle and liver

	Adipose tissue	Skeletal muscle (at rest)	Liver
Input	LP–TG ~ 45 g/day	NEFA ~ 20 g/day	NEFA ~ 20 g/day
	NEFA ~ 5 g/day	LP–TG ~ 10 g/day	Remnant-LP–TG ~ 25 g/day
			DNL ~ 1 g/day
Stimulation of uptake	Feeding/insulin	Fasting (high NEFA supply)	Delivery
		Exercise	
FA transporters	FAT	FAT	FAT
	FATP-1, 4	FATP-1, 4	FATP-2, 5
Typical whole-body TG store	15 kg	300 g	100 g
Half-life of store	250 days	24 h	100 h
Lipolysis of TG store	HSL - stimulated lipolysis	HSL ?	Unknown
	ATGL - basal lipolysis		
	MGL - monoacylglycerol hydrolysis		
Releases mainly	NEFA into plasma	FA for oxidation	FAs re-esterified in ER and released as VLDL-TG

Quantitative data involve some estimates and should be taken as representative only. ER, endoplasmic reticulum; FA, fatty acids; LP, lipoprotein; MGL, monoacylglycerol lipase; TG, triacylglycerol.

triacylglycerol and fatty acid metabolism in these organs, and of its relationship to health and disease.

There is a continual flow of fatty acids between the three tissues described above, outlined in Figure 1 with some quantitative estimates in Table 1. Dietary fat enters the plasma from the small intestine in the form of chylomicron-triacylglycerol. The chylomicrons are the largest of the lipoprotein particles and have a very fast turnover (the half-life of chylomicron-triacylglycerol in the circulation is around 5 min). They deliver triacylglycerol-fatty acids to tissues expressing the enzyme LPL (lipoprotein lipase), an enzyme bound to the endothelial cells lining capillaries of a number of tissues including adipose tissue, skeletal and cardiac muscle (more details are given in Figure 2).

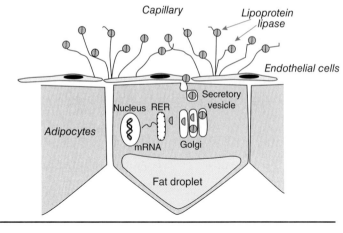

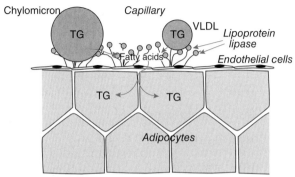

Figure 2. Regulation and action of LPL

This is shown for adipose tissue but aspects of the regulation and action are likely to be similar in other tissues. Top panel: LPL is synthesized in the rough endoplasmic reticulum (RER) and post-translationally modified, becoming active in the Golgi apparatus. An important aspect of activation is dimerization. From the Golgi, LPL is secreted via the vascular endothelial cells to proteoglycan chains attached to the endothelial cell membrane. The lipid droplet of the mature adipocytes has been reduced in size in this diagram for clarity. In principle, regulation of LPL activity could occur at many points. In fact, up-regulation of adipose tissue LPL activity in the fed state occurs with little change in mRNA or intracellular enzyme mass. It appears mainly to involve the mobilization of active enzyme to the capillary-luminal aspect of the endothelial cells. There is no evidence for reversible phosphorylation as a means of regulation of LPL activity. In fasting, more LPL becomes inactive (perhaps via monomerization). Note that, in contrast, LPL in skeletal and cardiac muscle is activated during fasting. Lower panel: LPL acts via binding to the triacylglycerol-rich lipoprotein particles, chylomicrons (carrying dietary fat) and VLDL (secreted from the liver). It hydrolyses the triacylglycerol to liberate fatty acids, that can be taken up by the adipocyte (or muscle cell) and esterified to form new triacylglycerol. In skeletal or cardiac muscle, these fatty acids might also be a substrate for oxidation. Lower panel taken from Frayn, K.N. (2003) *Metabolic Regulation : a Human Perspective*, 2nd edn. Published by Blackwell Publishing.

The remaining 'remnant' particles (that have lost perhaps two-thirds of their triacylglycerol) are mainly taken up by the liver. This is the starting point for fatty acid metabolism in the tissues.

Adipose tissue takes up fatty acids via the action of LPL. It releases fatty acids by the hydrolysis (lipolysis) of stored (intracellular) triacylglycerol, by the action of the enzyme known as HSL (hormone-sensitive lipase) and other lipases, to liberate NEFA (non-esterified fatty acids) into the plasma. Plasma NEFA circulate bound to albumin. The turnover of plasma NEFA is also rapid, with a half-life of 4–5 min. The liver takes up fatty acids in various forms and liberates triacylglycerol-fatty acids as VLDL (very-low-density lipoprotein) particles. In this scenario, skeletal and heart muscle (and other oxidative tissues not considered here) are the only pure consumers, taking up fatty acids either from lipoprotein-triacylglycerol or from the plasma NEFA pool and using them ultimately for oxidation.

Regulation of triacylglycerol and fatty acid metabolism at rest

Overview

The pattern of flow of fatty acids between the tissues changes with nutritional state. In the fed, or postprandial, state there is a drive to store excess nutrients and as part of this, adipose tissue LPL is up-regulated, probably by the action of insulin released in response to carbohydrate in the meal. This diverts chylomicron-fatty acids to adipose tissue rather than muscle, where LPL is somewhat down-regulated by insulin (muscle LPL becomes particularly active with physical training or during fasting, conditions when the muscle has a greater need for fatty acids). Since adipose tissue is acquiring fatty acids in the postprandial period, it makes sense that fat mobilization is suppressed at this time, again by the action of insulin. Both the liver and skeletal muscle take up fatty acids largely according to their availability. The rate of removal of plasma NEFA is, under most conditions, fairly closely proportional to their plasma concentration. The removal by the liver of remnant-particle triacylglycerol-fatty acids is also probably determined by their delivery in plasma. The abundance of the different sources of fatty acids in plasma varies with nutritional state, with the highest supply of NEFA in the fasting state and chylomicron-remnant triacylglycerol fatty acids becoming more prominent in the fed state. As mentioned earlier, muscle LPL is up-regulated during fasting although its activity does not seem to vary greatly during the normal day. The secretion of VLDL-triacylglycerol by the liver is undoubtedly subject to nutritional regulation. Insulin acutely suppresses hepatic VLDL-triacylglycerol secretion. VLDL particles are secreted with a range of sizes, and it is especially the secretion of the larger, more triacylglycerol-rich particles that is suppressed by insulin. The mechanism by which insulin suppresses VLDL-triacylglycerol secretion is 2-fold. First, it suppresses delivery of NEFA to the liver from adipose tissue as described above. But there is a further, and more important, effect on VLDL particle secretion from the hepatocytes. Whether insulin has this effect in the normal daily feeding situation is not so clear: it is difficult to study *in vivo* in humans because the non-steady state of feeding is not ideal for the tracer experiments that have mostly been used to study regulation of VLDL secretion.

Tissue-specific features of triacylglycerol and fatty acid metabolism

Adipose tissue

Adipose tissue triacylglycerol storage varies widely between individuals. The 'standard' adult female has approx. 30% of body weight as fat and the male approx. 20%, most of which is in adipocytes [1]. The adipocyte is a cell highly specialized for fat storage, although we now also appreciate that it has important protein secretory functions secreting hormones such as leptin, adiponectin and a range of other so-called 'adipokines'. The specific fatty acids stored in human adipose tissue (saturated, monounsaturated and unsaturated) reflect dietary intake. There is debate about the contribution of DNL (*de novo* lipogenesis) to adipose tissue fat stores but, at the whole-body level, DNL only operates significantly when carbohydrate intake exceeds energy requirements. Isotopic data suggest that approx. 10% of adipose tissue triacylglycerol fatty acids arise from DNL [2]. Most of the triacylglycerol-fatty acids in human adipose tissue therefore arise from plasma, mainly from the triacylglycerol fraction of plasma lipids with a small contribution of direct uptake from NEFAs [3].

The control of fatty acid uptake by adipocytes is not well understood. Up-regulation of adipose tissue LPL activity in the fed state is brought about by multiple mechanisms (Figure 2). LPL is synthesized within adipocytes and exported to its site of action, the luminal side of the capillary endothelial cells. Of the large pool of LPL in adipose tissue, only a portion becomes active endothelial-bound LPL. An important mechanism for up-regulation in the fed state is the diversion of LPL away from the degradative, into the secretory pathway [4]. LPL acts on circulating lipoprotein-triacylglycerol and generates fatty acids in the local area close to the endothelium. Chylomicrons are the pre-ferred substrate for adipose tissue LPL. Chylomicron-triacylglycerol is hydro-lysed considerably more rapidly than VLDL-triacylglycerol. Nevertheless, both substrates may contribute fatty acid under appropriate circumstances. The fatty acids released by LPL migrate across the endothelial wall and into the underlying adipocytes. The mechanisms involved in this process are not clear, although there is increasing evidence for the involvement of specific fatty acids transporters including FAT (fatty acid translocase, also known as CD36) in facilitating fatty acid movement across the adipocyte cell membrane. There is also non-regulated diffusion through the cell membrane. Within the adi-pocyte, fatty acids are 'activated' by esterification to CoA in an ATP-requiring process that seems to be intimately linked to fatty acid transport into the cell, at least when mediated by a member of the FATP (fatty acid transport protein) family (FATP1) [5].

Adipose tissue LPL generates an excess of fatty acids. The adipocytes then take up a proportion, depending upon nutritional state. There is always an 'overspill' of fatty acids into the plasma. Insulin increases the proportion of LPL-derived fatty acids taken up by the tissue but even in the postprandial state

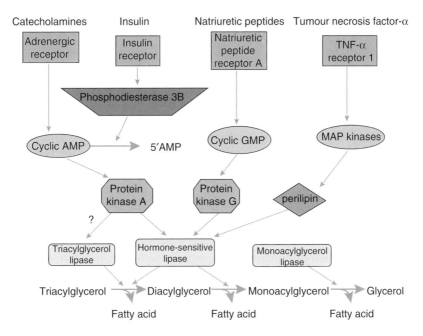

Figure 3. Regulation of lipolysis in white adipose tissue
For more detail please refer to the text.

typically approx. 50% may be released as NEFA, clearly shown by enrichment of the plasma NEFA pool with dietary fatty acids soon after a meal. These fatty acids are then available for uptake by other tissues including muscle and liver. The control of fatty acid uptake into the adipocyte may involve recruitment of the fatty acid transporters CD36 and FATP1 to the cell surface upon insulin stimulation [5]. It also involves stimulation of fatty acid esterification to make new triacylglycerol within the adipocyte. Regulation of the enzymes of triacylglycerol synthesis is still not understood in detail although the pathway as a whole is certainly stimulated by insulin [6]. In addition, insulin may stimulate glucose uptake and glycolysis, which supplies the glycerol 3-phosphate necessary for fatty acid esterification. The ability of fat cells to take up acylglycerols directly is very limited.

Adipose tissue fat mobilization has been studied in detail [7] and is summarized in Figure 3. Until recently it was considered that the only major regulatory point was the enzyme HSL. HSL has triacylglycerol-lipase activity directed at two fatty acids on a triacylglycerol molecule, but is not active against monoacylglycerols, whereas it is especially active against diacylglycerols. There is a separate, and unrelated, monoacylglycerol lipase that is consitutively expressed in adipose tissue and catalyses the last step in triacylglycerol hydrolysis. HSL is regulated in the long-term by transcriptional control: HSL mRNA abundance increases during starvation, and is decreased in obesity. But the most important aspect of HSL on a day-to-day basis is its regulation by reversible phosphorylation [7]. HSL has three phosphorylation sites that are substrates for PKA (protein kinase A), phosphorylation of which greatly increases its activity. Adipocyte fat mobilization is brought about by signals that increase the cAMP concentration. Typically, catecholamines would act by binding to β-adreno-ceptors in the cell membrane, linked by G-proteins to adenylate cyclase. Insulin suppresses HSL activity by activation of a particular phosphodieste-rase, PDE3B, which reduces the cAMP concentration. These effects are rapid and potent. However, the increased rate of lipolysis seen upon stimulation of fat cells with β-adrenergic agents is far greater than would be predicted from the increase in activity of HSL *in vitro*. It is now clear that phosphorylation of HSL is accompanied by phosphorylation of a protein, perilipin, that coats the adipocyte fat droplet. This dual phosphorylation allows HSL to translocate from the cytosol to the surface of the fat droplet to achieve lipolysis. Under non-stimulated conditions, HSL is excluded from the fat droplet surface.

A further system of human-specific regulation has been described, involv-ing the circulating peptides known as ANF (atrial natriuretic factor) and BNF (brain natriuretic factor) [8]. These factors are released during stress states including exercise and bind to specific cell-surface receptors that are cou-pled to synthesis of cGMP and activation of cyclic GMP-dependent protein kinase. Finally, there is an autocrine regulation of lipolysis by tumour necrosis factor-α. This cytokine acts on perilipin through MAPK (mitogen-activated protein kinase) signalling pathways.

The primary role of HSL in lipolysis has been challenged by findings in mice deficient in HSL. These mice have relatively normal adipose tissue mass, and lipolysis is preserved, although β-adrenergic responsiveness is almost or completely lost, depending upon the model. This has led to a search for other lipases in the adipocyte. One candidate, ATGL (adipose triglyceride lipase), has marked specificity for triacylglycerols compared with di- or mono-acylglycerols, and may be of great importance for lipolysis in rodents. It now seems likely that ATGL is responsible for 'basal' lipolysis in human adipose tissue, with HSL responsible for the majority of catecholamine- or ANF-stimulated lipolysis [9].

Liver

The normal triacylglycerol content of the liver is around 1–10% by weight [1] but can expand considerably in the condition generally called 'fatty liver'. The liver receives plasma fatty acids as NEFA, from hydrolysis of circulating triacylglycerol and from the uptake of remnant lipoprotein particles. Uptake of NEFA appears to be similar to the process described in adipose tissue: FAT/CD36, FATP2 and FATP5 are expressed in liver. The adult liver does not express LPL, but a related enzyme, HL (hepatic lipase) which acts preferentially upon smaller particles than LPL. It will remove triacylglycerol from small VLDL particles and from particles on their way to becoming LDL (low-density lipoprotein) and also from HDL (high-density lipoprotein) particles. It also has a major role in 'docking' with particles that are being internalized bound to specific receptors expressed in the liver. The liver is the main organ for uptake of the remnant particles formed from the action of LPL on triacylglycerol-rich chylomicrons and VLDL. The chylomicron remnant particle is thought to contain typically about one-third of its original triacylglycerol content. This is still appreciable (a typical chylomicron particle contains approx. 10^6 molecules of triacylglycerol), and would lead to delivery to the liver of around 20–30 g/day of dietary triacylglycerol.

In addition, the liver has the enzymatic capacity for DNL, the synthesis of fatty acids from glucose and other non-lipid precursors. DNL makes a small contribution in people on a typical, western relatively high-fat diet, but it becomes activated during a high-energy diet rich in carbohydrate [10]. The pathway involves export of acetyl-CoA formed in the mitochondrion (in the case of glucose as the precursor, by pyruvate dehydrogenase) to the cytosol (in the form of citrate), conversion of acetyl-CoA to malonyl-CoA by acetyl-CoA carboxylase and then sequential addition of two carbon units by fatty acid synthase.

Fatty acids taken up into the hepatocytes are activated by esterification to CoA. The long-chain acyl-CoA may then enter the mitochondria for oxidation or be a substrate for glycerolipid synthesis (triacylglycerol and phospholipids). This is a key regulatory point, determined largely by regulation of entry into the mitochondria, via the enzyme CPT 1 (carnitine palmitoyltransferase 1, the 'overt' isoform, expressed in the outer mitochondrial enzyme). This enzyme is allosterically regulated by the cytosolic malonyl-CoA concentration. Malonyl-CoA (an intermediate in fatty acid synthesis) is a very potent inhibitor of CPT 1. Its concentration is high when insulin levels are high and glucose is readily available, conditions when fatty acid synthesis should be favoured over fatty acid oxidation. In the fasting state, when insulin levels are low, fatty acid oxidation is therefore favoured. There is a further branch point in fatty acid oxidation when acetyl-CoA may either enter the tricarboxylic acid cycle or may be directed into ketone body synthesis. Less is known about regulation of this 'metabolic branch point'. A suggested regulation of ketone body synthesis is by reversible succinylation of the mitochondrial 3-hydroxy-3-methylglutaryl-CoA synthase [11].

The cytosolic triacylglycerol pool within the hepatocyte is the precursor for VLDL-triacylglycerol. Lipolysis of this cytosolic pool is necessary to generate fatty acids that are then esterified to make new triacylglycerol within the endoplasmic reticulum, where VLDL particles are assembled. The identity of the lipase responsible, and its regulation, are not clear. VLDL-triacylglycerol secretion is acutely inhibited by insulin, although hepatic fatty acids are preferentially stored as triacylglycerol when insulin levels are high. This implies that the hepatocyte triacylglycerol store fluctuates in size, increasing after meals and then discharging during fasting as VLDL are secreted. This has recently been visualized directly in healthy humans where approx. 10% of the fat from a meal was stored in the liver in the few hours following feeding [12].

Muscle

The total triacylglycerol store in a healthy human liver is approx. 100 g (or less). The typical triacylglycerol content in whole-body skeletal muscle might be approx. 300 g (estimated making various assumptions, see [13]).

There are two major triacylglycerol stores in muscle: in adipocytes interleaved with the muscle fibres (seen, for instance, as 'marbling' in a cut of meat) and triacylglycerol stored within the muscle fibre itself ('intramyocellular triacylglycerol'). Here we will discuss only the latter. It is still not clear whether there is any direct metabolic relationship between adipocytes and skeletal muscle fibres even when they are located in close proximity.

Intramyocellular triacylglycerol is present as lipid droplets, often in close contact with mitochondria. Some of the enzymatic machinery for fatty acid and triacylglycerol metabolism in the muscle fibre is similar to that in the adipocyte. Fatty acids can be taken up from the plasma, either from the albumin-bound NEFA pool or, as in adipose tissue, from the pool of fatty acids generated by the action of LPL on circulating triacylglycerol. In either case it seems that the fatty acids enter the cells at least in part by facilitated diffusion, as both FAT/CD36 and FATP1 are expressed in skeletal muscle. Muscle has the enzymatic machinery to synthesize malonyl-CoA from glucose utilization, the first stage of the biosynthesis of fatty acids. However, expression of fatty acid synthase (which makes fatty acids from malonyl-CoA) is very small or non-existent. Therefore the triacylglycerol present in muscle can be assumed to arise entirely from plasma fatty acids (NEFA or triacylglycerol). The role of malonyl-CoA appears to be in the regulation of fatty acid oxidation, as described above for the liver.

The intramyocellular triacylglycerol is hydrolysed to make fatty acids available for oxidation. HSL is likely to be the key lipase controlling this process, although there is no direct evidence for this other than the fact that HSL is expressed in muscle and becomes activated on muscle contraction [14]. This is reinforced by the accumulation of large lipid droplets in skeletal muscle of HSL-deficient mice [15]. Fatty acids made available from muscle triacylglycerol lipolysis would be a substrate for oxidation after activation and entry into the mitochondria. Muscle lipolysis is less sensitive to hormone regulation than adipocyte lipolysis, at least in humans. Insulin is not effective but catecholamines stimulate muscle lipolysis [14,16].

It is not clear whether, as in the adipocyte, fatty acids may be released from the cell into the plasma. Certainly this does not happen in a net sense: muscle always extracts NEFA from plasma, never adds them. Some measurements suggest that fatty acids are released from muscle beds, in larger amounts than could be accounted for by the adipocytes likely to be present [17]. Nevertheless, it is clear that adipose tissue is the only tissue that contributes NEFA to the plasma in a net sense.

The processes of fatty acid uptake by muscle, and of mobilization of muscle triacylglycerol stores, are covered in detail in Chapter 4 and will not be covered here in further detail.

The heart muscle (myocardium) is also involved in fatty acid metabolism; in fact, as a continuously contracting oxidative muscle, it has a very high demand for fatty acids. These fatty acids are acquired from plasma both as NEFA and through the LPL-route. Many features of myocardial fatty acid metabolism are similar to skeletal muscle, although the major isoform of the FATP family expressed in the heart is FATP6, which co-localizes on the plasma membrane with CD36.

Metabolic interactions during exercise

Fat is an important fuel for skeletal muscle during exercise. Its importance is greater at lower intensities of exercise and as the duration of exercise increases. In any exercise lasting more than approximately 2 h, fat becomes the major fuel (once muscle glycogen stores are exhausted). Most of the fatty acids oxidized in muscle during exercise come from the plasma NEFA pool. Hence coordination between adipose tissue (activation of lipolysis) and muscle (fatty acid utilization) is crucial. The contribution of VLDL-triacylglycerol fatty acids during exercise is small, but in the fed state chylomicron-triacylglycerol fatty acids might make a greater contribution [18]. Regarding the role of the intramuscular triacylglycerol store, early studies involving muscle biopsies before and after exercise were generally uninformative. New approaches have increased our understanding of muscle triacylglycerol. Isotope infusion studies show that muscle triacylglycerol utilization makes a substantial contribution to fatty acid oxidation at moderate intensity of exercise (approx. 55–65% VO_2max), almost equal to the contribution from plasma NEFA, but less at lesser or greater intensity [19,20]. The measurement of IMCL (intra-myocellular lipid) by magnetic resonance spectroscopy also shows muscle triacylglycerol utilization during exercise, at rates comparable with those observed with tracer techniques [21,22].

The activation of adipose tissue lipolysis during exercise is largely β-adrenergic, responding presumably to circulating adrenaline or perhaps activation of the sympathetic outflow to adipose tissue (studies in people with spinal cord injuries suggest mainly the former [23]). The technique of microdialysis of adipose tissue involves a small probe of semi-permeable membrane, which is used both to introduce agents and to sample the interstitial glycerol concentration (as a marker of lipolysis). Introduction of propanolol (a non-specific β-adrenergic blocker) largely, but not completely, inhibits the stimulation of lipolysis by exercise [24]. The remaining, non-β-adrenergic component, may represent activation by the ANF pathway [8].

If activation of adipose tissue lipolysis relies on signals that are part of the exercise response, how is it that the rate of fatty acid delivery so closely matches the rate of utilization by skeletal muscle? This would seem to require some direct signal from the muscle to the adipose tissue. If someone exercises whilst lipolysis is suppressed, e.g. using the drug acipimox which acts on the so-called nicotinic acid receptor on adipocytes and potently blocks NEFA release, then the muscles use more IMCL and also more glucose. That implies that NEFA delivery from adipose tissue is a 'preferred' fuel and the muscles will use other fuels to make up any lack of NEFA. An alternative view is that adipose tissue lipolysis normally operates at a greater rate than is necessary for fatty acid oxidation in other tissues. The 'excess' fatty acids are re-esterified, for instance in the liver, and returned to adipose tissue in VLDL. Then, at the onset of exercise, a greater proportion of the NEFA delivered from adipose tissue will be oxidized and a correspondingly lower portion re-esterified [25]. However, this view is not supported by all studies [17].

Tissue triacylglycerol metabolism in health and disease

The systems described above function efficiently in health to maintain appropriate delivery of fatty acids when they are needed. Dysfunction of these systems may underlie some specific disorders of lipid metabolism. For instance, in the relatively common condition known as familial combined hyperlipidaemia, there is evidence that the primary defect is an over-production of small VLDL particles from the liver. This may be combined with a low rate of lipolysis in adipose tissue [26].

We will discuss here one very common condition which may arise from a dysfunction of these systems: the 'metabolic syndrome' or 'insulin resistance syndrome'. This is a collection of inter-connected adverse metabolic changes including insulin resistance (with some degree of glucose intolerance), elevated blood triacylglycerol concentrations and low concentrations of the 'protective' HDL-cholesterol. This condition is usually associated with central (abdominal) obesity. It has become clear in recent years that insulin resistance is closely associated with increased concentrations of triacylglycerol in liver and skeletal muscle. An increase in triacylglycerol deposition in the pancreatic β-cell may lead, in time, to impairment of insulin secretion, therefore explaining why this syndrome is an important precursor to development of type 2 diabetes. This has been termed 'ectopic fat deposition', i.e. deposition of triacylglycerol in tissues other than adipose tissue. It may arise from a dysfunction of the adipose tissue, leading to exposure of other tissues to excess flux of fatty acids (both NEFA and triacylglycerol-rich remnant particles) [27]. One possible mechanism is that abdominal fat, including the visceral fat within the abdominal cavity, is less efficient than is lower-body adipose tissue at 'sequestering' excess dietary fat and thereby protecting other tissues. There is evidence for this view from tracer studies showing a high rate of turnover of triacylglycerol stores in abdominal, especially intra-abdominal adipose tissue [28] and indirectly from the strong protective effect of lower-body adipose tissue against insulin resistance, dyslipidaemia and hypertension [29].

Why should an increased triacylglycerol concentration in liver and skeletal muscle be associated with insulin resistance? The difficulty is in dissociating cause and effect. It is possible that the persistent high insulin concentrations that characterize insulin resistance lead to altered partitioning of fatty acids, with more going towards esterification at the expense of oxidation. In that view, ectopic fat deposition would be a consequence of insulin resistance rather than a cause. But there are also strong suggestions of a causal relationship. There are many demonstrations, especially in skeletal muscle (which is more accessible to study than the liver), that elevated fatty acid availability reduces the efficiency of insulin signalling (e.g. to stimulate glucose metabolism). The underlying mechanisms are discussed in Chapter 4 of this volume. The potential mechanisms by which regular exercise and training prevent insulin resistance despite large intramyocellular triacylglycerol stores in muscle are discussed in several of the essays in this volume.

It is also clear that treatments that reduce 'ectopic' fat content improve insulin resistance. For instance, the TZD (thiazolidinedione) insulin-sensitizing drugs that are now in clinical use for the treatment of type 2 diabetes improve insulin sensitivity and reduce hepatic fat content [30]. The interesting point is that the TZDs are agonists to the nuclear receptor/transcription factor PPARγ (peroxisome-proliferator-activated receptor γ), which is most highly expressed in adipose tissue and not expressed in liver. This suggests that TZDs reduce liver fat and improve hepatic insulin sensitivity by effects on adipose tissue, possibly increasing the capacity of adipose tissue to 'entrap' fatty acids and thus protect the liver.

There are further links between the tissues that are the subject of this chapter. It is now recognized that adipose tissue secretes a large number of peptides and other factors, some of which may function as hormones and affect metabolism in other tissues. One of these is a protein called adiponectin. It is abundant in the circulation (typical plasma concentration 10 mg/l). Adiponectin is most highly secreted by small adipocytes. As adipocytes increase in size, adiponectin expression and secretion are so highly down-regulated (the mechanism is unknown) that plasma concentrations are actually lower in obese than in lean people. There are strong relationships between high adiponectin concentrations and a 'healthy' metabolic profile, or conversely between low adiponectin and features of the metabolic syndrome. At least some of these effects may be mediated by adiponectin-induced reduction in liver fat content. The molecular mechanism may involve activation of the AMP-activated protein kinase [31]. It is also noteworthy that a strong effect of TZD administration is to raise adiponectin expression, secretion and plasma concentration, and that the reduction in liver fat content observed with TZD treatment is closely related to the increase in adiponectin concentration [30].

Summary

- *Fat is the most important stored fuel in mammals.*
- *Three tissues play major roles in fatty acid and triacylglycerol metabolism: adipose tissue, skeletal muscle and liver.*
- *Each of these tissues has a store of triacylglycerol that can be hydrolysed (mobilized) in a regulated way to release fatty acids.*
- *There is clearly cooperation amongst the tissues, so that, for instance, adipose tissue fat mobilization increases to meet the demands of skeletal muscle during exercise.*
- *When triacylglycerol accumulates excessively in skeletal muscle and liver, sometimes called ectopic fat deposition, then the condition of insulin resistance arises. This may reflect a lack of exercise and an excess of fat intake.*

The authors collaborate as part of the project 'Hepatic and adipose tissue and functions in the metabolic syndrome' (HEPADIP, http://www.hepadip.org/), which is supported by the European Commission as an Integrated Project under the 6th Framework Programme (Contract LSHM-CT-2005-018734).

References

1. Snyder, W.S. (1975) *Report of the task force on reference man,* Pergamon Press for the International Commission on Radiological Protection, Oxford
2. Strawford, A., Antelo, F., Christiansen, M. & Hellerstein, M.K. (2004) Adipose tissue triglyceride turnover, de novo lipogenesis, and cell proliferation in humans measured with ^2H_2O. *Am. J. Physiol. Endocrinol. Metab.* **286**, E577–E588
3. Coppack, S.W., Persson, M., Judd, R.L. & Miles, J.M. (1999) Glycerol and nonesterified fatty acid metabolism in human muscle and adipose tissue *in vivo. Am. J. Physiol.* **276**, E233–E240
4. Bergö, M., Olivecrona, G. & Olivecrona, T. (1996) Forms of lipoprotein lipase in rat tissues: in adipose tissue the proportion of inactive lipase increases on fasting. *Biochem. J.* **313**, 893–898
5. Stahl, A. (2004) A current review of fatty acid transport proteins (SLC27). *Pflügers Arch.* **447**, 722–727
6. Coleman, R.A. & Lee, D.P. (2004) Enzymes of triacylglycerol synthesis and their regulation. *Prog. Lipid Res.* **43**, 134–176
7. Holm, C. (2003) Molecular mechanisms regulating hormone-sensitive lipase and lipolysis. *Biochem. Soc. Trans.* **31**, 1120–1124
8. Lafontan, M., Moro, C., Sengenes, C., Galitzky, J., Crampes, F. & Berlan, M. (2005) An unsuspected metabolic role for atrial natriuretic peptides: the control of lipolysis, lipid mobilization, and systemic nonesterified fatty acids levels in humans. *Arterioscler. Thromb. Vasc. Biol.* **25**, 2032–2042
9. Langin, D., Dicker, A., Tavernier, G., Hoffstedt, J., Mairal, A., Rydén, M., Arner, E., Sicard, A., Jenkins, C.M., Viguerie, N. et al. (2005) Adipocyte lipases and defect of lipolysis in human obesity. *Diabetes* **54**, 3190–3197
10. Hellerstein, M.K., Schwarz, J.-M. & Neese, R.A. (1996) Regulation of hepatic de novo lipogenesis in humans. *Annu. Rev. Nutr.* **16**, 523–557
11. Hegardt, F.G. (1999) Mitochondrial 3-hydroxy-3-methylglutaryl-CoA synthase: a control enzyme in ketogenesis. *Biochem. J.* **338**, 569–582

12. Ravikumar, B., Carey, P.E., Snaar, J.E.M., Deelchand, D.K., Cook, D.B., Neely, R.D.G., English, P.T., Firbank, M.J., Morris, P.G. & Taylor, R. (2005) Real-time assessment of postprandial fat storage in liver and skeletal muscle in health and type 2 diabetes. *Am. J. Physiol. Endocrinol. Metab.* **288**, E789–E797

13. Frayn, K.N. & Blaak, E.E. (2005) Metabolic fuels and obesity: carbohydrate and lipid metabolism in skeletal muscle and adipose tissue, in: *Clinical Obesity in Adults and Children* (Kopelman, P., Caterson, I., Dietz, W., eds), pp. 102–122, Blackwell Publishing Ltd, Oxford

14. Donsmark, M., Langfort, J., Holm, C., Ploug, T. & Galbo, H. (2005) Hormone-sensitive lipase as mediator of lipolysis in contracting skeletal muscle. *Exerc. Sport. Sci. Rev.* **33**, 127–133

15. Hansson, O., Donsmark, M., Ling, C., Nevsten, P., Danfelter, M., Andersen, J.L., Galbo, H. & Holm, C. (2005) Transcriptome and proteome analysis of soleus muscle of hormone-sensitive lipase-null mice. *J. Lipid Res.* **46**, 2614–2623

16. Moberg, E., Sjöberg, S., Hagström-Toft, E. & Bolinder, J. (2002) No apparent suppression by insulin of in vivo skeletal muscle lipolysis in nonobese women. *Am. J. Physiol. Endocrinol. Metab.* **283**, E295–E301

17. van Hall, G., Sacchetti, M., Radegran, G. & Saltin, B. (2002) Human skeletal muscle fatty acid and glycerol metabolism during rest, exercise and recovery. *J. Physiol.* **543**, 1047–1058

18. Henriksson, J. (1995) Muscle fuel selection: effect of exercise and training. *Proc. Nutr. Soc.* **54**, 125–138

19. Romijn, J.A., Coyle, E.F., Sidossis, L.S., Gastaldelli, A., Horowitz, J.F., Endert, E. & Wolfe, R.R. (1993) Regulation of endogenous fat and carbohydrate metabolism in relation to exercise intensity and duration. *Am. J. Physiol.* **265**, E380–E391

20. van Loon, L.J.C., Greenhaff, P.L., Constantin-Teodosiu, D., Saris, W.H.M. & Wagenmakers, A.J.M. (2001) The effects of increasing exercise intensity on muscle fuel utilisation in humans. *J. Physiol.* **536**, 295–304

21. Watt, M.J., Heigenhauser, G.J. & Spriet, L.L. (2002) Intramuscular triacylglycerol utilization in human skeletal muscle during exercise: is there a controversy? *J. Appl. Physiol.* **93**, 1185–1195

22. van Baak, M.A., Mooij, J.M.V. & Wijnen, J.A.G. (1993) Effect of increased plasma non-esterified fatty acid concentrations on endurance performance during β-adrenoceptor blockade. *Int. J. Sports Med.* **14**, 2–8

23. Stallknecht, B., Lorentsen, J., Enevoldsen, L.H., Bülow, J., Biering-Sørensen, F., Galbo, H. & Kjaer, M. (2001) Role of the sympathoadrenergic system in adipose tissue metabolism during exercise in humans. *J. Physiol.* **536**, 283–294

24. Arner, P., Kriegholm, E., Engfeldt, P. & Bolinder, J. (1990) Adrenergic regulation of lipolysis in situ at rest and during exercise. *J. Clin. Invest.* **85**, 893–898

25. Wolfe, R.R., Klein, S., Carraro, F. & Weber, J.-M. (1990) Role of triglyceride-fatty acid cycle in controlling fat metabolism in humans during and after exercise. *Am. J. Physiol.* **258**, E382–E389

26. Reynisdottir, S., Eriksson, M., Angelin, B. & Arner, P. (1995) Impaired activation of adipocyte lipolysis in familial combined hyperlipidemia. *J. Clin. Invest.* **95**, 2161–2169

27. Frayn, K.N. (2002) Adipose tissue as a buffer for daily lipid flux. *Diabetologia* **45**, 1201–1210

28. Jensen, M.D., Sarr, M.G., Dumesic, D.A., Southorn, P.A. & Levine, J.A. (2003) Regional uptake of meal fatty acids in humans. *Am. J. Physiol. Endocrinol. Metab.* **285**, E1282–E1288

29. Lemieux, I. (2004) Energy partitioning in gluteal-femoral fat: does the metabolic fate of triglycerides affect coronary heart disease risk? *Arterioscler. Thromb. Vasc. Biol.* **24**, 795–797

30. Tiikkainen, M., Häkkinen, A.M., Korsheninnikova, E., Nyman, T., Mäkimattila, S. & Yki-Järvinen, H. (2004) Effects of rosiglitazone and metformin on liver fat content, hepatic insulin resistance, insulin clearance, and gene expression in adipose tissue in patients with type 2 diabetes. *Diabetes* **53**, 2169–2176

31. Yamauchi, T., Kamon, J., Minokoshi, Y., Ito, Y., Waki, H., Uchida, S., Yamashita, S., Noda, M., Kita, S., Ueki, K. et al. (2002) Adiponectin stimulates glucose utilization and fatty-acid oxidation by activating AMP-activated protein kinase. *Nat. Med.* **8**, 1288–1295

32. Frayn, K.N. (2003) *Metabolic regulation: A human perspective. 2nd edn*, Blackwell Publishing, Oxford

8

The anti-inflammatory effect of exercise: its role in diabetes and cardiovascular disease control

Bente Klarlund Pedersen[1]

The Centre of Inflammation and Metabolism, Department of Infectious Diseases and Copenhagen Muscle Research Centre, Copenhagen University Hospital, Rigshospitalet, University of Copenhagen, Faculty of Health Sciences, Denmark

Abstract

Chronic low-grade systemic inflammation is a feature of chronic diseases such as cardiovascular disease and type 2 diabetes. Regular exercise offers protection against all-cause mortality, primarily by protection against atherosclerosis and insulin resistance and there is evidence that physical training is effective as a treatment in patients with chronic heart diseases and type 2 diabetes.

Regular exercise induces anti-inflammatory actions. During exercise, IL-6 (interleukin-6) is produced by muscle fibres. IL-6 stimulates the appearance in the circulation of other anti-inflammatory cytokines such as IL-1ra (interleukin-1 receptor antagonist) and IL-10 (interleukin-10) and inhibits the production of the pro-inflammatory cytokine TNF-α (tumour necrosis factor-α). In addition, IL-6 enhances lipid turnover, stimulating lipolysis as well as fat oxidation. It is suggested that regular exercise induces suppression of TNF-α and thereby offers protection against TNF-α-induced insulin resistance. Recently, IL-6 was introduced as the first myokine, defined as a cytokine, that is produced

[1]*To whom correspondence should be addressed (email bkp@rh.dk).*

and released by contracting skeletal muscle fibres, exerting its effects in other organs of the body. Myokines may be involved in mediating the beneficial health effects against chronic diseases associated with low-grade inflammation such as diabetes and cardiovascular diseases.

Introduction

Cardiovascular disease and type 2 diabetes are not only leading causes of death and illness in developed countries, but these chronic diseases are becoming the dominating health problem worldwide [1]. Regular exercise offers protection against all-cause mortality, primarily by protection against atherosclerosis and type 2 diabetes [2]. In addition, physical training is effective in the treatment of patients with ischaemic heart disease and type 2 diabetes [3].

Over the past decade, there has been an increasing focus on the role of inflammation in the pathogenesis of atherosclerosis [4]. Further, inflammation has been suggested to be a key factor in insulin resistance [5]. Low-grade chronic inflammation is reflected by increased systemic levels of some cytokines [6] as well as CRP (C-reactive protein). Several reports investigating various markers of inflammation have confirmed an association between low-grade systemic inflammation on one hand and atherosclerosis and type 2 diabetes on the other [7]. Recent findings demonstrate that physical activity induces an increase in the systemic levels of a number of cytokines with anti-inflammatory properties [8]. Skeletal muscle has recently been identified as an endocrine organ, that produces and releases cytokines (termed myokines) [8–11].

Given that skeletal muscle is the largest organ in the human body, the discovery that contracting muscle is a cytokine producing organ opens a new paradigm: skeletal muscle is an endocrine organ that by contraction stimulates the production and release of cytokines, which can influence metabolism and modify cytokine production in tissue and organs (Figure 1).

This chapter reviews the evidence for physical training as a means to treat cardiovascular disease, insulin resistance and type 2 diabetes and discusses to what extent anti-inflammatory activity induced by regular exercise may exert the beneficial health effects in these disorders.

Clinical evidence for physical training in coronary heart disease, insulin resistance and type 2 diabetes

Coronary heart disease

The evidence for a beneficial effect of physical training in patients with coronary heart disease is strong. Physical training improves survival and is believed to have direct effects on the pathogenesis of the disease [3]. A meta-analysis was published in 2004 [12] based on 48 randomized controlled trials and 8940 patients. The patients were typically randomized at the time of

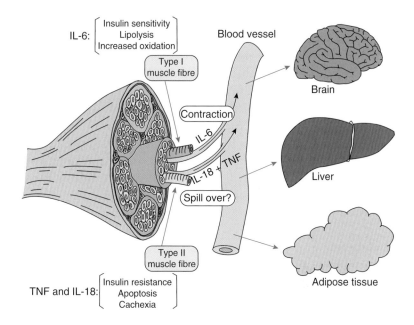

Figure 1. Skeletal muscle is an endocrine organ, that expresses and releases cytokines (also termed myokines) into the circulation and potentially influences metabolism and the inflammatory status in tissue and organs

acute myocardial infarction or up to six weeks thereafter. The exercise training was predominantly aerobic, but varied considerably as regards frequency, intensity and duration. Exercise-based cardiac rehabilitation reduced all-cause mortality by 20% (OR 0.80; 95% CI 0.68–0.93). Exercise-based cardiac rehabilitation reduced cardiac mortality by 26% (OR 0.74; 95% CI 0.61–0.96). Exercise-based cardiac rehabilitation in addition reduced total cholesterol, triglyceride levels and systolic blood pressure. More patients in the exercise-based cardiac rehabilitation group ceased smoking (OR 0.64; 95% CI 0.50–0.83). There was no effect on non-fatal myocardial infarction. In summary, exercise has pronounced health outcome effects in patients with cardiac diseases.

Insulin resistance

Few studies have examined the isolated effect of training on the prevention of diabetes in patients with impaired glucose tolerance, but there is good evidence for a beneficial effect of combined physical training and dietary modification. Two randomized controlled trials including people with impaired glucose tolerance have found that lifestyle modification protects against the development of type 2 diabetes. A Finnish trial randomized 522 overweight middle-aged people with impaired glucose tolerance to a physical training combined with diet group or to a control group and followed them for 3.2 years [13]. The risk of type 2 diabetes was reduced by

58% in the intervention group. The effect was greatest in the patients who made the greatest lifestyle modification. An American trial randomized 3234 people with impaired glucose tolerance to either treatment with metformin, lifestyle modification entailing dietary change and at least 150 min of physical exercise weekly, or placebo, and followed them for 2.8 years [14]. The lifestyle modification reduced the risk of type 2 diabetes by 58%. The reduction was thus the same as in the Finnish trial [13], whereas treatment with metformin only reduced the risk of diabetes by 31%. It is not possible to determine the isolated effect of exercise in these trials [13,14], in which the intervention was combined exercise and diet. In summary, there is strong evidence that exercise protects against development of type 2 diabetes in patients with insulin resistance.

Type 2 diabetes

The beneficial effect of training in patients with type 2 diabetes is very well documented, and there is international consensus that physical training comprises one of the three cornerstones of the treatment of diabetes together with diet and medicine. A meta-analysis published in 2001 examined the effect of at least eight weeks of physical training on glycaemic control [15]. The meta-analysis included 14 controlled clinical trials encompassing a total of 504 patients. Twelve of the trials examined the effect of aerobic training [mean (S.D.); 3.4 (0.9) times/week for 18 (15) weeks], whilst two examined the effect of strength conditioning [mean (S.D.); 10 (0.7) exercises, 2.5 (0.7) sets, 13 (0.7) repetitions, 2.5 (0.4) times/week for 15 (10) weeks]. No differences could be identified between the effect of aerobic training and strength conditioning. Neither could any dose–response effect be demonstrated relative to either the intensity or the duration of training. Post-intervention, HbA1c (haemoglobin A1c) was lower in the exercise groups than in the control groups (7.65% versus 8.31%; weighted mean difference, 0.66%; $P<0.001$). In comparison, intensive glycaemic control with metformin reduced HbA1c by 0.6%, whereas it reduced the risk of diabetes-related complications by 32% and the risk of diabetes-related mortality by 42% [16]. A meta-analysis encompassing 95 783 non-diabetic individuals showed that cardiovascular morbidity is strongly correlated to fasting blood glucose [17]. The effect of physical training on HbA1c is thus clinically relevant and there is evidence to support exercise recommendations in patients with type 2 diabetes.

The players in chronic low-grade inflammation and its link with chronic diseases

The local inflammatory response is accompanied by a systemic response known as the acute phase response [8]. This response includes the production of a large number of hepatocyte-derived acute phase proteins, such as CRP and can be mimicked by the injection of the cytokines TNF-α (tumour necrosis factor-α), IL-1β (interleukin-1β) and IL-6 (interleukin-6) into laboratory animals or humans. The initial cytokines in the cytokine cascade are (named in order): TNF -α, IL-1β, IL-6, IL-1ra (interleukin-1 receptor antagonist) and sTNF-R (soluble TNF-α-receptors). IL-1ra inhibits IL-1 signal transduction, and sTNF-R represents the naturally occurring inhibitors of TNF-α. In response to an acute infection or trauma, the cytokines and cytokine inhibitors may increase 3- to 4-fold and decrease after recovery. Chronic low-grade systemic inflammation has been introduced as a term for conditions in which a 2- to 3-fold increase in the systemic concentrations of TNF-α, IL-1, IL-6, IL-1ra, sTNF-R and CRP is reflected. In the latter case, the stimuli for the cytokine production are not known, but the likely origin of TNF-α in chronic low-grade systemic inflammation is mainly the adipose tissue.

The link between inflammation, insulin resistance and atherosclerosis

Ageing is associated with increased resting plasma levels of TNF-α, IL-6, IL-1ra, sTNF-R and CRP [18]. High levels of TNF-α are associated with dementia and atherosclerosis [19]. Also, elevated levels of circulating IL-6 are associated with several disorders. Increased levels of both TNF-α and IL-6 are observed in obese individuals, in smokers and in patients with type 2 diabetes mellitus. Plasma concentrations of IL-6 have been shown to predict all-cause mortality as well as cardiovascular mortality. Furthermore, plasma concentrations of IL-6 and TNF-α have been shown to predict the risk of myocardial infarction in several studies, and the CRP level is shown to be a stronger predictor of cardiovascular events than the low density lipoprotein cholesterol level.

Mounting evidence suggests that TNF-α plays a direct role in the metabolic syndrome [20]. Patients with diabetes demonstrate high mRNA and protein expression of TNF-α in skeletal muscle and increased TNF-α levels in plasma and it is likely that adipose tissue, which produces TNF-α, is the main source of the circulating TNF-α. Mounting evidence points to an effect of TNF-α on insulin signalling. TNF-α impairs insulin-stimulated rates of glucose storage in cultured human muscle cells and impairs insulin mediated glucose uptake in rats. Obese mice with a gene knockout of TNF-α are protected from insulin resistance and inhibition of TNF-α with an anti-TNF-α antibody treatment improves the insulin sensitivity in the insulin resistance rat model. *In vitro* studies demonstrate that TNF-α has direct inhibitory effects on insulin signalling. Recently, it was demonstrated that TNF-α infusion in healthy humans induces insulin resistance in skeletal muscle, without an effect on endogenous glucose production. TNF-α directly impaired glucose uptake and metabolism by altering insulin signal transduction. These data provide a direct molecular link between low-grade systemic inflammation and insulin resistance [20]. It has also been proposed that TNF-α indirectly causes insulin resistance *in vivo* by increasing the release of NEFAs (non-esterified fatty acids) from adipose tissue. TNF-α increases lipolysis in human, rat and 3T3-L1 adipocytes. Recently, it was found that TNF-α had no effect on muscle fatty acid oxidation, but increased fatty acid incorporation into diacylglycerol, which may be involved in the development of TNF-α-induced insulin resistance in skeletal muscle.

Recent evidence suggests that TNF-α plays a key role in linking insulin resistance to vascular disease. Several downstream mediators and signalling pathways seem to provide the crosstalk between inflammatory and metabolic signalling. These include the discovery of JNK (c-Jun N-terminal kinase) and IκK (IκB kinase) as critical regulators of insulin action activated by TNF-α [21]. In human TNF-α infusion studies, TNF-α increases phosphorylation of the p70 S6 kinase, extracellular signal-regulated kinase-1/2 and JNK, concomitant with increased serine and reduced tyrosine phosphorylation of insulin receptor substrate-1. These signalling effects are associated with impaired phosphorylation of Akt substrate 160, the most proximal step identified in the insulin signalling cascade regulating GLUT4 translocation and glucose uptake [22] (Figure 2).

With regard to IL-6, its role in insulin resistance is highly controversial. In humans, circulating IL-6 levels may or may not be associated with insulin resistance [23]. Infusion of recombinant human (rh) IL-6 into resting

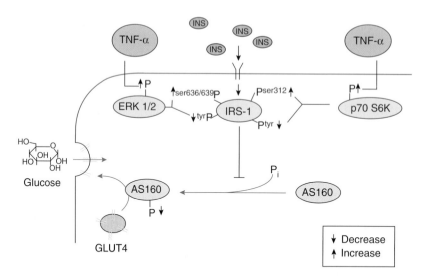

Figure 2. TNF-α represents a molecular link between low-grade systemic inflammation and the metabolic syndrome
TNF-α infusion to humans increases phosphorylation of p70 S6 kinase, ERK-1/2 (extracellular signal-regulated kinase-1/2) and JNK, concomitant with increased serine and reduced tyrosine phosphorylation of IRS (insulin receptor substrate)-1. These signalling effects are associated with impaired phosphorylation of AS160 (Akt substrate 160), the most proximal step identified in the insulin signalling cascade regulating GLUT4 translocation and glucose uptake. Thus excessive concentrations of TNF-α negatively regulate insulin signalling and whole-body glucose uptake in humans.

healthy humans does not impair whole body, lower limb or subcutaneous adipose tissue glucose uptake or EGP (endogenous glucose production), although IL-6 contributes to the contraction-induced increase in EGP. When diabetes patients were given an rhIL-6 infusion, plasma concentrations of insulin decreased to levels comparable with that in age and BMI (body mass index)-matched healthy controls, indicating that the IL-6 enhanced insulin sensitivity. *In vitro* studies demonstrate that IL-6 can induce insulin resistance in isolated 3T3-L1 adipocytes and in mice. However, the IL-6 dose applied in the latter studies was supraphysiological, and is therefore probably not relevant to human physiology. Interestingly, IL-6 knockout mice develop impaired glucose tolerance that is reverted by IL-6 [24]. Thus accumulating data suggest that IL-6 enhances glucose uptake in myocytes.

AMPK (AMP-activated protein kinase) activity stimulates a variety of processes that increases ATP generation including fatty acid oxidation and glucose transport in skeletal muscle [25]. Incubation with IL-6 increases the phosphorylation of AMPK (an indicator of its activation) and that of its target molecule, ACC (acetyl-CoA carboxylase) in skeletal muscles. In addition, AMPK activity and ACC levels are very low in IL-6 knockout mice, suggesting a role of IL-6 in the regulation of AMPK activity. These data suggest that IL-6 activation of AMPK is dependent on the presence of IL-6 [26].

A number of studies indicate that IL-6 enhances lipolysis [27–31], as well as fat oxidation [30]. Consistent with this idea, Wallenius et al. [24] demonstrated that IL-6 deficient mice developed mature-onset obesity and insulin resistance. In addition, when the mice were treated with IL-6, there was a significant decrease in body fat mass in the IL-6 knockout, but not in the wild-type mice. To determine whether physiological concentrations of IL-6 affected lipid metabolism, our group administered physiological concentrations of rhIL-6 to healthy young and elderly humans as well as patients with type 2 diabetes [30,32]. The latter studies identified IL-6 as a potent modulator of fat metabolism in humans, increasing lipolysis as well as fat oxidation without causing hypertriacylglycerolaemia.

Of note, whereas it is known that both TNF-α and IL-6 induce lipolysis, only IL-6 appears to induce fat oxidation [23]. High levels of IL-6 and TNF-α in patients with the metabolic syndrome is associated with truncal fat mass and both TNF-α and IL-6 are produced in adipose tissue. Given the different biological profiles of TNF-α and IL-6 and given that TNF-α can trigger IL-6 release, one theory holds that it is TNF-α derived from adipose tissue that actually is the 'driver' behind insulin resistance and cardiovascular diseases and that locally produced TNF-α causes increased systemic levels of IL-6.

The cytokine response to exercise

In sepsis and experimental models of sepsis, the cytokine cascade consists of (named in order): TNF-α, IL-1β, IL-6, IL-1ra, sTNF-R and IL-10 (interleukin-10) [33]. The first two cytokines in the cytokine cascade are TNF-α and IL-1β, which are produced locally. These cytokines are usually referred to as pro-inflammatory cytokines. TNF-α and IL-1β stimulate the production of IL-6, which has been classified as both a pro- and an anti-inflammatory cytokine. The cytokine response to exercise differs from that elicited by severe infections [34–37]. The fact that the classical pro-inflammatory cytokines, TNF-α and IL-1β, in general do not increase with exercise indicates that the cytokine cascade induced by exercise markedly differs from the cytokine cascade induced by infections. Typically, IL-6 is the first cytokine released into the circulation during exercise. The level of circulating IL-6 increases in an exponential fashion (up to 100-fold) in response to exercise, and declines in the post-exercise period [34–37] (Figure 3).

The circulating levels of well-known anti-inflammatory cytokines and cytokine inhibitors such as IL-1ra and sTNF-R also increase after exercise.

Taken together, exercise provokes an increase primarily in IL-6, followed by an increase in IL-1ra and IL-10. The appearance of IL-6 in the circulation is by far the most marked and its appearance precedes that of the other cytokines. The IL-6 response to exercise has recently been reviewed [10,23,34–36]. A marked increase in circulating levels of IL-6 after exercise without muscle damage has been a remarkably consistent finding. Plasma IL-6 increases in an exponential fashion with exercise and is related to exercise intensity, duration, the mass of muscle recruited and one's endurance capacity [10,34–36]. In 2000, Steensberg et al. [38] published the first article demonstrating that most of the IL-6 seen in the circulation was likely to be derived from the contracting limb. Using a single-legged kicking model and measuring arteriovenous difference and blood flow across the contracting and non-contracting limb, it was clear that net release from the contracting limb was marked. This study has been followed by many others that confirmed the net limb release of IL-6 is marked and that the IL-6 mRNA levels in biopsy samples taken from the contracting limb rapidly increases above baseline values. However, it was only recently confirmed that the myocytes themselves produce IL-6. A qualitative elevation in IL-6 protein measured in muscle cells within human muscle biopsy sections using immunohistochemistry has been reported. In a follow-up study, however, definitive evidence was found that myocytes themselves are a major source of contraction-induced IL-6. In addition to immunohistochemistry techniques, *in situ* hybridization assays were performed on muscle cross-sections before and after exercise. Consistent with the immunohistochemical data, IL-6 mRNA was almost absent in cross-sections before exercise, but prominent after contraction.

The cytokine IL-6 exerts it actions via the IL-6R (IL-6 receptor) in conjunction with the ubiquitously expressed gp130 receptor. IL-6 is regulated in an autocrine fashion [39]. In accordance, acute exercise induces IL-6R expression in the post-exercise period after exercise suggesting a post-exercise-sensitizing mechanism to IL-6. We further demonstrated, that after a ten week training

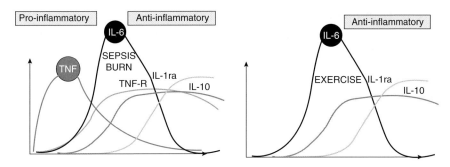

Figure 3. In sepsis, the cytokine cascade within the first few hours consists of TNF-α, IL-6, IL-1ra, sTNF-R and IL-10
The cytokine response to exercise does not include TNF-α but does show a marked increase in IL-6, which is followed by IL-1ra, sTNF-R and IL-10. Increased CRP levels do not appear until 8–12 h later.

period, IL-6R mRNA production was increased in skeletal muscle, suggesting a sensitization of skeletal muscle to IL-6 at rest.

Studies have reported that carbohydrate ingestion attenuates elevations in plasma IL-6 during both running and cycling. Low muscle glycogen concentration further enhances IL-6 mRNA and the transcription rate for IL-6. Therefore, pre-exercise intramuscular glycogen content appears to be an important stimulus for IL-6 gene transcription. It appears that muscle-derived IL-6 acts as an energy sensor.

Most studies of muscle-derived IL-6 have been performed in healthy young volunteers, exercised at high intensities. However, the clinical relevance of muscle-derived IL-6 is supported by the findings that even moderate exercise has major effects on muscle-derived IL-6. Young healthy individuals performed 3 h of dynamic two-legged knee-extensor exercise at 50% of their individual maximal power output. This exercise induced an only moderate increase in heart rate (from 113 to 122 beats·min^{-1}), but induced a 16-fold increase in IL-6 mRNA, a 20-fold increase in plasma IL-6 and a marked IL-6 release from working muscle. When the same model was applied in elderly healthy untrained subjects, even higher amounts of IL-6 were released from working muscle during exercise at the same relative intensity.

Studies have demonstrated that monocytes are not major contributors to the IL-6 response to exercise. However, small amounts of IL-6 are also produced and released from adipose tissue, and studies indicate that also the brain and peritendon tissue may release IL-6 in response to exercise. Although we have yet to determine the precise biological action of muscle-derived IL-6, accumulating data support the hypothesis that the role of IL-6 released from contracting muscle during exercise is to act in a hormone-like manner to mobilize extracellular substrates and/or augment substrate delivery during exercise. In addition, IL-6 has important anti-inflammatory effects.

The anti-inflammatory effects of IL-6

A couple of studies suggest that IL-6 may exert inhibitory effects on TNF-α [8]. IL-6 inhibits lipopolysaccharide-induced TNF-α production both in cultured human monocytes and in the human monocytic line U937. Furthermore, levels of TNF-α are markedly elevated in anti-IL-6-treated mice and in IL-6 deficient knockout mice, indicating that circulating IL-6 is involved in the regulation of TNF-α levels. In addition, rhIL-6 infusion inhibits the endotoxin-induced increase in circulating levels of TNF-α in healthy humans. Lastly, IL-6 stimulates the release of soluble TNF-α receptors, but not IL-1β and TNF-α, and appears to be the primary inducer of the hepatocyte derived acute-phase proteins, many of which have anti-inflammatory properties.

The anti-inflammatory effects of IL-6 are also demonstrated by the fact that IL-6 stimulates the production of IL-1ra and IL-10. The appearance of IL-10 and IL-1ra in the circulation following exercise also contributes to mediating the anti-inflammatory effects of exercise. IL-10 inhibits the production of IL-1α, IL-1β and TNF-α as well as the production of chemokines, including IL-8 and macrophage inflammatory protein-α from lipopolysaccharide-activated human monocytes. These cytokines and chemokines play a critical role in the activation of granulocytes, monocytes/macrophages and lymphocytes and in their recruitment to the sites of inflammation. Whereas IL-10 influences multiple cytokines, the biological role of IL-1ra is to inhibit signal transduction through the IL-1 receptor complex.

The anti-inflammatory effects of acute exercise and regular training

An association between physical inactivity and low-grade systemic inflammation has been demonstrated in cross-sectional studies including healthy younger individuals, elderly people, as well as in patients with intermittent claudication [40]. These data, however, do not provide any information with regard to a possible causal relationship. Longitudinal studies show that regular training induces a reduction in CRP levels and suggest that physical activity may suppress systemic low-grade inflammation. To study whether acute exercise induces a true anti-inflammatory response, a model of 'low grade inflammation' was established in which we injected a low dose of *Escherichia coli* endotoxin to healthy volunteers, who had been randomized to either rest or exercise prior to endotoxin administration. In resting subjects, endotoxin induced a 2- to 3-fold increase in circulating levels of TNF-α. In contrast, when the subjects performed 3 h of ergometer cycling and received the endotoxin bolus at 2.5 h, the TNF-α response was totally blunted.

Following exercise, the high circulating levels of IL-6 are followed by an increase in IL-1ra and IL-10, and the latter two anti-inflammatory cytokines can be induced by IL-6. Therefore, IL-6 induces an anti-inflammatory environment by inducing the production of IL-1ra and IL-10, but it also inhibits

TNF-α production as suggested by *in vitro* and animal studies. In addition, rhIL-6 infusion inhibited the endotoxin-induced increase in plasma TNF-α in humans. The possibility exists that with regular exercise, the anti-inflammatory effects of an acute bout of exercise will protect against chronic systemic low-grade inflammation, but such a link between the acute effects of exercise and the long-term benefits has not yet been proven. Given that the atherosclerotic process is characterized by inflammation, one alternative explanation would be that regular exercise, which offers protection against atherosclerosis, indirectly offers protection against vascular inflammation and hence systemic low-grade inflammation.

Conclusion

The long-term effect of exercise on the progression of disease may be ascribed to the anti-inflammatory response elicited by an acute bout of exercise, which in part is mediated by muscle-derived IL-6. These anti-inflammatory effects of exercise may offer protection against TNF-induced insulin resistance. It is suggested that muscle contraction-induced factors, so-called myokines, may be involved in mediating the health benefits of exercise and play important roles in the protection against diseases associated with low-grade inflammation such as cardiovascular diseases and type 2 diabetes.

Summary

- *Low-grade chronic systemic inflammation accompanies chronic diseases such as cardiovascular disease and type 2 diabetes.*
- *Regular exercise induces an anti-inflammatory response.*
- *During exercise, skeletal muscle releases IL-6.*
- *IL-6 has anti-inflammatory actions and modulates glucose and lipid metabolism.*
- *Muscle-derived cytokines, termed myokines, are likely to mediate the health benefits against chronic diseases.*

The Centre of Inflammation and Metabolism is supported by a grant from the Danish National Research Foundation (# 02-512-55). The study was further supported by the Danish Medical Research Council (# 22-01-0019) and from the Commission of the European Communities (Contract No LSHM-CT-2004-005272 EXGENESIS). The Copenhagen Muscle Research Centre is supported by grants from The Copenhagen Hospital Corporation, The University of Copenhagen and The Faculties of Science and of Health Sciences at this University.

References

1. Murray, C.J. & Lopez. A.D. (1997) Global mortality, disability, and the contribution of risk factors: Global Burden of Disease Study. *Lancet* **349**, 1436–1442
2. Blair, S.N., Cheng, Y. & Holder, J.S. (2001) Is physical activity or physical fitness more important in defining health benefits? *Med. Sci. Sports Exercise* **33**, S379–S399
3. Pedersen, B.K. & Saltin, B. (2006) Evidence for prescribing exercise as therapy in chronic disease. *Scand. J. Med. Sci. Sports* **16** (Suppl 1), 3–63
4. Libby, P. (2002) Inflammation in atherosclerosis. *Nature* **420**, 868–874
5. Dandona, P., Aljada, A. & Bandyopadhyay, A. (2004) Inflammation: the link between insulin resistance, obesity and diabetes. *Trends Immunol.* **25**, 4–7
6. Ross, R. (1999) Atherosclerosis: an inflammatory disease. *N. Engl. J. Med.* **340**, 115–126
7. Festa, A., D'Agostino, Jr, R., Tracy, R.P. & Haffner, S.M. (2002) Elevated levels of acute-phase proteins and plasminogen activator inhibitor-1 predict the development of type 2 diabetes: the insulin resistance atherosclerosis study. *Diabetes* **51**, 1131–1137
8. Petersen, A.M. & Pedersen, B.K. (2005) The anti-inflammatory effect of exercise. *J. Appl. Physiol.* **98**, 1154–1162
9. Pedersen, B.K. & Febbraio, M. (2005) Muscle-derived interleukin-6: A possible link between skeletal muscle, adipose tissue, liver, and brain. *Brain Behav. Immun.* **19**, 371–376
10. Pedersen, B.K., Steensberg, A., Fischer, C., Keller, C., Keller, P., Plomgaard, P., Febbraio, M. & Saltin, B. (2003) Searching for the exercise factor: is IL-6 a candidate. *J. Muscle Res. Cell Motil.* **24**, 113–119
11. Pedersen, B.K., Steensberg, A., Fischer, C., Keller, C., Keller, P., Plomgaard, P., Wolsk-Petersen, E. & Febbraio, M. (2004) The metabolic role of IL-6 produced during exercise: is IL-6 an exercise factor? *Proc. Nutr. Soc.* **63**, 263–267
12. Taylor, R.S., Brown, A., Ebrahim, S., Jolliffe, J., Noorani, H., Rees, K., Skidmore, B., Stone, J.A., Thompson, D.R. & Oldridge, N. (2004) Exercise-based rehabilitation for patients with coronary heart disease: systematic review and meta-analysis of randomized controlled trials. *Am. J. Med.* **116**, 682–692
13. Tuomilehto, J., Lindstrom, J., Eriksson, J.G., Valle, T.T., Hamalainen, H., Ilanne-Parikka, P., Keinanen-Kiukaanniemi, S., Laakso, M., Louheranta, A., Rastas, M. et al. (2001) Prevention of type 2 diabetes mellitus by changes in lifestyle among subjects with impaired glucose tolerance. *N. Engl. J. Med.* **344**, 1343–1350
14. Knowler, W.C., Barrett-Connor, E., Fowler, S.E., Hamman, R.F., Lachin, J.M., Walker, E.A. & Nathan, D.M. (2002) Reduction in the incidence of type 2 diabetes with lifestyle intervention or metformin. *N. Engl. J. Med.* **346**, 393–403
15. Boule, N.G., Haddad, E., Kenny, G.P., Wells, G.A. & Sigal, R.J. (2001) Effects of exercise on glycemic control and body mass in type 2 diabetes mellitus: a meta-analysis of controlled clinical trials. *J. Am. Med. Assoc.* **286**, 1218–1227
16. UK Prospective Diabetes Study (UKPDS) Group. (1998) Effect of intensive blood-glucose control with metformin on complications in overweight patients with type 2 diabetes (UKPDS 34). *Lancet* **352**, 854–865
17. Coutinho, M., Gerstein, H.C., Wang, Y. & Yusuf, S. (1999) The relationship between glucose and incident cardiovascular events. A metaregression analysis of published data from 20 studies of 95783 individuals followed for 12.4 years. *Diabetes Care* **22**, 233–240
18. Bruunsgaard, H. (2005) Physical activity and modulation of systemic low-level inflammation. *J. Leukocyte Biol.* **78**, 819–835
19. Bruunsgaard, H., Andersen-Ranberg, K., Jeune, B., Pedersen, A.N., Skinhoj, P. & Pedersen, B.K. (1999) A high plasma concentration of TNF-α is associated with dementia in centenarians. *J. Gerontol. Ser. A* **54**, M357–M364
20. Plomgaard, P., Bouzakri, K., Krogh-Madsen, R., Mittendorfer, B., Zierath, J.R. & Pedersen, B.K. (2005) Tumor necrosis factor-α induces skeletal muscle insulin resistance in healthy human subjects via inhibition of Akt substrate 160 phosphorylation. *Diabetes* **54**, 2939–2945

21. Hotamisligil, G.S. (2003) Inflammatory pathways and insulin action. *Int. J. Obes. Relat. Metab. Disord.* **27** (Suppl 3), S53–S55

22. Plomgaard, P., Keller, P., Keller, C. & Pedersen, B.K. (2005) TNF-α, but not IL-6, stimulates plasminogen activator inhibitor-1 expression in human subcutaneous adipose tissue. *J. Appl. Physiol.* **98**, 2019–2023

23. Febbraio, M.A. & Pedersen, B.K. (2005) Contraction-induced myokine production and release: is skeletal muscle an endocrine organ? *Exerc. Sport Sci. Rev.* **33**, 114–119

24. Wallenius, V., Wallenius, K., Ahren, B., Rudling, M., Carlsten, H., Dickson, S.L., Ohlsson, C. & Jansson, J.O. (2002) Interleukin-6-deficient mice develop mature-onset obesity. *Nat. Med.* **8**, 75–79

25. Carling, D. (2004) The AMP-activated protein kinase cascade-a unifying system for energy control. *Trends Biochem. Sci.* **29**, 18–24

26. Kelly, M., Keller, C., Avilucea, P.R., Keller, P., Luo, Z., Xiang, X., Giralt, M., Hidalgo, J., Saha, A.K. & Pedersen, B.K. (2004) AMPK activity is diminished in tissues of the IL-6 knockout mice: the effect of exercise. *Biochem. Biophys. Res. Commun.* **320**, 449–454

27. Bruce, C.R & Dyck, D.J. (2004) Cytokine regulation of skeletal muscle fatty acid metabolism: effect of interleukin-6 and tumor necrosis factor-α. *Am. J. Physiol. Endocrinol. Metab.* **287**, E616–E621

28. Nonogaki, K., Fuller, G.M., Fuentes, N.L., Moser, A.H., Staprans, I., Grunfeld, C. & Feingold, K.R. (1995) Interleukin-6 stimulates hepatic triglyceride secretion in rats. *Endocrinology* **136**, 2143-2149

29. Path, G., Bornstein, S.R., Gurniak, M., Chrousos, G.P., Scherbaum, W.A. & Hauner, H. (2001) Human breast adipocytes express interleukin-6 (IL-6) and its receptor system: increased IL-6 production by β-adrenergic activation and effects of IL-6 on adipocyte function. *J. Clin. Endocrinol. Metab.* **86**, 2281–2288

30. Petersen, E.W., Carey, A.L., Sacchetti, M., Steinberg, G.R., Macaulay, S.L., Febbraio, M.A. & Pedersen, B.K. (2005) IL-6 treatment increases fatty acid turnover in elderly humans *in vivo* and in tissue culture *in vitro*: evidence that IL-6 acts independently of lipolytic hormones. *Am. J. Physiol.* **288**, E155–E162

31. Stouthard, J.M., Romijn, J.A., van der P.T., Endert, E., Klein, S., Bakker, P.J., Veenhof, C.H. & Sauerwein, H.P. (1995) Endocrinologic and metabolic effects of interleukin-6 in humans. *Am. J. Physiol.* **268**, E813–E819

32. Van Hall, G., Steensberg, A., Sacchetti, M., Fischer, C., Keller, C., Schjerling, P., Hiscock, N., Moller, K., Saltin, B., Febbraio, M.A. & Pedersen, B.K. (2003) Interleukin-6 stimulates lipolysis and fat oxidation in humans. *J. Clin. Endocrinol. Metab.* **88**, 3005–3010

33. Akira, S., Taga, T. & Kishimoto, T. (1993) Interleukin-6 in biology and medicine. *Adv. Immunol.* **54**, 1–78

34. Febbraio, M.A. & Pedersen, B.K. (2002) Muscle-derived interleukin-6: mechanisms for activation and possible biological roles. *FASEB J.* **16**, 1335–1347

35. Pedersen, B.K. & Hoffman-Goetz, L. (2000) Exercise and the immune system: regulation, integration and adaption. *Physiol. Rev.* **80**, 1055–1081

36. Pedersen, B.K., Steensberg, A. & Schjerling, P. (2001) Muscle-derived interleukin-6: possible biological effects. *J. Physiol. (London)* **536**, 329–337

37. Suzuki, K., Nakaji, S., Yamada, M., Totsuka, M., Sato, K. & Sugawara, K. (2002) Systemic inflammatory response to exhaustive exercise. Cytokine kinetics. *Exercise Immun. Rev.* **8**, 6–48

38. Steensberg, A., Keller, C., Starkie, R.L., Osada, T., Febbraio, M.A. & Pedersen, B.K. (2002) IL-6 and TNF-α expression in, and release from, contracting human skeletal muscle. *Am. J. Physiol. Endocrinol. Metab.* **283**, E1272–E1278

39. Keller, P., Keller, C., Carey, A.L., Jauffred, S., Fischer, C.P., Steensberg, A. & Pedersen, B.K. (2003) Interleukin-6 production by contracting human skeletal muscle: Autocrine regulation by IL-6. *Biochem. Biophys. Res. Commun.* **319**, 550–554

40. Tisi, P.V., Hulse, M., Chulakadabba, A., Gosling, P. & Shearman, C.P. (1997) Exercise training for intermittent claudication: does it adversely affect biochemical markers of the exercise-induced inflammatory response? *Eur. J. Vasc. Endovasc. Surg.* **14**, 344–350

9

Vascular nitric oxide: effects of physical activity, importance for health

Richard M. McAllister[1] and M. Harold Laughlin

Department of Biomedical Sciences and Dalton Cardiovascular Research Center, University of Missouri, Columbia, 65211 MO, U.S.A.

Abstract

NO (nitric oxide), formed in the vascular endothelium and derived from a biochemical reaction catalysed by eNOS (endothelial NO synthase), appears to play a role in exercise-induced dilation of blood vessels supplying cardiac and skeletal muscle. Endothelium-dependent, NO-mediated vasodilation is augmented by exercise training. Increases in eNOS gene transcription, eNOS mRNA stability and eNOS protein translation appear to contribute to increased NO formation and, consequently, enhanced NO-mediated vasodilation after training. Enhanced endothelial NO formation may also have a role(s) in the prevention and management of atherosclerosis because several steps in the atherosclerotic disease process are inhibited by NO. A growing body of work suggests that exercise training, perhaps via increased capacity for NO formation, retards atherosclerosis. This has significant implications for human health, given that atherosclerosis is the leading killer in Western society.

Introduction

In the 25 years following the discovery of NO (nitric oxide)-mediated dilation of blood vessels by Furchgott and Zawadski [1], a wealth of knowledge has accumulated concerning vascular NO. The driving force for this study

[1]*To whom correspondence should be addressed (email mcallisterr@missouri.edu).*

---

was the discrepancy between vascular responses to acetylcholine *in vivo* (vasodilation) and those observed when vessels were isolated from an animal and acetylcholine administered *in vitro* (frequently vasoconstriction). Furchgott and Zawadski astutely hypothesized that the latter was due to unintentional vessel damage during isolation. These investigators demonstrated that vasodilation induced by the agent acetylcholine requires an intact endothelium (Figure 1). The endothelium consists of a single layer of endothelial cells, with one or more layers of smooth muscle cells underlying it in the vascular wall. The requirement for endothelium led to the term endothelium-dependent vasodilation. Subsequent research revealed that acetylcholine administration leads to formation of NO from the amino acid L-arginine in the endothelium which, in turn, results in cGMP formation in vascular smooth muscle cells and relaxation of those cells. In addition, a host of other pharmacological agents, as well as physiological stimuli, were subsequently reported to induce NO formation in the vascular endothelium [2].

Given that vasodilation is a key component of the cardiovascular response to acute exercise (i.e. a single bout of exercise [3]), there has been considerable interest in determining whether endothelium-dependent, NO-mediated vasodilation occurs during exercise. Animal studies are generally supportive of such a role [4], whereas human studies are more equivocal [5]. Further, given that exercise training (i.e. regular physical activity) induces numerous

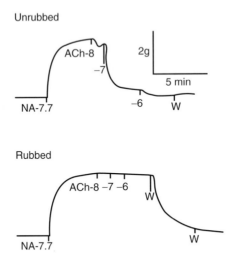

Figure 1. Effect of removing endothelium from rabbit aortic rings by rubbing
Aortic rings were studied using myograph preparations. The ordinate represents isometric tension development by rings. NA (noradrenaline) was used to induce a contractile response. Ach (acetylcholine) was used to induce vasorelaxation. The concentrations of NA and ACh are given in log molar units. W indicates the washing out of the vasoactive agent. Note that the rubbed aortic ring fails to relax in response to ACh, in contrast to the unrubbed ring with intact endothelium. Reproduced by permission from Macmillan Publishers Ltd: *Nature* (1980) vol. 288, pages 373–376. Copyright (1980); www.nature.com/nature.

adaptations in the cardiovascular system [3], it has also been of interest to determine whether training augments endothelium-dependent vasodilation. A principal focus of this review will be on exercise-training-induced adaptations in endothelium-dependent, NO-mediated dilation of the coronary and skeletal muscle circulations. These two vascular beds would benefit from enhanced endothelium-dependent dilation because the tissues they supply with blood flow, cardiac and skeletal muscle, are the most metabolically active tissues during exercise. Augmented vasodilation would serve to deliver more oxygen and other nutrients to these tissues. Although we will primarily refer to exercise training studies involving humans or animals, some reference will be made to studies involving cultured endothelial cells. Such studies, although limited by their *in vitro* nature, involve tight experimental control and therefore permit more definitive conclusions. These studies have typically applied laminar shear stress, a physiological stimulus for the endothelium to generate NO, to mono-layers of endothelial cells.

A second focus of this review will be on the potential role of NO in preventing and/or managing chronic disease. Atherosclerosis, specifically its associated events such as myocardial infarction, is the leading killer in Western society. There is, however, evidence that vascular NO retards several aspects of the atherosclerotic process [6]. Our focus will be, therefore, on how exercise training may modulate this specific disease process. Given that atherosclerosis in the coronary and skeletal muscle vascular beds (coronary artery disease and peripheral arterial disease respectively) constitute a majority of human patients with this disease, we will again focus on these two circulations.

Biochemistry of NO formation in the endothelium

Superficially, NO formation appears to be a simple biochemical reaction in which L-arginine is converted into L-citrulline and NO. It is, however, a more complex reaction (Figure 2) catalysed by multiple isoforms of a protein. Three isoforms of the protein NOS (NO synthase), including eNOS (endothelial NOS), nNOS (neuronal NOS) and iNOS (inducible NOS), catalyse NO formation in various tissues/cell types. It appears that iNOS, expressed in macrophages, is only present in the vasculature under pathological conditions.

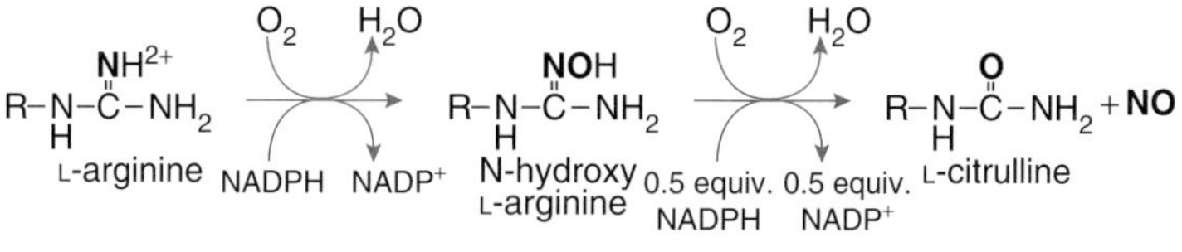

Figure 2. Detailed representation of the NOS reaction
Note that the conversion of the guanidino group on L-arginine into a carbonyl group (relevant atoms bolded) results in the formation of L-citrulline, with the evolution of NO. Reproduced from *Methods in Nitric Oxide Research* (Feelisch, M. and Stamler, J.S., eds.), 1999, with permission from John Wiley & Sons.

The nNOS isoform, whilst reported to be present in normal vascular smooth muscle [7], has an uncertain role in vascular function. We will therefore restrict our discussion to the eNOS isoform.

Many enzymes require a coenzyme(s) for their function, and NOS is such an enzyme as reflected by the number of participants in Figure 2. A key coenzyme of the NO-generating reaction is NADPH. Oxidation of NADPH is coupled to conversion of the guanidino group of L-arginine into a carbonyl group and, consequently, evolution of L-citrulline and NO. Several additional coenzymes are required, primarily for electron shuttling from NADPH to the haem iron of NOS, including FAD, FMN and tetrahydrobiopterin (BH_4). Calmodulin, a Ca^{2+}-binding protein, is yet another requisite coenzyme by virtue of its delivery of the cofactor Ca^{2+} to NOS [9]. Both eNOS and nNOS are Ca^{2+}-dependent isoforms of NOS.

Although we will restrict this review to NO production, it is important to recognize that NO availability is also governed by its inactivation. ROS (reactive oxygen species), such as the superoxide anion, quench NO, rendering it inactive [10]. Several endogenous antioxidant systems oppose these ROS, and there is emerging evidence that certain nutritional supplements and exercise training can bolster these endogenous antioxidants, thereby increasing NO availability. This is an area of intense research interest [11].

Adaptations of endothelium-dependent vasodilation to exercise training

Exercise training is a potent stimulus for adaptations of the cardiovascular system [3]. Numerous studies in both humans [12] and animals [13] have demonstrated augmented endothelium-dependent dilation of both conductance (i.e. larger, low-resistance) and resistance (i.e. smaller, high-resistance) blood vessels, specifically those supplying skeletal muscle with blood flow, following a period of endurance exercise training. Endurance training consists of lower intensity, more prolonged sessions of physical activity such as walking, running or swimming, and is that typically used in preventive and rehabilitative programmes with humans. Studies have also demonstrated an augmentation of endothelium-dependent dilation of vessels in the coronary circulation [14]. The majority of these studies concluded, based on pharmacological blockade experiments, that enhanced NO formation accounted for increased vasodilatory responses in the coronary and skeletal muscle circulations.

Adaptations of eNOS to exercise training

Since it appears that augmented endothelium-dependent dilation associated with exercise training is primarily due to enhanced NO formation in the vascular endothelium, most mechanistic research has focused on eNOS. An increase in NO formation could result from increased activity of pre-existing eNOS and/or an increase in the amount of eNOS protein present in the endothelium. As detailed below, there is considerable evidence for the latter possibility; that is, regular physical activity leads to increases in expression of the eNOS gene and, subsequently, eNOS protein.

mRNA for eNOS

The question of whether an increase in mRNA for eNOS is associated with exercise training is important in understanding the mechanism(s) responsible for enhancement of endothelial NO formation. An increase in eNOS mRNA quantity could indicate that exercise training induces increased transcription of the eNOS gene. Early studies involving cultured endothelial cells suggested that this possibility underlies training-induced increases in endothelium-dependent vasodilation. In 1992, Nishida et al. [15] reported that when cultured endothelial cells were exposed to 24 h of a sustained increase in shear stress, increased eNOS mRNA levels were observed. Increases in eNOS transcription have been attributed to a shear stress-responsive element that has been demonstrated to be present in the promoters of several endothelial-specific genes [16]. In addition to increasing transcription of the eNOS gene, exercise training may lead to elevated eNOS mRNA levels via post-transcriptional mechanisms. One such mechanism is increased mRNA stability. Recent work by Harrison et al. has shown that cultured endothelial cells increase poly(A) tail length in response to shear stress, conferring a prolonged half-life on eNOS mRNA [17].

The first study to demonstrate that these endothelial adaptations occurred with exercise training was that of Sessa et al., who reported that a brief period of treadmill run training (10 days) led to increased eNOS mRNA levels in canine aorta [18]. This finding has since been replicated in murine aorta [19], as well as resistance vessels from both rat skeletal muscle [20] and the porcine coronary circulation [21].

Collectively, these studies indicate that exercise training, perhaps due to increases in shear stress on the vascular endothelium during exercise training sessions, induces increased transcription of the eNOS gene and increases in stability of eNOS mRNA. These events would be predicted to lead, in turn, to increased translation of eNOS protein.

eNOS protein

Studies utilizing cultured endothelial cells have also been helpful in understanding how exercise training modulates eNOS protein expression. The 1992 study by Nishida et al. [15] that showed increases in eNOS mRNA with shear stress (see above) also demonstrated increased eNOS protein content. An increase in translation of eNOS protein would be an anticipated outcome of increased eNOS mRNA availability. Exercise training studies examining the aorta have uniformly reported that increased eNOS protein content is

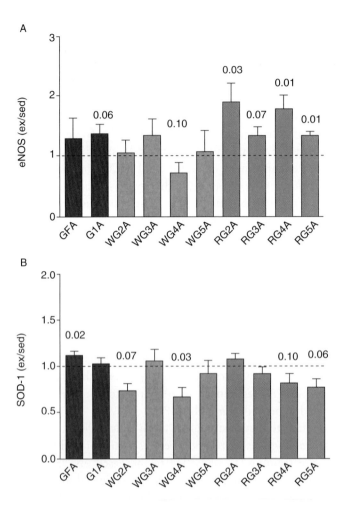

Figure 3. eNOS protein content of various orders of arterioles from rat gastrocnemius muscle
Rats either underwent endurance exercise training (ex) or remained sedentary (sed). FA, feed artery; 1A–5A, various orders of arterioles from proximal to distal. Values above bars are P-values for ex versus sed (sed=1.00). Note that arterioles from red, but not white, sections of muscle exhibit significant increases in eNOS protein content. Reproduced from *Journal of Applied Physiology* (2005) vol. 98, pages 753–761, with permission from The American Physiological Society.

associated with training [19,22,23]. This adaptation has been extended to the resistance vasculature of the coronary [24] and skeletal muscle circulations [20,25], although it does not appear to be uniformly distributed in either vascular bed (Figure 3). In the gastrocnemius muscle, 2A through 5A arterioles in the red section, but not the white section, exhibit increased eNOS content. This is likely because endurance exercise training sessions would be predicted to increase blood flow through vessels supplying the red, but not white, section of this muscle. These findings for resistance vessels are important because these vessels play a large role in determining tissue blood flow.

eNOS activity

An expected outcome of increased eNOS gene and protein expression would be increased eNOS activity and, consequently, greater capacity for NO formation in vascular endothelium. Selected studies have confirmed that exercise-trained animals with an increase in eNOS protein expression exhibit increased eNOS activity [18,19].

Post-translational mechanisms

It has become appreciated in recent years that eNOS activity can be acutely modulated by interactions with other endothelial proteins, most notably protein kinase B (also known as Akt) and Hsp (heat shock protein) 90 [9]. It appears that increased eNOS activity can be realized upon phosphorylation of certain amino acid residues; this phosphorylation is mediated by Akt, with Hsp90 playing a facilitating role. Several studies have demonstrated that cultured endothelial cells respond to shear stress by increasing the extent of eNOS phosphorylation, with unchanged eNOS protein content [26]. It is unknown whether acute exercise, like shear stress, induces eNOS phosphorylation; further, effects of exercise training on eNOS phosphorylation are uncertain. One study in which human patients with coronary atherosclerosis were subjected to an exercise training programme demonstrated an increase in phosphorylated eNOS content of the internal mammary artery [27]. This study also reported increased total cNOS protein content in the same artery. Importantly, this study demonstrated augmented endothelium-dependent dilation of internal mammary arteries from exercise-trained patients, suggesting that increases in phosphorylated eNOS and total eNOS protein were of functional significance.

Substrate and coenzyme availability

No data are available concerning either substrate (i.e. L-arginine) or coenzyme (e.g. BH_4) availability following a period of exercise training. It is an important question, however, because of the so-called arginine paradox. The essence of this paradox is that although the intracellular concentration of L-arginine is well in excess of that required for the eNOS reaction to proceed, L-arginine supplementation is frequently effective in augmenting endothelium-dependent vasodilation [28]. This effect has been reported for patient populations; it is uncertain whether exercise-trained humans and/or animals also exhibit the L-arginine paradox. It is conceivable that a relative lack of substrate is present, given the exercise training-induced increase in eNOS protein expression (see above).

Exercise training, NO and the prevention and management of atherosclerosis

Exercise training is a powerful measure for both prevention and management of atherosclerosis. In a recent study, Myers et al. [29] divided approx. 2500

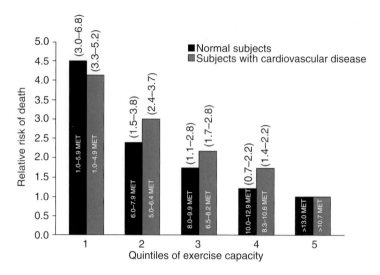

Figure 4. Risk of death over 6 year follow-up as a function of exercise capacity in normal subjects (black bars) and patients with cardiovascular disease (blue bars)
MET, metabolic equivalents, fold increase over resting metabolic rate at maximal exercise. Highest exercise capacity quintiles set to risk of 1.0. Range of exercise capacity given within each quintile bar; 95% confidence intervals given above each quintile bar. Note increasing risk of death with decreasing exercise capacity, in both normal subjects and patients with cardiovascular disease. Reproduced, with permission, from Myers, J. Prakash, M., Froelicher, V., Do, D., Partington, S. and Atwood, J.E. (2002) Exercise capacity and mortality among men referred for exercise testing. New England Journal of Medicine, **346**, 793–801. Copyright © 2002 Massachusetts Medical Society.

individuals without cardiovascular disease into quintiles based on exercise capacity, which presumably reflected exercise training status. At the end of a 6 year follow-up period, risk of death in the individuals comprising the lowest quintile of exercise capacity was more than four times that of individuals in the highest quintile (Figure 4). These findings were paralleled by approx. 3500 individuals with cardiovascular disease (Figure 4). It is important to note that risk of death was arbitrarily set to 1.0 in the groups of healthy individuals and those with cardiovascular disease; the latter were, of course, at higher risk of death than the former in any given quintile. These epidemiological data suggest that exercise training confers both preventive and rehabilitative effects on atherosclerosis. The mechanisms underlying these beneficial effects are poorly understood, but as explained below it is likely that NO is involved.

It is well-established that the endothelium is dysfunctional in athero-sclerosis, at least in part due to decreased NO availability [30]. In contrast to normal vessels, in which endothelium-dependent dilation is augmented by exercise training (see above), it appears that training merely normalizes dilation of atherosclerotic vessels in humans and animals [14]. This effect may not be trivial, however, given that dysfunctional endothelium has been proposed to play a central role in atherosclerosis [30].

Evidence for modulation of the atherosclerotic disease process by exercise training is available in the areas of adhesion molecule expression, smooth muscle cell migration and proliferation, and platelet aggregation. Regarding adhesion molecules, tethering of leukocytes to the vascular endothelium via these molecules and the subsequent migration of leukocytes into the subendothelial space are important preliminary events in foam cell formation [31]. Foam cells are cholesterol-laden macrophages that are significant constituents of atherosclerotic plaques; macrophages are derived from monocytes, a subset of the leukocyte population. Vascular smooth muscle cell migration to or proliferation in the subendothelium is a later event in the atherosclerotic process [31]. Platelet aggregation is a late and often terminal event (in the case of fatal myocardial infarction) in this disease process [31].

Leukocyte adhesion is promoted by expression of endothelial proteins such as P-selectin and VCAM-1 (vascular cell adhesion molecule-1) [31]. NO inhibits leukocyte adhesion [6] and raises the possibility that greater NO formation, an outcome of exercise training-induced increases in eNOS expression, inhibits this aspect of atherosclerosis. Recent findings from Chen and co-workers lend support for this hypothesis [32]. In this study, cholesterol-fed rabbits were assigned to either a sedentary or an exercise-trained group. Exercise training consisted of treadmill walking for up to 6 weeks. Cholesterol feeding led to areas of atherosclerosis in the aortic wall of sedentary rabbits (approx. one-third of the wall area after 6 weeks), along with expression of adhesion molecules such as P-selectin and VCAM-1. Exercise training retarded both the extent of atherosclerosis and expression of the adhesion molecules, P-selectin and VCAM-1. These investigators did not examine eNOS protein expression or activity, but they did determine aortic endothelium-dependent dilation, a functional surrogate of eNOS expression. Endothelium-dependent vasodilation was significantly greater in the exercise-trained rabbits compared with their sedentary counterparts, suggesting that reduced atherosclerosis in the trained animals was, at least in part, due to enhanced NO availability.

In another study examining the impact of exercise training on atherosclerosis, Indolfi et al. [33] examined vascular wall remodelling consequent to angioplasty in the carotid artery. This intervention induces vascular wall injury, with de-endothelialization being a prominent feature. In this study, some carotid-injured rats remained sedentary whereas other rats were subjected to swim training for up to 4 weeks. Angioplasty-induced vascular smooth muscle cell proliferation was dramatically reduced in trained animals, as was the neointima/media ratio, an index of the extent of smooth muscle cell migration/proliferation. Importantly, carotid eNOS expression and activity were determined and found to be increased in trained rats. Inhibition of eNOS by chronic administration of an eNOS inhibitor eliminated beneficial effects of training on smooth muscle cell proliferation and neointima/media ratio. The authors speculated that accelerated re-endothelialization of the carotid artery subsequent to vascular injury was a mechanism underlying the beneficial effects of exercise training.

These data for expression of adhesion molecules [32] and smooth muscle cell proliferation [33] may contribute to findings from studies of coronary artery disease patients. Exercise training in both American [34] and European populations [35] has been reported to decrease the number of patients exhibiting progression in severity of coronary atherosclerosis; indeed, patients showing regression of atherosclerotic lesions were frequently observed in the trained groups of these studies but only rarely in their respective sedentary groups. These results, whilst confounded by other lifestyle changes made simultaneously (e.g. nutritional), nonetheless hint at a beneficial effect of physical activity on established atherosclerosis.

Platelet aggregation, whilst important for normal haemostatic function, can be lethal in advanced atherosclerosis [31]. It is well-established that aggregation is inhibited by NO via cGMP-mediated actions in platelets [6]. Furthermore, reduced platelet aggregatory potential is associated with exercise training [36]. Swim-trained rats in the study of Indolfi et al. [33] exhibited reduced platelet aggregation, relative to sedentary animals, in an *in vitro* assay. Such changes in platelet aggregation may contribute to a lower cardiac event rate observed in exercise-trained human atherosclerotic patients compared with sedentary control patients [34].

Conclusion

Animal-based research is supportive of a role for endothelium-derived NO in mediating exercise-induced vasodilation, although parallel evidence in humans is scarce. The reason(s) for this discordance is unclear, but needs to be elucidated. On the other hand, studies in both animals and humans have demonstrated that endothelium-dependent, NO-mediated vasodilation is greater after exercise training. Transcriptional, post-transcriptional and translational mechanisms leading to increased eNOS expression appear to contribute to enhanced NO-mediated vasodilation in trained individuals. Post-translational modification(s) of eNOS (e.g. phosphorylation) may be an additional mechanism underlying enhanced eNOS function after exercise training; this is, however, a largely uninvestigated possibility. Training-induced adaptations involving eNOS are likely to be clinically relevant, given that NO inhibits several steps of the atherosclerotic disease process. This is another area worthy of additional investigation, given that atherosclerosis is the leading killer in Western society.

Summary

- *NO derived from the eNOS-catalysed reaction appears to play a role in exercise-induced vasodilation.*
- *Endothelium-dependent, NO-mediated vasodilation is augmented by exercise training.*

- *Increases in eNOS gene transcription, eNOS mRNA stability and eNOS protein translation likely underlie increased NO formation in the endothelium and, consequently, enhanced endothelium-dependent, NO-mediated vasodilation after training.*
- *Enhanced endothelial NO formation may also have a role(s) in the prevention and management of atherosclerosis by exercise training because several steps in the atherosclerotic disease process are inhibited by NO. A growing body of work suggests that exercise training, in part via increased capacity for NO formation, retards atherosclerosis.*

The authors gratefully acknowledge the important technical contributions of numerous technical staff to research by the authors that is cited in this review. The authors' research was supported by the National Institutes of Health (HL36088, HL52490, HL57226 and RR18276) and by the American Heart Association (AHA-KS-98-GB-25).

References

1. Furchgott, R.F. & Zawadski, J.V. (1980) The obligatory role of endothelial cells in the relaxation of arterial smooth muscle by acetylcholine. *Nature* **288**, 373–376

2. Moncada, S., Palmer, R.M.J., & Higgs, E.A. (1991) Nitric oxide: physiology, pathophysiology, and pharmacology. *Pharmacol. Rev.* **43**, 109–142

3. Laughlin, M.H., Korthuis, R.J., Duncker, D.J., & Bache, R.J. (1996) Control of blood flow to cardiac and skeletal muscle during exercise, in *Handbook of Physiology. Exercise: Regulation and Integration of Multiple Systems. Control of Respiratory and Cardiovascular Systems* (Rowell, L.B. & Shepherd, J.J., eds), pp. 705–769, American Physiological Society, Bethesda, U.S.A.

4. Sheriff, D.D., Nelson, C.D. & Sundermann, R.K. (2000) Does autonomic blockade reveal a potent contribution of nitric oxide to locomotion-induced vasodilation? *Am. J. Physiol. Heart Circ. Physiol.* **279**, H726–H732

5. Joyner, M.J. & Dietz, N.M. (1997) Nitric oxide and vasodilation in human limbs. *J. Appl. Physiol.* **83**, 1785–1796

6. Gewaltig, M.T. & Kojda, G. (2002) Vasoprotection by nitric oxide: mechanisms and therapeutic potential. *Cardiovasc. Res.* **55**, 250–260

7. Brophy, C.M., Knoepp, L., Xin, J. & Pollock, J.S. (2000) Functional expression of NOS 1 in vascular smooth muscle. *Am. J. Physiol. Heart Circ. Physiol.* **278**, H991–H997

8. Stamler, J.S. & Feelisch, M. (1996) Biochemistry of nitric oxide and redox-related species, in *Methods in Nitric Oxide Research* (Feelisch, M. & Stamler, J.S., eds.), pp.19–27, John Wiley & Sons, New York

9. Fulton, D., Gratton, J.-P. & Sessa, W.C. (2001) Post-translational control of endothelial nitric oxide synthase: why isn't calcium/calmodulin enough? *J. Pharmacol. Exp. Ther.* **299**, 818–824

10. Stocker, R. & Keaney, J.F. (2004) Role of oxidative modifications in atherosclerosis. *Physiol. Rev.* **84**, 1381–1478

11. Kojda, G. & Hambrecht, R. (2005) Molecular mechanisms of vascular adaptations to exercise. Physical activity as an effective antioxidant therapy? *Cardiovasc. Res.* **67**, 187–197

12. Clarkson, P., Montgomery, H.E., Mullen, M.J., Donald, A.E., Powe, A.J., Bull, T., Jubb, M., World, M. & Deanfield, J.E. (1999) Exercise training enhances endothelial function in young men. *J. Am. Coll. Cardiol.* **33**, 1379–1385

13. Jasperse, J.L. & Laughlin, M.H. (2006) Endothelial function and exercise training: evidence from studies using animal models. *Med. Sci. Sports Exerc.* **38**, 445–454

14. Laughlin, M.H. (2004) Physical activity in prevention and treatment of coronary disease: the battle line is in exercise vascular cell biology. *Med. Sci. Sports Exerc.* **36**, 352–362

15. Nishida, K., Harrison, D.G., Navas, J.P., Fisher, A.A., Dockery, S.P., Uematsu, M., Nerem, R.M., Alexander, R.W. & Murphy, T.J. (1992) Molecular cloning and characterization of the constitutive bovine aortic endothelial cell nitric oxide synthase. *J. Clin. Invest.* **90**, 2092–2096

16. Resnick, N., Collins, T., Atkinson, W., Bonthron, D.T., Dewey, C.F. & Gimbrone, M.A. (1993) Platelet-derived growth factor B chain promotor contains a cis-acting fluid shear-stress-responsive element. *Proc. Natl. Acad. Sci. U.S.A.* **90**, 4591–4595

17. Weber, M., Hagedorn, C.H., Harrison, D.G., & Searles, C.D. (2005) Laminar shear stress and 3? polyadenylation of eNOS mRNA. *Circ. Res.* **96**, 1161–1168

18. Sessa, W.C., Pritchard, K., Seyedi, N., Wang, J. & Hintze, T.H. (1994) Chronic exercise in dogs increases coronary vascular nitric oxide production and endothelial cell nitric oxide synthase gene expression. *Circ. Res.* **74**, 349–353

19. Kojda, G., Cheng, Y.C., Burchfield, J. & Harrison, D.G. (2001) Dysfunctional regulation of endothelial nitric oxide synthase (eNOS) expression in response to exercise in mice lacking one eNOS gene. *Circulation* **103**, 2839–2844

20. Spier, S.A., Delp, M.D., Meininger, C.D., Donato, A.J., Ramsey, M.W. & Muller-Delp, J.M. (2004) Effects of aging and exercise training on endothelium-dependent vasodilation and structure of rat skeletal muscle arterioles. *J. Physiol.* **556**, 947–958

21. Woodman, C.R., Muller, J.M., Laughlin, M.H., & Price, E.M. (1997) Induction of nitric oxide synthase mRNA in coronary resistance vessels isolated from exercise-trained pigs. *Am. J. Physiol. Heart Circ. Physiol.* **273**, H2575–H2579

22. Delp, M.D. & Laughlin, M.H. (1997) Time course of enhanced endothelium-mediated dilation of aorta of trained rats. *Med. Sci. Sports Exerc.* **29**, 1454–1461

23. Fukai, T., Siegfried, M.R., Ushio-Fukai, M., Cheng, Y., Kojda, G. & Harrison, D.G. (2000) Regulation of the vascular extracellular superoxide dismutase by nitric oxide and exercise training. *J. Clin. Invest.* **105**, 1631–1639

24. Laughlin, M.H., Pollock, J.S., Amann, J.F., Hollis, M.L., Woodman, C.R. & Price, E.M. (2001) Training induces nonuniform increases in eNOS content along the coronary arterial tree. *J. Appl. Physiol.* **90**, 501–510

25. McAllister, R.M., Jasperse, J.L. & Laughlin, M.H. (2005) Nonuniform effects of endurance exercise training on vasodilation in rat skeletal muscle. *J. Appl. Physiol.* **98**, 753–761

26. Boo, J.C. & Jo, H. (2003) Flow-dependent regulation of endothelial nitric oxide synthase: role of protein kinases. *Am. J. Physiol. Cell Physiol.* **285**, C499–C508

27. Hambrecht, R., Adams, V., Erbs, S., Linke, A., Krankel, N., Shu, Y., Baither, Y., Gielen, S., Thiele, H., Gummert, J.F. et al. (2003) Regular physical activity improves endothelial function in patients with coronary artery disease by increasing phosphorylation of endothelial nitric oxide synthase. *Circulation* **107**, 3152–3158

28. Loscalzo, J. (2000) What we know and don't know about L-arginine and NO. *Circulation* **101**, 2126–2129

29. Myers, J., Prakash, M., Froelicher, V., Do, D., Partington, S. & Atwood, J.E. (2002) Exercise capacity and mortality among men referred for exercise testing. *N. Engl. J. Med.* **346**, 793–801

30. Vita, J.A. & Keaney, J.F. (2002) Endothelial function: a barometer for cardiovascular risk. *Circulation* **106**, 640–642

31. Berliner, J.A., Navab, M., Fogelman, A.M., Frank, J.S., Demer, L.L., Edwards, P.A., Watson, A.D. & Lusis, A.J. (1995) Atherosclerosis: basic mechanisms. *Circulation* **91**, 2488–2496

32. Yang, A.-L., Jen, C.J. & Chen, H.-I. (2003) Effects of high-cholesterol diet and parallel exercise training on the vascular function of rabbit aortas: a time course study. *J. Appl. Physiol.* **95**, 1194–1200

33. Indolfi, C., Torella, D., Coppola, C., Curcio, A., Rodriguez, F., Bilancio, A., Leccia, A., Arcuccia, O., Falco, M., Leosco, D. & Chiariello, M. (2002) Physical training increases eNOS vascular

expression and activity and reduces restenosis after balloon angioplasty or arterial stenting in rats. *Circ. Res.* **91**, 1190–1197

34. Ornish, D., Scherwitz, L.W., Billings, J.H., Gould, K.L., Merritt, T.A., Sparler, S., Armstrong, W.T., Ports, T.A., Kirkeeide, R.L., Hogeboom, C. & Brand, R.A. (1998) Intensive lifestyle changes for reversal of coronary heart disease. *J. Am. Med. Assoc.* **280**, 2001–2007

35. Hambrecht, R., Niebauer, J., Marburger, C., Grunze, M., Kalberer, B., Hauer, K., Schlierf, G., Kubler, W. & Schuler, G. (1993) Various intensities of leisure time physical activity in patients with coronary artery disease: effects on cardiorespiratory fitness and progression of coronary atherosclerotic lesions. *J. Am. Coll. Cardiol.* **22**, 468–477

36. Womack, C.J., Nagelkirk, P.R. & Coughlin, A.M. (2003) Exercise-induced changes in coagulation and fibrinolysis in healthy populations and patients with cardiovascular disease. *Sports. Med.* **33**, 795–807

10

Muscle metabolism and control of capillary blood flow: insulin and exercise

Stephen Rattigan[1], Eloise A. Bradley,
Stephen M. Richards and Michael G. Clark

*University of Tasmania, Biochemistry, School of Medicine, Hobart,
Tasmania, Australia.*

Abstract

The evidence that muscle metabolism is determined by available capillary surface area is examined. From newly developed methods it is clear that exercise and insulin mediate capillary recruitment as part of their actions *in vivo*. In all insulin-resistant states examined thus far, insulin-mediated capillary recruitment is impaired with little or no change to the exercise response. Control mechanisms for capillary recruitment for exercise and insulin are considered, and the failure of the microvasculature to respond to insulin is examined for possible mechanisms that might account for impaired vascular responses to insulin in insulin resistance.

Introduction

The study of muscle metabolism by biochemists has traditionally involved the reductionist approach so that much of what is known has emerged from experiments involving isolated incubated muscles, single cells (in culture), organelles and homogenates. Unfortunately, when such knowledge gained from this approach is put back into a physiological context it is often found wanting.

[1]*To whom correspondence should be addressed (email s.rattigan@utas.edu.au).*

The main reason for this is the complexities of the vascular system and its unique relationship with skeletal muscle. Often the vascular system of muscle has been assumed to play a passive role delivering nutrients and hormones and removing waste products. In addition, it has been assumed that the vascular system is solely regulated by metabolic demand of the skeletal muscle. Recent evidence paints a different picture and suggests that the vasculature may play a large part in controlling muscle metabolism and contraction. Thus the muscle vasculature can respond directly to stimuli to change the pattern of microvascular perfusion, which by controlling delivery, influences muscle metabolism. Hormones such as insulin are now known to control their own, as well as substrate, delivery to muscle by vascular effects. Furthermore, there is growing evidence that insulin-resistant diabetes may originate from impaired vascular control with diminished delivery for both insulin and glucose to muscle.

The objective of this review is to examine the impact of the vasculature in controlling muscle metabolism and contraction largely through the manner in which the vascular system regulates nutrient delivery and removal.

Capillary recruitment

Transition from rest to exercise

There is evidence that, at rest, muscle is only partly perfused with autonomic vasomotion responsible for switching flow between different regions of the microvascular network to ensure relative normoxia. Thus at any one time (i.e. if one were to take a snapshot) under basal or resting conditions a relatively small proportion of the available capillaries in muscle is perfused (albeit there is both temporal and spatial heterogeneity). With the onset of contraction (muscle work) the 'snapshot' number of perfused capillaries increases several times, ranging from a three- to fourteen-fold increase, depending on the conditions and muscle type. A direct result of the increase in perfused capillaries is the increase in nutrient delivery, providing the additional substrates required to fuel the aerobic work done by contraction.

Normal action of insulin

Being able to measure changes in capillary surface area has been a significant step forward in understanding the *in vivo* vascular actions of hormones such as insulin and of exercise. To this end, a biochemical marker method using 1-MX (1-methylxanthine) has been developed for assessing capillary recruitment in muscle (Figure 1). Infused 1-MX was found to be converted stoichiometrically by rat hindlimb to 1-methylurate by xanthine oxidase, which others have shown to be largely concentrated in the capillary endothelial cells [1]. The method for measuring relative nutritive (capillary) flow was established and checked in the constant (total) flow perfused rat hindlimb system, where the proportion of total flow that is nutritive, could be varied. For example,

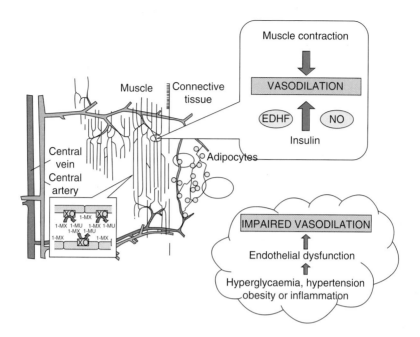

Figure 1. Vascular blood flow routes in skeletal muscle

Skeletal muscle microvascular blood flow is controlled by vasodilation at the terminal arterioles that enables perfusion of capillaries in contact with muscle myocytes (nutritive flow). Capillaries contain XO (xanthine oxidase) which can metabolize 1-MX and provide an indication of the extent of perfusion. The illustration is based upon the vascular arrangement of the rabbit tenuissimus muscle observed by Borgstrom et al. [32].

serotonin, a vasoconstrictor that reduces nutritive flow in this preparation, decreased 1-MX conversion into 1-methylurate but did so without altering either total flow or individual muscle flow rates (as determined by 15 μm microspheres) (see review [2] and references therein). In another example, electrical stimulation of the gastrocnemius-plantaris-soleus muscle group (to simulate exercise) of the pump-perfused rat hindlimb system increased 1- MX conversion into 1-methylurate. Thus, these findings strongly suggested that 1-MX conversion is an indicator of muscle nutritive flow and changes in metabolism of 1-MX could reasonably be assumed to reflect changes in capillary recruitment. With this as background, 1-MX was infused under conditions of steady state in the anaesthetized, *ad lib.* fed rat *in vivo* and metabolism of 1-MX determined from blood samples taken across the hindlimb. It was found that insulin (at doses which increased basal plasma insulin levels 4-fold, equivalent to a maximal physiological dose) increased 1-MX metabolism approximately 80% [3] in association with increased glucose uptake in muscle of the same hindlimb. The increase in 1-MX metabolism was indicative of capillary recruitment.

Whilst the first of the two methods for assessing capillary recruitment or nutritive flow relied on the metabolism of an infused exogenous substrate, the second approach was based on imaging of the change in perfusion by CEU (contrast enhanced ultrasound). The technique is derived from that described for the heart in which microbubbles of albumin (phospholipid microbubbles can also be used) provide the contrast medium. Essentially the technique involves simultaneously imaging and destroying all microbubbles within the ultrasound beam with the use of a high energy ultrasound pulse. The time between successive ultrasound pulses is progressively extended, allowing the tissue within the beam to be replenished with microbubbles. Eventually, the tissue will be fully replenished and further increases in time between each pulse will not alter the microbubble acoustic signal returning from the muscle. Preliminary assessment was made to ensure that the energy settings (> 4 MHz) used to destroy the microbubbles did not damage the endothelium (< 3 MHz). Once the images are collected a background subtraction (representing large rapidly filling vessels) is made to isolate effects on capillaries and allow calculation of the microvascular volume. Using this approach, changes in capillary blood volume in response to insulin and exercise have been assessed in skeletal muscle of the rat hindlimb *in vivo* and the CEU data have been found to correlate well with 1-MX metabolism data. Capillary blood volume increased approx. 100% during physiologic doses of insulin; with exercise slightly more of an increase. Data from these two approaches indicate that insulin mediates changes in muscle microvascular perfusion consistent with capillary recruitment. The response to administered insulin has been found in muscle of anaesthetized rats [3] and conscious humans [4] and to mixed meal and light exercise in conscious humans [5]. Furthermore, by using a number of interventions in rats, a tight link between insulin-mediated capillary recruitment and glucose uptake in the same muscle beds has begun to emerge, suggesting that capillary recruitment accounts for approximately half of the insulin-mediated muscle glucose uptake *in vivo*. Such a relationship raises the possibility that any impairment in capillary recruitment may also cause impairment in glucose uptake by muscle.

Insulin resistant states

A number of insulin resistant states have been studied in the rat and insulin-mediated muscle capillary recruitment from 1-MX metabolism has been compared with glucose uptake in each (see review [2] and references therein). These include insulin resistance induced by the acute administration of TNF-α (tumour necrosis factor-α) for 4 h, where a hyperinsulinaemic euglycaemic clamp was conducted over the last 2 h. In that study, it was noted that insulin-mediated capillary recruitment and limb blood flow (which occurs with this high physiological dose) were completely blocked by TNF-α. Total blockade of insulin's haemodynamic responses was accompanied by a 50% inhibition of muscle glucose uptake and an 18% inhibition of whole body glucose uptake. Another model involved infusion of the serotonergic agonist, α-methyl serotonin, which from perfused rat hindlimb studies reduced capillary recruitment as a result of its vasoconstriction. In the study *in vivo* [6], α-methyl serotonin was infused shortly before and throughout an insulin clamp. Mean arterial blood pressure was increased by 25% and insulin-mediated capillary recruitment as well as limb blood flow were completely inhibited. Muscle glucose uptake was inhibited by 50% and whole body glucose uptake was inhibited by 28%. It is interesting as this study represents the first demonstration of a model of muscle insulin resistance associated with hypertension, where vasoconstriction was very likely the cause of both [6]. Two other models of fatty acid- [7] and glucosamine-induced [8] insulin resistance gave similar outcomes with complete inhibition of capillary recruitment, as measured by-1 MX metabolism across the hindlimb muscle, and loss of approx. 50% of muscle glucose uptake due to insulin. In addition, in the genetically obese insulin-resistant Zucker rat, hyperinsulinaemia was unable to either increase muscle capillary recruitment (by 1-MX metabolism) or glucose uptake in hindlimb muscle [9]. One recent study has compared obese and lean human subjects using ultrasound and microbubbles as the means of assessing capillary recruitment [10]. In this study, physiologic insulin administered systemically failed to increase forearm microvascular perfusion (capillary recruitment), glucose uptake or brachial artery flow in obese subjects when compared with lean controls. In total, impaired microvascular recruitment was in each case associated with a decline in skeletal muscle insulin-mediated glucose disposal and is thus suggestive of insulin resistance. This would be expected if, as discussed by Renkin et al. (references 19 and 20 in [10]), endothelial surface area is an important factor limiting delivery of substrates (and hormones) to muscle tissue.

Mechanisms by which capillary perfusion is controlled

To summarize the position at this stage would be to conclude that muscle metabolism is very much dependent on the extent of microvascular perfusion. At rest, muscle is minimally perfused with vasomotion responsible for periodic redistribution so that hypoxia is avoided. However, as the metabolic demand of the muscle increases, such as in exercise, microvascular perfusion is enhanced commensurate with demand and, although the mechanism for this increased perfusion is still largely unknown, it is clearly controlled by the working myocytes themselves. A signal of myocyte or associated neuromuscular junction origin is undoubtedly responsible as only the actively contracting fibres, but not mechanically moved fibres [11], receive the benefit of increased capillary flow (recruitment). It appears that the initial rapid onset vasodilation (< 1 s) is due to muscarinic receptor activation, but the prolonged vasodilation involves other mechanisms [12]. Although insulin also produces capillary recruitment, the effect is more global with large groups of muscles affected. The question is where does the signal for insulin initiate? It would seem unlikely that capillary recruitment is controlled by a mechanism similar to that used by exercise involving a signal emanating from the initially accessible myocytes that spreads outwards. Rather, the data favours the view that the signal arises outside the under-perfused myocytes. For example, the time course for insulin action *in vivo* shows that insulin-mediated capillary recruitment precedes activation of muscle Akt or glucose uptake by this tissue [13]. In addition, insulin dose curves conducted *in vivo* show that muscle capillary recruitment is more sensitive than muscle glucose uptake to insulin action [14]. These studies [13,14] would thus suggest that insulin acts externally to the myocytes, probably at the endothelium adjacent to smooth muscle cells constituting the terminal arterioles to achieve a dilatation into capillary units that are not at that time perfused. There is also indirect evidence that constriction of arterioles leading to nearby functional shunts occurs concomitantly.

However, the detailed mechanism by which insulin-mediated capillary recruitment occurs is unresolved. Insulin-mediated capillary recruitment is blocked by systemically infused L-NAME (N^{ω}-nitro-L-arginine methyl ester), an inhibitor of NOS (nitric oxide synthase) [15]. The insulin-mediated action does appear to involve the phosphatidylinositol 3-kinase branch of the insulin signalling pathway as it is inhibited *in vivo* by wortmannin (Figure 2). This is consistent with the pathway in cultured endothelial cells that insulin uses to stimulate NO production (e.g. see [16] and [17] and references therein). However, NOS mediates numerous responses in a multitude of cell types, and global NOS inhibition *in vivo* is likely to produce complex effects. For example, systemic L-NAME administration causes elevated blood pressure, which

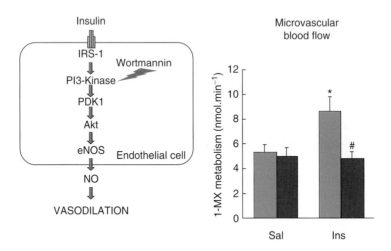

Figure 2. *In vivo* effects of wortmannin in the rat hindlimb
Wortmannin, which inhibits PI3 Kinase (phosphatidylinositol 3-kinase) activity in endothelial cells and prevents insulin mediated NO release [33], was administered to rats during either saline or insulin infusion. Muscle capillary recruitment was measured in hindlimbs of untreated (blue bars) or wortmannin treated (black bars) animals. * Insulin treatment significantly different (*P*<0.05) from saline treatment; # wortmannin plus insulin treatment significantly different (*P*<0.05) from insulin treatment. IRS-1, insulin receptor substrate-1; PDK1, phosphoinositol-dependent protein kinase 1; Akt, protein kinase B.

may be the result of central effects [18], that increase neural outputs, which are capable of inhibiting capillary recruitment. Also EDHF (endothelial-derived hyperpolarizing factor) factors, such as H_2O_2, may also be inhibited when nitric oxide synthase (NOS) is inhibited [19]. Methacholine, a NO producer, but also an EDHF producer, augments insulin-mediated capillary recruitment and muscle glucose uptake [20], and it too is inhibited by L-NAME. Furthermore, TEA (tetraethylammonium chloride), an EDHF inhibitor when used at low doses (0.5 mM) blocks insulin-mediated capillary recruitment (unpublished observation). Thus the evidence supporting NO involvement in insulin action is not conclusive even though the data overall appear to favour the notion that capillary perfusion controls muscle metabolism. Finally, there is the possibility that insulin acts to increase low frequency vasomotion, as has been reported using impaled laser Doppler flowmetry probes in human muscle [21]. An increase in vasomotion would have the net effect of extending the interval during which each capillary is perfused and reduce the interval during which blood cells are stationary in each capillary. This would translate to an increase in effective capillary surface area and is consistent with increased 1-MX metabolism and microvascular blood volume measured by contrast enhanced ultrasound. Just how insulin would act to increase low frequency vasomotion is hard to guess, but neural input is likely.

Vascular dysfunction and its consequences for muscle metabolism

It is clear that a unique intimacy exists between skeletal muscle and its vasculature. Factors such as exercise and insulin that control the capillary surface area available for nutrient and hormone delivery, as well as product removal, dictate the extent of metabolism that can be engaged by muscle. However, having said that, it is important to define the critical elements of the vasculature controlling recruitment. Because of the separation of total (limb) blood flow from metabolism by muscle at rest noted by a number of researchers, including ourselves (e.g. see review [2] and references therein), macrovascular dysfunction may prove to have little bearing on the control of muscle metabolism. Thus failure of large vessels to show vasodilatory response to cholinergic vasodilators or insulin may not necessarily have implications for muscle perfusion, metabolism and insulin's action on metabolism. This point becomes eminently visible when the total flow is manipulated by vasodilator infusion (e.g. see review [2] and references therein). Thus the focus moves to the microvasculature (Figure 1), where functional control may depend on a number of factors yet to be identified. Most consider impaired endothelial function of the microvasculature to be the key, where this may contribute to insulin resistance regardless of the presence of diabetes [22]. Thus far, causes of this dysfunction include direct effects of hyperglycaemia on the endothelial cells, indirect effects of growth factors, cytokines or vasoactive agents produced by other cells, or the impact of components of the metabolic syndrome acting on the endothelial cells [22]. All of the mechanisms assume that insulin's action to increase capillary surface area is NO-dependent where this is a logical extension from findings where large vessel and feed artery dilatation by insulin are clearly NO-dependent (e.g. see review [2] and references therein). However, as discussed above, other factors such as EDHFs and neural input, may also be necessary for microvascular actions of insulin.

Hyperglycaemia

A number of mechanisms have been proposed to explain how hyperglycaemia may interact directly with the endothelial cells and lead to vascular dysfunction. Some, if not all of these, may impact on microvascular control of muscle perfusion. Excessive glucose, even acutely following a meal, may cause a number of metabolic disturbances. Increased flux in the polyol pathway has been attributed to increased accumulation of intracellular glucose leading in turn to sorbitol accumulation, which may cause damage due to osmotic effects and reduced oxygen free radical scavenging due to $NADP^+$ depletion by aldose reductase. However, the relatively low expression of aldose reductase in endothelial cells may not be sufficient to cause significant sorbitol formation (e.g. see [22] and references therein). Increased intracellular glucose may also cause an increase in glucosamine 6-phosphate via the hexosamine pathway and this may be the mechanism by which glucosamine itself causes the loss of insulin-mediated capillary recruitment [8]. A key issue seems to be the accumulation of N-acetylglucosamine which by the addition to serine and threonine residues results in O-linked glycosylation. One such crucial enzyme that can be altered in this way is eNOS where O-linked glycosylation of the Akt phosphorylation site leads to decreased enzyme activity [23]. Another possible impact of hyperglycaemia is the activation of PKC (protein kinase C) via *de novo* synthesis of diacylglycerol from the excess intracellular glucose. The activation of PKC has a number of consequences particularly since activation may not necessarily only occur in the endothelial cells. For example, activation of PKC in the vascular smooth muscle cells nearby can lead to the induction of vascular endothelial growth factor which in turn causes dysregulation of endothelial cell permeability (e.g. see [22] and references therein). Activated endothelial PKC may act to decrease eNOS activity and/or increase the synthesis of endothelin-1. There may also be a PKC-mediated increase in oxidative stress by the regulation of a number of NADPH oxidases [22]. The accumulation of excessive amounts of glucose and glycolytic intermediates within the endothelial cell may also induce the overproduction of superoxide anions by uncoupled mitochondria. Some authors regard this as a key event which alone could be responsible for activation of the aldose reductase and hexosamine pathways, PKC activation, and AGE (advanced glycation end-products) formation by methylglyoxal [22].

Finally hyperglycaemia may induce non-enzymic glycosylation to form AGEs. In endothelial cells methylglyoxal is probably the main AGE formed, but AGEs either in the extracellular matrix, or formed by binding to the AGE receptors can impact on endothelial cell function [24].

Cytokines and vasoactive agent effects

The most prominent of the cytokines that has been reported to have deleterious effects on endothelial NO production is TNF-α. This cytokine when incubated with cultured endothelial cells inhibits insulin signalling by activating an opposing protein kinase system [16,17]. Acute administration of TNF-α into rats *in vivo* completely blocks insulin's haemodynamic effects [25] which very likely involves endothelial NO production in the microvasculature, causing a state of acute insulin resistance resulting in diminished insulin-mediated muscle glucose uptake [25]. Indeed there is some evidence in experimental animals that blockade or lowering of TNF-α ameliorates the insulin resistance [26]. Another important potential antagonist of capillary recruitment is angiotensin II, which impacts on NO bioavailability by increasing vascular NAD(P)H oxidases, superoxide production and NO scavenging [27]. There are also other aspects of endothelial dysfunction that may be independent of NO production. One example is endothelin-1, which is produced predominantly by the endothelium [28], and is elevated in the plasma of diabetes. When over produced, endothelin-1 may cause the redistribution of flow, reducing the nutritive component and increasing functional shunting [29]. Such a scenario could lead to decreased insulin delivery and insulin resistance.

Impact of components of the metabolic syndrome

The endothelium can control the initiation of atherosclerosis and its progression. Contributing issues may include elevated plasma cholesterol, elevated fatty acids and triglycerides, smoking and diabetes. Each of these decrease endothelial NO bioavailability, whether through decreased production or through increased degradation. One mechanism is through free radical attack, in particular via the increased production of ROS (reactive oxygen species). Increased plasma levels of low-density lipoprotein-cholesterol increases the production of ROS as well as decreasing the level of NOS, the enzyme responsible for NO production. Increased production of ROS quenches NO also reducing its concentration. Elevated non-esterified fatty acids are another component of the metabolic syndrome that bears on NO production. Fatty acids may do so by acting to inhibit the insulin signalling process, preventing insulin-mediated activation of Akt and thus the phosphorylation and activation of eNOS [16,17].

Comparing insulin- and exercise-mediated capillary recruitment

In all of the models of insulin resistance studied thus far there appears to be corroborative data from cellular studies to account for the basis by which the insulin resistance has occurred. In cultured endothelial cells acutely administered TNF-α blocked insulin-mediated NO production (see commentaries [16,17] and references therein). Non-esterified fatty acids may act similarly to TNF-α to cause insulin resistance through loss of the vascular action of insulin and loss of NO production at the endothelium [16,17]. The elevated TNF-α and nonesterified fatty acids in plasma of the obese Zucker rat may account for the impairment of capillary recruitment by insulin in this model. It is important to note, however, that acutely administered TNF-α does not inhibit exercise-mediated capillary recruitment [30] and the insulin resistant obese Zucker rat, which exhibits a complete loss of insulin-mediated capillary recruitment and has elevated plasma levels of TNF-α, responds normally in terms of exercise-mediated capillary recruitment [31]. This suggests that the loss of capillary recruitment, as measured by 1-MX metabolism, in obesity may result from impaired insulin signalling or endothelial vasodilator mechanisms and these defects do not exert significant effects on the response to exercise. Notwithstanding the impaired response to insulin in obesity there are perfusion limitations during exercise *in vivo* that reduce exercise capacity. This is dealt with elsewhere in this series.

Conclusions

Insulin, by enhancing total blood flow and capillary recruitment in muscle, enhances delivery of itself and glucose for optimal glucose metabolism within the muscle myocyte. The process insulin uses is independent of skeletal muscle metabolism and probably involves the endothelial cell. Muscle contraction, which has similar microvascular actions, uses processes that are dependent on skeletal muscle metabolism and thus differ from insulin. Further elucidation of the mechanisms and interactions between contraction- and insulin-mediated capillary recruitment is important to provide insight into how insulin resistance can be overcome.

Summary

- *Total flow reaching the muscle may not necessarily affect the extent of capillary recruitment.*
- *Newly developed methods demonstrate that exercise and insulin each mediate capillary recruitment as part of their actions in vivo.*
- *In all insulin resistant states examined thus far the action of insulin to recruit capillary flow is impaired; exercise induced recruitment seems to be less affected.*
- *Control mechanisms for capillary recruitment are different for contraction and insulin.*

This work was supported by National Institutes of Health (U.S.A.) Grant DK-58787, National Health and Medical Research Council Australia, National Heart Foundation of Australia. Stephen Rattigan is a Heart Foundation Career Fellow. We thank our many colleagues whose research we have summarized here and we regret that space limitations prevented us citing directly the many researchers whose published research we have summarized in this article.

References

1. Jarasch, E.D., Bruder, G. & Heid, H.W. (1986) Significance of xanthine oxidase in capillary endothelial cells. *Acta Physiol. Scand. Suppl.* **548**, 39–46

2. Clark, M.G., Wallis, M.G., Barrett, E.J., Vincent, M.A., Richards, S.M., Clerk, L.H. & Rattigan, S. (2003) Blood flow and muscle metabolism: a focus on insulin action. *Am. J. Physiol. Endocrinol. Metab.* **284**, E241–E258

3. Rattigan, S., Clark, M.G. & Barrett, E.J. (1997) Hemodynamic actions of insulin in rat skeletal muscle: evidence for capillary recruitment. *Diabetes* **46**, 1381–1388

4. Coggins, M., Lindner, J., Rattigan, S., Jahn, L., Fasy, E., Kaul, S. & Barrett, E. (2001) Physiologic hyperinsulinemia enhances human skeletal muscle perfusion by capillary recruitment. *Diabetes* **50**, 2682–2690

5. Vincent, M.A., Clerk, L.H., Lindner, J.R., Price, W.J., Jahn, L.A., Leong-Poi, H. & Barrett, E.J. (2006) Mixed meal and light exercise each recruit muscle capillaries in healthy humans. *Am. J. Physiol. Endocrinol. Metab.* **290**, E1191–E1197

6. Rattigan, S., Clark, M.G. & Barrett, E.J. (1999) Acute vasoconstriction-induced insulin resistance in rat muscle *in vivo*. *Diabetes* **48**, 564–569

7. Clerk, L.H., Rattigan, S. & Clark, M.G. (2002) Lipid infusion impairs physiologic insulin-mediated capillary recruitment and muscle glucose uptake *in vivo*. *Diabetes* **51**, 1138–1145

8. Wallis, M.G., Smith, M.E., Kolka, C.M., Zhang, L., Richards, S.M., Rattigan, S. & Clark, M.G. (2005) Acute glucosamine-induced insulin resistance in muscle *in vivo* is associated with impaired capillary recruitment. *Diabetologia* **48**, 2131–2139

9. Wallis, M.G., Wheatley, C.M., Rattigan, S., Barrett, E.J., Clark, A.D. & Clark, M.G. (2002) Insulin-mediated hemodynamic changes are impaired in muscle of Zucker obese rats. *Diabetes* **51**, 3492–3498

10. Clerk, L.H., Vincent, M.A., Jahn, L.A., Liu, Z., Lindner, J.R. & Barrett, E.J. (2006) Obesity blunts insulin-mediated microvascular recruitment in human forearm muscle. *Diabetes* **55**, 1436–1442

11. Sarelius, I.H., Cohen, K.D. & Murrant, C.L. (2000) Role for capillaries in coupling blood flow with metabolism. *Clin. Exp. Pharmacol. Physiol.* **27**, 826–829

12. VanTeeffelen, J.W. & Segal, S.S. (2006) Rapid dilation of arterioles with single contraction of hamster skeletal muscle. *Am. J. Physiol. Heart Circ. Physiol.* **290**, H119–H127

13. Vincent, M.A., Clerk, L.H., Lindner, J.R., Klibanov, A.L., Clark, M.G., Rattigan, S. & Barrett, E.J. (2004) Microvascular recruitment is an early insulin effect that regulates skeletal muscle glucose uptake *in vivo*. *Diabetes* **53**, 1418–1423

14. Zhang, L., Vincent, M.A., Richards, S.M., Clerk, L.H., Rattigan, S., Clark, M.G. & Barrett, E.J. (2004) Insulin sensitivity of muscle capillary recruitment *in vivo*. *Diabetes* **53**, 447–453

15. Vincent, M.A., Barrett, E.J., Lindner, J.R., Clark, M.G. & Rattigan, S. (2003) Inhibiting NOS blocks microvascular recruitment and blunts muscle glucose uptake in response to insulin. *Am. J. Physiol. Endocrinol. Metab.* **285**, E123–E129

16. Kim, F., Tysseling, K.A., Rice, J., Pham, M., Haji, L., Gallis, B.M., Baas, A.S., Paramsothy, P., Giachelli, C.M., Corson, M.A. & Raines, E.W. (2005) Free fatty acid impairment of nitric oxide production in endothelial cells is mediated by IKKβ. *Arterioscler. Thromb. Vasc. Biol.* **25**, 989–994

17. Kim, J.A., Koh, K.K. & Quon, M.J. (2005) The union of vascular and metabolic actions of insulin in sickness and in health. *Arterioscler. Thromb. Vasc. Biol.* **25**, 889–891

18. Shankar, R., Zhu, J.S., Ladd, B., Henry, D., Shen, H.Q. & Baron, A.D. (1998) Central nervous system nitric oxide synthase activity regulates insulin secretion and insulin action. *J. Clin. Invest.* **102**, 1403–1412

19. Shimokawa, H. & Morikawa, K. (2005) Hydrogen peroxide is an endothelium-derived hyperpolarizing factor in animals and humans. *J. Mol. Cell. Cardiol.* **39**, 725–732

20. Mahajan, H., Richards, S.M., Rattigan, S. & Clark, M.G. (2004) Local methacholine but not bradykinin potentiates insulin-mediated glucose uptake in muscle *in vivo* by augmenting capillary recruitment. *Diabetologia* **47**, 2226–2234

21. De Jongh, R.T., Clark, A.D., IJzerman, R.G., Serne, E.H., De Vries, G. & Stehouwer, C.D. (2004) Physiological hyperinsulinaemia increases intramuscular microvascular reactive hyperaemia and vasomotion in healthy volunteers. *Diabetologia* **47**, 978–986

22. Schalkwijk, C.G. & Stehouwer, C.D. (2005) Vascular complications in diabetes mellitus: the role of endothelial dysfunction. *Clin. Sci.* **109**, 143–159

23. Musicki, B., Kramer, M.F., Becker, R.E. & Burnett, A.L. (2005) Inactivation of phosphorylated endothelial nitric oxide synthase (Ser-1177) by O-GlcNAc in diabetes-associated erectile dysfunction. *Proc. Natl. Acad. Sci. U.S.A.* **102**, 11870–11875

24. Stern, D.M., Yan, S.D., Yan, S.F. & Schmidt, A.M. (2002) Receptor for advanced glycation endproducts (RAGE) and the complications of diabetes. *Ageing Res. Rev.* **1**, 1–15

25. Youd, J.M., Rattigan, S. & Clark, M.G. (2000) Acute impairment of insulin-mediated capillary recruitment and glucose uptake in rat skeletal muscle *in vivo* by TNF-α. *Diabetes* **49**, 1904–1909

26. Borst, S.E. & Bagby, G.J. (2002) Neutralization of tumor necrosis factor reverses age-induced impairment of insulin responsiveness in skeletal muscle of Sprague–Dawley rats. *Metabolism* **51**, 1061–1064

27. Cheng, Z.J., Vapaatalo, H. & Mervaala, E. (2005) Angiotensin II and vascular inflammation. *Med. Sci. Monit.* **11**, RA194–RA205

28. Luscher, T.F. & Barton, M. (2000) Endothelins and endothelin receptor antagonists: therapeutic considerations for a novel class of cardiovascular drugs. *Circulation* **102**, 2434–2440

29. Kolka, C.M., Rattigan, S., Richards, S. & Clark, M.G. (2005) Metabolic and vascular actions of endothelin-1 are inhibited by insulin-mediated vasodilation in perfused rat hindlimb muscle. *Br. J. Pharmacol.* **145**, 992–1000

30. Zhang, L., Wheatley, C.M., Richards, S.M., Barrett, E.J., Clark, M.G. & Rattigan, S. (2003) TNF-α acutely inhibits vascular effects of physiological but not high insulin or contraction. *Am. J. Physiol. Endocrinol. Metab.* **285**, E654–E660

31. Wheatley, C.M., Rattigan, S., Richards, S.M., Barrett, E.J. & Clark, M.G. (2004) Skeletal muscle contraction stimulates capillary recruitment and glucose uptake in insulin-resistant obese Zucker rats. *Am. J. Physiol. Endocrinol. Metab.* **287**, E804–E809

32. Borgstrom, P., Lindbom, L., Arfors, K.E. & Intaglietta, M. (1988) β-adrenergic control of resistance in individual vessels in rabbit tenuissimus muscle. *Am. J. Physiol.* **254**, H631–H635

33. Montagnani, M., Chen, H., Barr, V.A. & Quon, M.J. (2001) Insulin-stimulated activation of eNOS is independent of Ca^{2+} but requires phosphorylation by Akt at Ser(1179). *J. Biol. Chem.* **276**, 30392–30398

11

Vascular function in the metabolic syndrome and the effects on skeletal muscle perfusion: lessons from the obese Zucker rat

Jefferson C. Frisbee*† and Michael D. Delp*‡

*Center for Interdisciplinary Research in Cardiovascular Sciences, West Virginia School of Medicine, Morgantown, WV, U.S.A., †Department for Physiology and Pharmacology, West Virginia School of Medicine, Morgantown, WV, U.S.A., and ‡Division of Exercise Physiology, West Virginia School of Medicine, Morgantown, WV,U.S.A.

Abstract

The increased prevalence of obesity in Western society has been well established for many years, and with this trend, the prevalence of other associated pathologies including insulin resistance, dyslipidaemia, hypertension and the genesis of a proinflammatory and prothrombotic environment within individuals is also rapidly increasing, resulting in a condition known as the metabolic syndrome. From a physiological perspective, one of the most severe consequences of the metabolic syndrome is a progressive inability of the cardiovascular system to adequately perfuse tissues and organs during either elevated metabolic demand and, if sufficiently severe, under basal levels of demand. For the study of the metabolic syndrome, the OZR (obese Zucker rat) represents an important tool in this effort, as the metabolic syndrome in these animals results from a chronic hyperphagia, and thus can be an

[1]To whom correspondence should be addressed (email jfrisbee@hsc.wvu.edu).

excellent representation of the human condition. As in afflicted humans, OZR experience an attenuated functional and reactive hyperaemia, and can ultimately experience an ischaemic condition in their skeletal muscles at rest. The source of this progressive ischaemia appears to lie at multiple sites, as endothelium-dependent vasodilator responses are strongly impaired in OZR, and specific constrictor processes (e.g. adrenergic tone) may be enhanced. Whilst these active processes may contribute to a reduction in blood flow under resting conditions or with mild elevations in metabolic demand, an evolving structural alteration to individual microvessels (reduced distensibility) and microvascular networks (reduced microvessel density) also develop and may act to constrain perfusion at higher levels of metabolic demand. Given that constrained muscle perfusion in the metabolic syndrome appears to reflect a highly integrated, multi-faceted effect in OZR, and probably in humans as well, therapeutic interventions must be designed to address each of these contributing elements.

What constitutes the metabolic syndrome?

Whilst numerous challenges to public health exist within Western society, one of the most problematic in this regard is the increased prevalence and incidence of overweight and obesity. Using guidelines established by the Centers for Disease Control, overweight is considered to be represented by a BMI (body mass index) between 25 and 30 kg/m^2 in adults, or body mass in excess of the 95th percentile in paediatric populations, with obesity being defined as a BMI in excess of 30 kg/m^2 in adults [1]. Based on 1999–2002 NHANES (National Health and Nutrition Examination Survey) data, approx. 135 million American adults are classified as overweight, with approx. 63 million of these individuals classified as obese [1]. What is even more of a concern than the prevalence of overweight and obesity in Western society are recent trends demonstrating an increased incidence of these conditions. Comparisons between the 1971–1974 and 1999–2002 NHANES data sets, shows the incidence of obesity increased from 12.1% to 27.6% in men, whilst women demonstrated an increase from 16.6% to 33.2% over that same period, with comparable patterns evident in paediatric populations [1,2].

Whilst an increased prevalence of obesity represents a profound challenge for public health, a major concern over the development of the overweight/obese condition is that it predisposes individuals for the development of established cardiovascular disease risk factors, including dyslipidaemia, hypertension and impaired glycemic control. When combined, these myriad conditions create a multi-pathology state known as the metabolic syndrome (also termed Syndrome 'X' or insulin resistance syndrome). Specifically, the metabolic syndrome is defined as the combined presentation of three or more of: (i) abdominal obesity (waist circumference ≥102 cm in males; ≥88 cm in females), (ii) atherogenic dyslipidaemia (triglycerides ≥ 150 mg/dl; high-density lipoprotein cholesterol ≤ 40 mg/dl; 50 mg/dl in women), (iii) elevated blood pressure

(≥130/85 mmHg), (iv) insulin resistance or glucose intolerance (fasting glucose ≥110 mg/dl), (v) the presence of a prothrombotic state (e.g. high fibrinogen), and (vi) the presence of a proinflammatory state (e.g. elevated C-reactive peptide).

A recent study has demonstrated that the prevalence of the full metabolic syndrome is also increasing consistently within the American population, as between NHANES III (1988–1994) and NHANES IV (1999–2002), the age-adjusted prevalence of the metabolic syndrome increased from 24% to 27%, with the most dramatic increases identified among the female population, where the increase was 23.5% [3].

What are the implications of the metabolic syndrome for outcomes in human populations?

For cardiovascular health, the most profound implication of evolution of the metabolic syndrome is an increased likelihood for the development of peripheral vascular disease [4], a condition associated with compromised perfusion of the affected limbs and tissues, leading to impaired function and a progressive deterioration in tissue viability. Within humans, the numbers of studies that have focused on the vascular consequences of the full metabolic syndrome, and on mechanisms underlying identified impairments, are limited. As such, it is necessary to examine previous studies wherein a 'reduced' model of the metabolic syndrome is present (i.e. specific elements of the metabolic syndrome only) and to draw inferences from these results. Almost universally, previous studies have identified that with the progression of the metabolic syndrome, as well as with each of the contributing elements to it, perfusion of multiple tissues can be profoundly compromised [5,6]. In humans, the skeletal muscle constitutes approx. 40% of body mass and is a principle determinant of peripheral insulin sensitivity [7]. Consequently, deficits in skeletal muscle perfusion and the corresponding diminution of insulin and substrate diffusion from the intravascular space have been identified as a primary factor in the pathogenesis of the metabolic syndrome [5,6,8].

Vasodilation

One of the most commonly identified dysfunctions within vascular tissue with either the metabolic syndrome, or the contributing elements to it, is a compromised vasodilation in response to an imposed physiological (e.g. reactive hyperaemia, elevated metabolic demand) or pharmacological (e.g. infusion of endothelium-dependent agonists) challenge. As an example, Hamdy et al. [9] demonstrated in patients with the metabolic syndrome that brachial artery flow-mediated dilation was impaired relative to normal subjects, whereas responses to an exogenous NO (nitric oxide) donor was normal. Partial alleviation of the severity of the metabolic syndrome through weight reduction and chronic exercise improved brachial arterial flow-mediated dilation, although these effects were not associated with an improvement in microvascular reactivity [9]. Likewise, others have shown that infusion of endothelium-dependent vasodilators, such as acetylcholine, methacholine and insulin, result in blunted increases in limb perfusion in patients with the metabolic syndrome relative to control subjects, whereas vasodilator responses via endothelium-independent mechanisms were intact [10]. Importantly, whilst this impairment in endothelium-dependent vasodilation in humans afflicted with the metabolic syndrome is via a NO signalling mechanism, this impairment in NO signalling can adversely impact vascular smooth muscle cell proliferation/migration, platelet aggregation/thrombosis, monocyte/macrophage adhesion and inflammation throughout the circulation.

Vasoconstriction

In conjunction with depressed endothelium-dependent vasodilation, enhanced vasoconstriction could also limit skeletal muscle perfusion during the metabolic syndrome. For example, it has been suggested that in addition to decreased bioavailability of NO, there is a corresponding increase in the production of the potent vasoconstrictor ET-1 (endothelin-1). Indeed, higher circulating concentrations of ET-1 are reported to occur in patients with the metabolic syndrome [11], and Cardillo et al. [12] reported that there is an increased vasoconstrictor tone mediated through endogenous ET-1 in type II diabetic patients. In addition, previous studies have suggested that an increased production of vasoconstrictor prostanoids and angiotensin II [13], as well as activation of the sympathoadrenal system [14], have also been postulated as mechanisms constraining skeletal muscle perfusion in the metabolic syndrome.

Vascular structure

Several lines of evidence indicate that there are changes in arterial vascular structure in the metabolic syndrome that could serve to limit skeletal muscle perfusion. Clinical studies have demonstrated that increases in arterial pulse wave velocity are positively correlated with the cluster of features associated with the metabolic syndrome, and are frequently indicative of increases in the mechanical stiffness of arteries [15]. Further, increased arterial wall thickness is likely to be partially related to elevated concentrations of insulin through direct trophic effects on smooth muscle cells, as well as by the generation of reactive oxygen species, protein kinase C and activation of nuclear factor-κB to stimulate vascular smooth muscle cell growth, migration and proliferation. Further, Fossum et al. [6] reported a positive association between the appearance of peripheral structural vascular changes in the forearm and insulin resistance that could limit perfusion. This effect could clearly be mediated by decreases in arterial diameter and microvessel density.

Validity of the Zucker rat as a model of the metabolic syndrome

The OZR (obese Zucker rat; *fa/fa*) represents a key animal model in the study of the metabolic syndrome. The *fa* mutation represents an autosomal recessive locus on chromosome 5, and with both copies present, the leptin receptor gene is not properly encoded [16]. Heterozygotes (*fa*/+) exhibit no phenotypic anomaly, and are not distinguishable from the control lean Zucker rat (+/+). Owing to this dysfunctional leptin receptor gene, the OZR demonstrates an impaired satiety reflex and a chronic elevation in food intake. As a result, OZR rapidly develop profound obesity, exhibited through both hypertrophy and hyperplasia of adipocytes, as well as many of the subsequent disease states associated with chronic obesity, including insulin resistance and profound hypertriglyceridaemia [16]. Additionally, OZR can develop a moderate, clinically relevant form of hypertension [17–19], and ongoing studies suggest that OZR exist in a profound proinflammatory and prothrombotic [20] state, with expressions of plasminogen, plasminogen activator inhibitor-1 and C-reactive peptide all consistently elevated above that in controls.

Given that OZR develops its systemic pathologies through a chronic hyperphagia, this genesis of the metabolic syndrome is highly relevant to the human condition. Further, OZR experience a prolonged period of hypertriglyceridaemia and insulin resistance prior to the overt development of type II diabetes mellitus, as is frequently the case in obese humans. The degree of hypertension that does develop in OZR can best be described as mild to moderate, which is also in keeping with the levels of hypertension identified in most humans afflicted with the metabolic syndrome. Finally, the recent identification of a proinflammatory and prothrombotic environment within OZR has also demonstrated striking parallels to the conditions of the human metabolic syndrome. Taken together, these elements support the contention that OZR represent an appropriate model for studying the genesis, outcomes and potential treatment for the metabolic syndrome in humans.

Perfusion abnormalities in the OZR

Under resting conditions, skeletal muscle arteriolar perfusion in OZR has consistently been demonstrated to be reduced versus levels determined in controls, and this has been demonstrated in both trans-illuminated cremaster [21] and spinotrapezius muscle preparations [22]. These observations have translated to bulk perfusion of *in situ* whole skeletal muscles. Work from Frisbee's group has consistently demonstrated that perfusion of gastrocnemius muscle was reduced in OZR as compared with that identified in the lean Zucker rat counterparts [23,24].

As one of the hallmark characteristics of the metabolic syndrome in humans afflicted with this condition is the progressive inability to match muscle perfusion with metabolic demand, hyperaemic responses in skeletal muscle of OZR in response to physiological and pharmacological stimuli has received additional attention in recent years and is a vital avenue for ongoing investigation. In a recent study of reactive hyperaemia in skeletal muscle of OZR, it was suggested that the total perfusion response following removal of the occlusive stimulus was reduced in obese animals relative to that in controls [25].

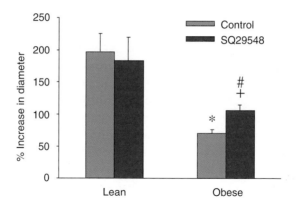

Figure 1. Impairment in functional vasodilation of spinotrapezius muscle arterioles in OZR compared with lean Zucker rats (controls)
SQ-29548 treatment partially restores the vasodilatory response to muscle stimulation in arterioles from OZR. * P <0.05 versus LZR (lean Zucker rat) control. Reproduced from Xiang et al. (2006) *Am. J. Physiol. Regul. Integr. Comp. Physiol.* vol. 290, pages R134–R138, with permission from The American Physiological Society.

The investigation of functional or active hyperaemia, points directly to the ability of the skeletal muscle circulation to alter perfusion appropriately to match convective and diffusive substrate exchange with metabolic intensity. Using *in situ* spinotrapezius muscle, Hester's group has determined that functional hyperaemia within single arterioles of OZR is attenuated as compared with that in lean Zucker rats (Figure 1), and that these impairments were correlated with impaired dilator responses to acetylcholine [26]. Ongoing studies using the *in situ* gastrocnemius muscle preparation have demonstrated that this constrained active hyperaemia is also evident at the level of bulk perfusion to skeletal muscle [23,24 and (Figure 2)]. When taken together, these results suggest that impaired active hyperaemia within skeletal muscle of OZR may be present regardless of the severity of metabolic demand and may also be independent of the type of muscle contraction imposed [23,24]. However, given that OZR continue to grow and that daily activity levels are not markedly different between lean Zucker rats and OZR at 14 weeks of age [10], it is unlikely that this ischaemia is sufficient to compromise growth or normal daily activity. However, with stronger elevations in metabolic demand, impaired perfusion of skeletal muscle in OZR may contribute to the genesis of premature fatigue development [24].

Vascular basis for perfusion abnormalities

Vasodilator reactivity
One of the most consistent observations regarding altered vascular function within OZR is an impaired endothelium-dependent vasodilation within not only the skeletal muscle circulation, but also within resistance arterioles of other multiple organs [27,28], suggesting the likelihood of common

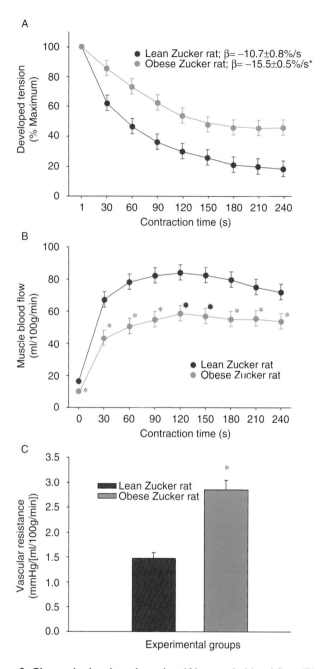

Figure 2. Change in developed tension (A), muscle blood flow (B) and mean vascular resistance during contraction (C) of *in situ* gastrocnemius muscle of LZR and OZR

Muscles were stimulated to contract via the sciatic nerve at 60 isometric titanic contractions/min (2003 ms, 503 Hz). Data are presented as means ± S.E. *P < 0.05 versus LZR control. Reproduced from Frisbee (2003) *Am. J. Physiol. Regul. Integr. Comp. Physiol.* vol. 285, pages R1124–R1134, with permission from The American Physiological Society.

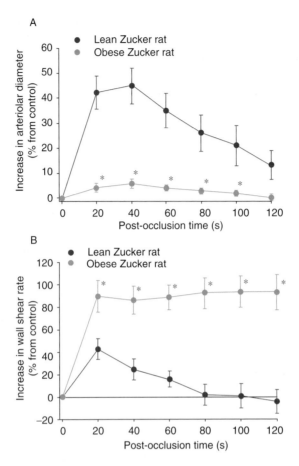

Figure 3. The change in arteriolar diameter (A) and wall shear rate (B) for *in situ* cremasteric arterioles of LZR and OZR after 120 s of physical occlusion of a parallel arteriole
*$P < 0.05$ versus LZR. Reproduced from Frisbee and Stepp (2001) *Am. J. Physiol. Heart Circ. Physiol.* vol. 281, pages H1304–H1311, with permission from The American Physiological Society.

mechanisms underlying this compromised behaviour. As examples, within cremaster or spinotrapezius muscles of OZR, dilator responses to elevated wall shear rate [21 and (Figure 3)] and challenge with acetylcholine [21,26] or arachidonic acid [21,22], have consistently been demonstrated to be reduced below that determined in lean rats. The impairments to endothelium-dependent dilation have also been verified using isolated skeletal muscle arterioles by several investigators. Johnson et al. [18] demonstrated that gracilis muscle resistance arterioles from OZR manifest an impaired dilation to application of acetylcholine and elevated perfusate flow rate, results that are consistent with previous studies demonstrating an impaired endothelium-dependent dilation of isolated arterioles in response to acetylcholine, reduced oxygen tension and arachidonic acid [21,23] in OZR versus lean rats. Whilst isolated reports of an impaired vasodilation in response to endothelium-independent stimuli exist [23], the overwhelming majority of the literature suggests that dilator reactivity following direct activation of the smooth muscle is near normal across vascular beds within OZR [18,26,27].

As many of the studies cited above have employed shear-induced and acetylcholine-induced dilation, both highly dependent on the appropriate production and bioavailability of NO from the endothelium, several studies have targeted these processes in terms of elucidating mechanisms of the impaired response in OZR. Fulton et al. [29] demonstrated that eNOS expression patterns, phosphorylation and binding to Hsp90 (heat shock protein 90) are not altered in OZR relative to controls, and concluded that mechanisms underlying the reduced vascular reactivity to endothelium- and NO-dependent stimuli must lie elsewhere, citing possible cofactor or substrate bioavailability limitations or elevated scavenging actions of superoxide anion. As an elevation in vascular oxidant stress in OZR manifesting the metabolic syndrome has been well documented, several investigators have pursued this avenue of investigation, treating these animals with an array of oxidative radical scavengers in an attempt to restore NO bioavailability and vascular reactivity. In general, treatment of OZR with antioxidants has improved vasodilator responses to NO-dependent stimuli in isolated microvessels [21,24] and using *in situ* preparations [21], suggesting that endothelium-dependent dilator reactivity can be improved by acute treatment with oxidative radical scavengers which, by extension, implicates oxidative radical scavenging of endothelium-derived NO as a key contributor to compromised dilator responses in OZR. Interestingly, a recent study by Geakelman et al. [30] provided insight into this area as they determined that chronic treatment of Zucker diabetic fatty rats (which develop type II diabetes mellitus more rapidly than do OZR), with a peroxynitrite scavenger improved acetylcholine-induced dilation of renal arteries/arterioles. These results raise an important issue of which process is more relevant to the reduced dilator reactivity in OZR, a reduction in NO bioavailability or the generation of peroxynitrite. This may be a key consideration in that Brzezinska et al. [31] identified that peroxynitrite can selectively antagonize the calcium-activated potassium (K_{Ca}) channels in smooth muscle cells, preventing membrane hyperpolarization in the face of elevated calcium and impairing the ability of the muscle cell to relax. The importance of oxidant stress-based reductions in NO bioavailability in terms of the regulation of functional hyperaemia and the matching of muscle perfusion with metabolic demand has recently been brought into question. Whole body acute reductions in vascular oxidant stress (via intravenous infusion of antioxidants), whilst improving depressor responses to methacholine, had no discernible impact on metabolic demand-induced increases in skeletal muscle perfusion [24].

A number of other mechanisms have been investigated in OZR that could contribute to a reduction in NO bioavailability and compromised arterial/arteriolar dilator reactivity, including increased expression and activity of protein

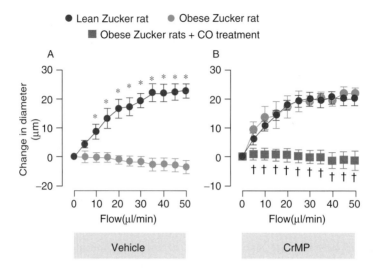

Figure 4. Flow-induced changes in internal diameter of first-order gracilis muscle arterioles isolated from LZR or OZR
Arterioles were acutely pretreated *in vitro* with vehicle (**A**), with an inhibitor of haem oxygenase, 15 μmol/l CrMP (chromium mesoporphyrin), or simultaneously with CrMP and a haem oxygenase product, 100 μmol/l carbon monoxide for 20 min before initiation of flow. Data are expressed as means ± SE. *$P < 0.05$ relative to lean group; †$P < 0.05$ relative to obese CrMP-pretreated arterioles. Reproduced from Johnson et al. (2006) *Am. J. Physiol. Regul. Integr. Comp. Physiol.*, vol. 290, pages R601–R608, with permission from The American Physiological Society.

kinase βII acting to constrain stimulus-induced NO formation [27], the role of haem oxygenase derived carbon monoxide production as a contributor to inhibiting NO synthase [18 and (Figure 4)].

In terms of arachidonic acid metabolism, whereas comparable evidence supporting an oxidant stress-based mechanism for NO scavenging has also been postulated to exist with regard to eicosanoid bioavailability [24], a recent study has demonstrated that the reduced dilation of *in situ* spinotrapezius muscle arterioles with arachidonic acid in OZR was partially restored following treatment of the muscle with the PGH$_2$–TxA$_2$ (prostaglandin H$_2$–thromboxane A$_2$) receptor antagonist SQ-29548 [22], suggesting that an inappropriate activation of vasoconstrictor pathways may contribute to the impaired dilator responses determined in these animals.

Vasoconstrictor reactivity
Although having received considerably less attention, there is evidence that pathways associated with vasoconstriction may also be markedly altered in OZR and that these may exhibit a much stronger influence on the evolving ischaemia in skeletal muscle of these animals than do pathways of vasodilation. Whilst isolated reports of increased vascular tone exist due to an increased myogenic activation [24] and an elevated expression and activity of serotonin [32] and endothelin receptors [33] and in skeletal muscle have

been reported, it is unclear how these results would impact skeletal muscle perfusion, as the necessary analyses have not been performed.

With development of obesity, an increased adrenergic activity is frequently observed [34], which can have a profound impact of the perfusion of tissues which are sensitive to adrenergic modulation. Carlson et al. [35] demonstrated that, with development of the metabolic syndrome in OZR, sympathetic nervous system activity was elevated as compared with levels in control animals. Building from this, Stepp and Frisbee [36] determined that norepinephrine-induced constriction of skeletal muscle resistance arterioles was increased in OZR relative to that in lean animals, and that intravenous infusion of the α_1-adrenoreceptor antagonist prazosin caused a pronounced dilation of *in vivo* arterioles, significantly greater than in controls. Further, Schreihofer et al. [37] determined that phenylephrine-induced elevation in vascular resistance in the hindlimb of OZR was greater than that in lean Zucker rats. Attempts at elucidating the mechanism underlying this increased adrenergic reactivity of skeletal muscle resistance arterioles in OZR have only recently been undertaken, although Naik et al. [38] has provided evidence suggesting that RhoA-kinase may play a significant role in increasing the sensitivity of the contractile machinery of the vascular smooth muscle cell of OZR in response to elevations in intracellular calcium levels.

Recent studies have begun to elucidate the significance of this increased adrenergic reactivity of the skeletal muscle microvessel of OZR for muscle perfusion. In *in situ* gastrocnemius muscle of OZR, the increased adrenergic vasoconstriction contributes to reduced skeletal muscle perfusion at rest, and in response to mild and moderate elevations in metabolic demand, as intravenous infusion of adrenergic antagonists restored perfusion in OZR to levels that were near those in control animals [23]. This study also clearly demonstrated that with high metabolic demand, adrenergic constraint on functional hyperaemia was not present. Additional recent studies have provided evidence suggesting the increased adrenergic reactivity of the skeletal muscle resistance arterioles contributes to both a premature reduction in skeletal muscle perfusion with incremental haemorrhage [39] and a reduced reactive hyperaemic response following removal of brief periods of serial vascular occlusion [25] in OZR.

Structural remodeling

Several studies have consistently determined that passive (i.e. pressurized in a calcium-free environment) diameter of skeletal muscle resistance arterioles of OZR was reduced below that in lean animals [40,41]; not a surprising observation given that many of the contributing elements to the metabolic syndrome have been previously identified as being associated with altered arteriolar wall mechanics. In OZR manifesting the metabolic syndrome, these alterations include significant reductions in arteriolar wall incremental distensibility and left-shifting of the circumferential wall stress versus strain relationship {[40] and (Figure 5)}. The skeletal muscle microcirculation of OZR

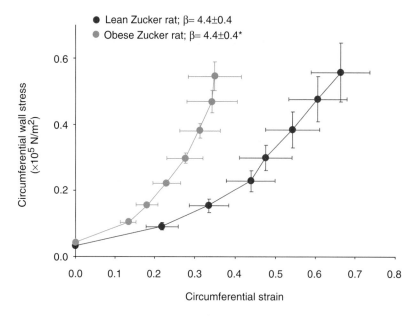

Figure 5. Circumferential wall stress versus strain relationship of isolated gracilis muscle first-order arterioles from LZR and OZR under Ca²⁺-free conditions
*P < 0.05 versus the slope coefficient (β) describing this relationship for arterioles from LZR. Reproduced from Frisbee (2003) *Am. J. Physiol. Heart Circ. Physiol.*, vol. 285, pages H104–H111, with permission from The American Physiological Society.

is also altered at the network level of resolution, as capillary density in muscle of these animals is significantly reduced versus that in controls [17,40,42].

When taken together, reduced vascular distensibility and microvascular rarefaction result not only in an increased minimum vascular resistance of the skeletal muscle of OZR {[40] and (Figure 6)}, but can also contribute to a blunted functional hyperaemia of skeletal muscle at higher levels of metabolic demand [24]. Recent studies exploring mechanisms underlying skeletal muscle microvascular rarefaction in OZR suggest that this reduction in microvessel density is closely associated with the severity of insulin resistance, and may be independent of the development of hypertension [17]. Further, whilst it has been suggested that rarefaction in OZR is closely aligned with a chronic reduction in vascular NO bioavailability [43], recent observations from Geakelman et al. [30] suggest that the generation of peroxynitrite from the scavenging of NO by superoxide could underlie the pattern of reduced microvessel density in these animals, as chronic treatment with a peroxynitrite scavenger prevented renal microvascular rarefaction in OZR.

Systemic cardiovascular control
A recent study has identified additional elements to the global cardiovascular system within OZR that may contribute to the ischaemic perfusion of skeletal muscle at rest and with elevated metabolic demand. Schreihofer et al. [37] made an initial observation that blood and plasma volumes of

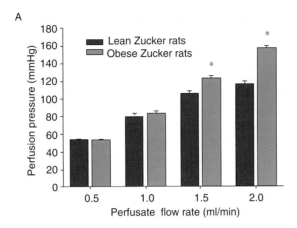

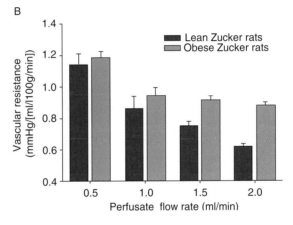

Figure 6. Perfusion pressure (A) and calculated vascular resistance (B) within pump-perfused gastrocnemius muscles of LZR and OZR
Gastrocnemius muscle mass was not different between LZR (2.35±0.13 g) and OZR (2.29±0.15 g). Data (means ± S.E.) are presented from perfusion of a maximally dilated microvascular bed at a constant volume flow rate of 0.5, 1.0, 1.5 or 2.0 ml/min. *$P < 0.05$ versus LZR at that perfusion rate. Reproduced from Frisbee (2003) *Am. J. Physiol. Heart Circ. Physiol.*, vol. 285, pages H104–H111, with permission from The American Physiological Society.

OZR are reduced as compared with lean Zucker rats, despite corrections for the increased adiposity. In addition to this, Frisbee demonstrated that the ability of OZR to tolerate incremental haemorrhage, largely dependent on rapid sympathetic neural responses, was impaired relative to that in lean Zucker rats [39]. Further, data presented in this study [39] suggest that the impaired ability to tolerate incremental haemorrhage may have been a function of the reduced circulating blood volume and an imbalance in the sympathetic neural responses to the hypovolaemia. Specifically, the skeletal muscle circulation received an immediate and pronounced elevation in vasoconstrictor tone of adrenergic origin, whilst in contrast adrenergic constriction of the splanchnic circulation was both delayed and blunted in magnitude [39]. It is possible that this reduction in circulating blood volume in OZR, acting in combination with an altered distribution of sympathetic neural tone may contribute to the underperfusion of skeletal muscle at rest and with elevated metabolic demand.

Clinical implications and therapeutic interventions

Several tentative conclusions can be drawn regarding processes that negatively impact muscle perfusion in OZR. Foremost, impaired endothelium-dependent dilation has been clearly demonstrated in skeletal muscle arterioles of OZR. However, whilst it is clear that acute interventions such as correcting oxidant stress, inhibiting protein kinase βII, antagonizing PGH_2–TxA_2 receptors, or blocking endogenous carbon monoxide production can improve arteriolar dilation in response to specific pharmacological stimuli, the importance of these processes in terms of the matching of perfusion with metabolic demand is less clear.

With regard to constrictor reactivity, the impact of enhanced responses to adrenergic stimulation may reduce resting perfusion and constrain functional hyperaemia at low to moderate elevations in metabolic demand in OZR. Whilst recent studies have implicated specific signalling pathways increasing the sensitivity of the smooth muscle contractile machinery to elevated calcium concentration as contributing to this enhanced adrenergic vascular tone, this is an area of investigation that warrants future investment. Additional investigation into other pathways of constrictor reactivity in OZR which, although identified, have not been fully verified with regard to the regulation of skeletal muscle perfusion, including increased myogenic activation, increased constrictor prostanoid generation, increased serotonin receptor expression and increased endothelin receptor expression and activity, require future validation.

Investigation into vascular structural alterations with genesis of the metabolic syndrome and the role of these alterations into the regulation of tissue perfusion has recently come under more intense investigation. However, it has rapidly become clear that skeletal muscle circulation of OZR experiences numerous alterations to its structure, including a reduced resistance arteriolar distensibility and a progressive rarefaction of microvascular networks. Whilst treatments designed to improve vascular wall stiffness are not uncommon in the clinical setting (e.g., angiotensin converting enzyme inhibitors) [19], therapeutic interventions designed to improve tissue vascularity and blunt microvascular rarefaction have been less well explored. However, given the potential importance of a maintained vascular NO bioavailability for the maintenance of microvessel density, developing therapeutic interventions into the protection of microvessel network structure, and not simply dilator reactivity or wall stiffness may prove to be a highly beneficial avenue for future investigation.

Conclusions

As both the prevalence and the incidence of the full metabolic syndrome, and the individual systemic pathologies that comprise it, are growing rapidly in Western society, the impact of this trend on afflicted individual mortality and morbidity will also become more severe. Given that one of the most clearly demonstrated outcomes of the metabolic syndrome is the progressive development of peripheral vascular disease, ongoing study into the nature of this evolving dysfunction and the interaction of specific mechanisms that underlie it will continue to be critical arenas for future investigation. Further, an understanding of how vascular reactivity (both dilator and constrictor) combines with vascular structure (at the individual vessel and vascular network levels of resolution) for the integrated regulation of perfusion will be vital for the development of effective interventional strategies and therapeutic regimens.

Summary

- *Owing to chronic hyperphagia, the OZR represents an excellent model of the metabolic syndrome in humans, as it progressively develops obesity, insulin resistance dyslipidaemia, moderate hypertension and represents a proinflammatory and prothrombotic environment.*

- *In OZR, resting skeletal muscle blood flow is reduced below that in normal control animals. Functional and reactive hyperaemic responses in skeletal muscle are also blunted, with a myriad of contributing mechanisms.*

- *Endothelium-dependent dilation of skeletal muscle microvessels is impaired in OZR, although dilation in response to endothelium-independent stimuli appears to be intact. The consequences of this impairment to dilator reactivity for skeletal muscle perfusion are presently unclear.*

- *Skeletal muscle microvessel constriction in response to adrenergic agonists is enhanced in OZR manifesting the full metabolic syndrome, and this has the potential to constrain skeletal muscle perfusion at rest and with mild to moderate elevations in metabolic demand.*

- *Structural alterations to the skeletal muscle microcirculation in the OZR, including reduced microvessel wall distensibility and microvessel density elevate minimum vascular resistance and may constrain blood flow with higher elevations in metabolic demand.*

References

1.   Center for Disease Control Information Pages, 'Overweight and Obesity' (2006). http://www.cdc.gov/nccdphp/dnpa/obesity/

2.   Hedley, A.A., Ogden, C.L., Johnson, C.L., Carroll, M.D., Curtin, L.R. & Flegal, K.M. (2004) Prevalence of overweight and obesity among US children, adolescents, and adults, 1999–2002. *J. Am. Med. Assoc.* **291**, 2847–2850

3.   Ford, E.S., Giles, W.H. & Dietz, W.H. (2002) Prevalence of the metabolic syndrome among US adults: findings from the third National Health and Nutrition Examination Survey. *J. Am. Med. Assoc.* **287**, 356–359

4. Mensah, G.A., Mokdad, A.H., Ford, E., Narayan, K.M., Giles, W.H., Vinicor, F. & Deedwania, P.C. (2004) Obesity, metabolic syndrome, and type 2 diabetes: emerging epidemics and their cardio-vascular implications. *Cardiol. Clin.* **22**, 485–504

5. Baron, A.D., Brechtel-Hook, G., Johnson, A. & Hardin, D. (1993) Skeletal muscle blood flow: a possible link between insulin resistance and blood pressure. *Hypertension* **21**, 129–135

6. Fossum, E., Høieggen, A., Moan, A., Rostrup, M., Nordby, G. & Kjeldsen, S.E. (1998) Relationship between insulin sensitivity and maximal forearm blood flow in young men. *Hypertension* **32**, 838–843

7. Capaldo, B., Lembo, G., Napoli, R., Rendina, V., Albano, G., Sacca, L. & Trimarco, B. (1991) Skeletal muscle is a primary site of insulin resistance in essential hypertension. *Metabolism* **40**, 1320–1322

8. Lind, L. & Lithell, H. (1993) Decreased peripheral blood flow in the pathogenesis of the metabolic syndrome comprizing hypertension, hyperlipidemia, and hyperinsulinemia. *Am. Heart J.* **125**, 1494–1497

9. Hamdy, O., Ledbury, S., Mullooly, C., Jarema, C., Porter, S., Ovalle, K., Moussa, A., Caselli, A., Caballero, A.E., Economides, P.A. et al. (2003) Lifestyle modification improves endothelial function in obese subjects with the insulin resistance syndrome. *Diabetes Care.* **26**, 2119–2125

10. Steinberg, O.H., Chaker, H., Leaming, R., Johnson, A., Brechtel, G. & Baron, A.D. (1996) Obesity/insulin resistance is associated with endothelial dysfunction: implications for the syndrome of insulin resistance. *J. Clin. Invest.* **97**, 2601–2610

11. Ferri, C., Bellini, C., Desideri, G., Baldoncini, R., Properzi, G., Santucci, A. & De Mattia G. (1997) Circulating endothelin-1 levels in obese patients with the metabolic syndrome. *Exp. Clin. Endocrinol. Diabetes* **105** (Suppl 2), 38–40

12. Cardillo, C., Campia, U., Bryant, M.B. & Panza, J.A. (2002) Increased activity of endogenous endothelin in patients with type II diabetes mellitus. *Circulation* **106**, 1783–1787

13. Prasad, A., Husain, S. & Quyyumi, A.A. (1999) Effect of enalaprilat on nitric oxide activity in coronary artery disease. *Am. J. Cardiol.* **84**, 1–6

14. Egan, B.M. (2003) Insulin resistance and the sympathetic nervous system. *Curr. Hypertens. Rep.* **5**, 247–254

15. Feener, E.P. & King, G.L. (1997) Vascular dysfunction in diabetes mellitus. *Lancet* **350** (Suppl 1), S9–S13

16. Bray, G.A. (1977) The Zucker-fatty rat: a review. *Fed. Proc.* **36**, 148–153

17. Frisbee, J.C. (2005) Hypertension-independent microvascular rarefaction in the obese Zucker rat model of the metabolic syndrome. *Microcirculation.* **12**, 383–392

18. Johnson, F.K., Johnson, R.A., Durante, W., Jackson, K.E., Stevenson, B.K. & Peyton, K.J. (2006) Metabolic syndrome increases endogenous carbon monoxide production to promote hypertension and endothelial dysfunction in obese Zucker rats. *Am. J. Physiol. Regul. Integr. Comp. Physiol.* **290**, R601–R608

19. Toblli, J.E., Cao, G., DeRosa, G., Di Gennaro, F. & Forcada, P. (2004) Angiotensin-converting enzyme inhibition and angiogenesis in myocardium of obese Zucker rats. *Am. J. Hypertens.* **17**, 172–180

20. Vaziri, N.D., Xu, Z.G., Shahkarami, A., Huang, K.T., Rodriguez-Iturbe, B. & Natarajan, R. (2005) Role of AT-1 receptor in regulation of vascular MCP-1, IL-6, PAI-1, MAP kinase, and matrix expressions in obesity. *Kidney Int.* **68**, 2787–2793

21. Frisbee, J.C. & Stepp, D.W. (2001) Impaired NO-dependent dilation of skeletal muscle arterioles in hypertensive diabetic obese Zucker rats. *Am. J. Physiol. Heart Circ. Physiol.* **281**, H1304–H1311

22. Xiang, L., Naik, J.S., Hodnett, B.L. & Hester, R.L. (2006) Altered arachidonic acid metabolism impairs functional vasodilation in metabolic syndrome. *Am. J. Physiol. Regul. Integr. Comp. Physiol.* **290**, R134–R138

23. Frisbee, J.C. (2004) Enhanced arteriolar α-adrenergic constriction impairs dilator responses and skeletal muscle perfusion in obese Zucker rats. *J. Appl. Physiol.* **97**, 764–772

24. Frisbee, J.C. (2003) Impaired skeletal muscle perfusion in obese Zucker rats. *Am. J. Physiol. Regul. Integr. Comp. Physiol.* **285**, R1124–R1134

25. Frisbee, J.C. (2006) Vascular adrenergic tone and structural narrowing constrain reactive hyperaemia in skeletal muscle of obese Zucker rats. *Am. J. Physiol. Heart Circ. Physiol.* **290**, H2066–H2074

26. Xiang, L., Naik, J. & Hester, R.L. (2005) Exercise-induced increase in skeletal muscle vasodilatory responses in obese Zucker rats. *Am. J. Physiol. Regul. Integr. Comp. Physiol.* **288**, R987–R991

27. Bohlen, H.G. (2004) Protein kinase βII in Zucker obese rats compromises oxygen and flow-mediated regulation of nitric oxide formation. *Am. J. Physiol. Heart Circ. Physiol.* **286**, H492–H497

28. Phillips, S.A., Sylvester, F.A. & Frisbee, J.C. (2005) Oxidant stress and constrictor reactivity impair cerebral artery dilation in obese Zucker rats. *Am. J. Physiol. Regul. Integr. Comp. Physiol.* **288**, R522–R530

29. Fulton, D., Harris, M.B., Kemp, B.E., Venema, R.C., Marrero, M.B. & Stepp, D.W. (2004) Insulin resistance does not diminish eNOS expression, phosphorylation, or binding to HSP-90. *Am. J. Physiol. Heart Circ. Physiol.* **287**, H2384–H2393

30. Geakelman, O., Brodsky, S.V., Zhang, F., Chander, P.N., Friedli, C., Nasjletti, A. & Goligorsky, M.S. (2004) Endothelial dysfunction as a modifier of angiogenic response in Zucker diabetic fat rat: amelioration with Ebselen. *Kidney Int.* **66**, 2337–2347

31. Brzezinska, A.K., Gebremedhin, D., Chilian, W.M., Kalyanaraman, B. & Elliott, S.J. (2000) Peroxynitrite reversibly inhibits $Ca(2+)$-activated $K(+)$ channels in rat cerebral artery smooth muscle cells. *Am. J. Physiol. Heart Circ. Physiol.* **278**, H1883–H1890

32. Janiak, P., Lainee, P., Grataloup, Y., Luyt, C.E., Bidouard, J.P., Michel, J.B., O'Connor, S.E. & Herbert, J.M. (2002) Serotonin receptor blockade improves distal perfusion after lower limb ischaemia in the fatty Zucker rat. *Cardiovasc. Res.* **56**, 293–302

33. Wu, S.Q., Hopfner, R.L., McNeill, J.R., Wilson, T.W. & Gopalakrishnan, V. (2000) Altered paracrine effect of endothelin in blood vessels of the hyperinsulinemic, insulin resistant obese Zucker rat. *Cardiovasc. Res.* **45**, 994–1000

34. van Baak, M.A. (2001) The peripheral sympathetic nervous system in human obesity. *Obes. Rev.* **2**, 3–14

35. Carlson, S.H., Shelton, J., White, C.R. & Wyss, J.M. (2000) Elevated sympathetic activity contributes to hypertension and salt sensitivity in diabetic obese Zucker rats. *Hypertension* **35**, 403–408

36. Stepp, D.W. & Frisbee, J.C. (2002) Augmented adrenergic vasoconstriction in hypertensive diabetic obese Zucker rats. *Am. J. Physiol. Heart Circ. Physiol.* **282**, H816–H820

37. Schreihofer, A.M., Hair, C.D. & Stepp, D.W. (2005) Reduced plasma volume and mesenteric vascular reactivity in obese Zucker rats. *Am. J. Physiol. Regul. Integr. Comp. Physiol.* **288**, R253–R261

38. Naik, J.S., Xiang, L. & Hester, R.L. (2006) Enhanced role for RhoA-associated kinase in adrenergic-mediated vasoconstriction in gracilis arteries from obese Zucker rats. *Am. J. Physiol. Regul. Integr. Comp. Physiol.* **290**, R154–R161

39. Frisbee, J.C. (2006) Impaired hemorrhage tolerance in the obese Zucker rat model of metabolic syndrome. *J. Appl. Physiol.* **100**, 465–473

40. Frisbee, J.C. (2003) Remodeling of the skeletal muscle microcirculation increases resistance to perfusion in obese Zucker rats. *Am. J. Physiol. Heart Circ. Physiol.* **285**, H104–H111

41. Stepp, D.W., Pollock, D.M. & Frisbee, J.C. (2004) Low-flow vascular remodeling in the metabolic syndrome X. *Am. J. Physiol. Heart Circ. Physiol.* **286**, H964–H970

42. Lash, J.M, Sherman, W.M. & Hamlin, R.L. (1989) Capillary basement membrane thickness and capillary density in sedentary and trained obese Zucker rats. *Diabetes* **38**, 854–860

43. Frisbee, J.C. Reduced nitric oxide bioavailability contributes to skeletal muscle microvessel rarefaction in the metabolic syndrome. (2005) *Am. J. Physiol. Reg. Integr. Comp. Physiol.* **289**, R307–R316

12

Microvascular dysfunction: causative role in the association between hypertension, insulin resistance and the metabolic syndrome?

Erik H. Serné*[1], Renate T. de Jongh*,
Etto C. Eringa†, Richard G. Ijzerman*,
Michiel P. de Boer* and Coen D.A. Stehouwer‡

*Department of Internal Medicine, VU Medical Center, PO Box 7057, 1007MB Amsterdam, The Netherlands, †Laboratory for Physiology, Institute for Cardiovascular Research, VU Medical Center, Amsterdam, The Netherlands, and ‡Department of Internal Medicine, Academic Hospital Maastricht, PO Box 5800, 6202 AZ Maastricht, The Netherlands

Abstract

The metabolic syndrome defines a clustering of metabolic risk factors that confers an increased risk for type 2 diabetes and cardiovascular disease. The metabolic syndrome seems to have multiple etiological factors and microvascular dysfunction may be one potential factor explaining the clustering of multiple metabolic risk factors including hypertension, obesity, insulin resistance and glucose intolerance. Microvascular dysfunction may increase not only peripheral vascular resistance and blood pressure, but may also decrease insulin-mediated glucose uptake in muscle. The present article summarizes some of the data concerning the role of microvascular dysfunction in the metabolic syndrome.

[1]To whom correspondence should be addressed (email e.serne@vumc.nl).

Introduction

The metabolic syndrome defines a clustering of metabolic risk factors that confers an increased risk for type 2 diabetes and cardiovascular disease [1]. Obesity and a central body fat distribution, hypertension, insulin resistance, glucose intolerance, dyslipidaemia and proinflammatory and prothrombotic factors are all part of the metabolic syndrome. Previously, a large amount of research has been aimed at elucidating the pathophysiology underlying this clustering of risk factors, since a better understanding may lead to new therapeutic approaches that specifically target underlying causes of the metabolic syndrome.

Recently it has become clear that microvascular dysfunction, by affecting both pressure and flow patterns, may have consequences not only for peripheral vascular resistance, but also for insulin-mediated changes in muscle perfusion and glucose metabolism, shedding new light on the association between hypertension, obesity and impaired insulin-mediated glucose disposal [2–4]. An important consequence of this concept is that any condition that impairs microvascular function will predispose to both insulin resistance and hypertension. The present article examines some of the data concerning the role of microvascular dysfunction as an explanation for the association between hypertension, obesity and impaired insulin-mediated glucose disposal.

Description of the microcirculation

The microcirculation is widely taken to encompass vessels < 150 μm in diameter. It therefore includes arterioles, capillaries and venules. Nowadays, a definition based on arterial vessel physiology rather than diameter or structure has been proposed, depending on the response of the isolated vessel to increased internal pressure [3]. By this definition, all those arterial vessels that respond to increasing pressure by a myogenic reduction in lumen diameter would be included in the microcirculation. Such a definition would include the smallest arteries and arterioles in the microcirculation in addition to capillaries and venules. Small arterial and arteriolar components should, therefore, be considered a continuum rather than distinct sites of resistance control.

A primary function of the microcirculation is to optimize nutrient and oxygen supply within the tissue in response to variations in demand. A second important function is to avoid large fluctuations in hydrostatic pressure at the level of the capillaries causing disturbances in capillary exchange. Finally, it is at the level of the microcirculation that a substantial proportion of the drop in hydrostatic pressure occurs. The microcirculation is therefore extremely important in determining the overall peripheral resistance.

Microvascular function is impaired in hypertension and obesity

In hypertension, the structure and function of the microcirculation are altered in at least three ways [3,5]. First, the mechanisms regulating vasomotor tone are abnormal, leading to enhanced vasoconstriction or reduced vasodilator responses. Secondly, there are anatomical alterations in the structure of individual precapillary resistance vessels, such as an increase in their wall-to-lumen ratio. Finally, there are changes at the level of the microvascular network involving a reduction in the number of arterioles or capillaries within vascular beds of various tissues (e.g. muscle and skin), so called vascular rarefaction [3,5,6]. In obese individuals similar defects in the microcirculation can be demonstrated [7]. Enhanced vasoconstriction and reduced vasodilator responses can be demonstrated in the microcirculation of obese subjects [7]. Rarefaction of arterioles and capillaries within vascular beds of various tissues (e.g. muscle and skin) can also be demonstrated [7]. In addition, measures of obesity in healthy individuals are strongly related to skin microvascular function [2,7].

Taken together, microvascular dysfunction in different tissues has been established in both hypertension and obesity.

Hypertension as a result of microvascular dysfunction

In most forms of experimental and clinical hypertension, cardiac output is close to normal and the peripheral vascular resistance is increased in proportion to the increase in blood pressure [3]. There is general agreement that there is relatively little pressure loss within the large conduit arteries and that the drop in pressure occurs predominantly in vessels ranging from 10 to 300 μm in diameter. The increase in total peripheral vascular resistance therefore, is likely to reflect changes in these vessels. Whereas it has been known for many years that increased wall-to-lumen ratio and microvascular rarefaction can be secondary to sustained elevation of blood pressure [3], there is also evidence that abnormalities in the microcirculation precede and thus may be a causal component of high blood pressure. Microvascular rarefaction similar in magnitude to the rarefaction observed in patients with established hypertension can already be demonstrated in subjects with mild intermittent hypertension, and in normotensive subjects with a genetic predisposition to high blood pressure [3,5,6]. In several tissues capillary density has been found to correlate inversely with peripheral vascular resistance and blood pressure in hypertensive, normotensive lean and normotensive obese subjects [2,6,7]. Moreover, in hypertensive subjects, capillary rarefaction in muscle has been shown to predict the increase in mean arterial pressure over two decades [8]. More recently, a smaller retinal arteriolar diameter has been shown to predict the occurrence and development of hypertension in a

© 2006 The Biochemical Society

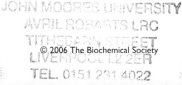

prospective, population-based study of normotensive middle-aged persons [9]. In addition, mathematical modelling of *in vivo* microvascular networks predicts an exponential relationship between capillary and arteriolar number and vascular resistance. Total vessel rarefaction up to 42% (within the range observed in hypertensive humans) can increase tissue vascular resistance by 21%. Thus it seems likely that microvascular abnormalities can both result from and contribute to hypertension, and a 'vicious cycle' may exist in which the microcirculation maintains or even amplifies an initial increase in blood pressure. It has been demonstrated that an initial small increase in pressure can lead to larger structural increases in pressure and flow resistance by a mechanism involving the tendency of vessels to reduce their luminal diameter in response to increased intraluminal pressure [3]. This argument could be taken a step further to suggest that microvascular abnormalities causing an increase in peripheral resistance might initiate the pathogenic sequence in primary hypertension. However, according to the Borst-Guyton concept, chronic hypertension can only occur if renal function is abnormal with a shift in the renal pressure–natriuresis relationship. In the absence of the latter, increased peripheral resistance only temporarily raises blood pressure, to be followed by an increase in renal sodium excretion restoring blood pressure towards normal. Importantly, therefore, subtle renal microvascular disease [10] as well as a reduced number of nephrons [11] may reconcile the Borst-Guyton concept with the putative role of vessel rarefaction in the etiology of high blood pressure. This may also explain the relationship between salt sensitivity of blood pressure, a characteristic of hypertension associated with the metabolic syndrome and insulin resistance [12].

It is important to realize that a decreased capillary density also affects the spatial pattern of flow in the microvascular bed, causing a non-uniform distribution of blood flow among exchange vessels. This non-uniform distribution of flow among vessels, which can be defined as some vessels receiving more and some less of their appropriate fraction of total flow, has been invoked to explain phenomena such as flow-limited muscular performance [13] and sub-optimal capillary transport of small solutes [14]. In addition, it may contribute to various kinds of end-organ damage (e.g. retinopathy, lacunar stroke, microalbuminuria and heart failure) [3].

In summary, microvascular dysfunction, in particular rarefaction, by affecting both pressure and flow patterns, may have consequences not only for peripheral vascular resistance and blood pressure, but also for muscle perfusion and metabolism.

Insulin resistance as a result of microvascular dysfunction

Insulin resistance is typically defined as decreased sensitivity and/or responsiveness to metabolic actions of insulin that promote glucose disposal. A major action of insulin in muscle tissue involves translocation of glucose transporters to the plasma membrane and activation of downstream pathways of glucose metabolism [15]. The glucose transporter protein is considered to be rate-limiting for insulin-stimulated glucose uptake in the muscle [15]. However, before insulin interacts with the receptor on the plasma membrane, insulin and glucose must be delivered to the muscle cells at normal levels and at the correct time. Recently, there has been a surge of interest in these pre-cellular steps, in particular with regard to the possible contribution of insulin-mediated changes in muscle blood flow to insulin-mediated glucose uptake.

Insulin increases total blood flow and blood volume in skeletal muscle [4]. Principally because the ability of insulin to dilate skeletal muscle vasculature is impaired in a wide range of insulin-resistant states (e.g. hypertension, obesity and type 2 diabetes), it has been hypothesized that insulin's vasodilatory and metabolic actions (i.e. glucose disposal) are functionally coupled [4,16,17]. However, despite the compelling nature of these findings, the concept that insulin might control its own access and that of other substances, particularly glucose, has been vigorously challenged. By approaching the experiments differently, in particular with lower doses of insulin and shorter time courses, it was shown that insulin-mediated changes in total blood flow appear to have time kinetics and a dose dependence on insulin different from those for the effect on glucose uptake. In addition, studies in which glucose uptake has been measured during hyperinsulinaemia and manipulation of total limb blood flow with different vasodilators have shown that total limb blood flow could be increased in either normal or insulin-resistant individuals, yet there was no increase in insulin-mediated glucose uptake [4]. The discrepancy in these findings has been ascribed to the fact that various vasoactive agents may change total flow but have distinct effects on the microcirculation and on the distribution of blood flow in nutritive compared with non-nutritive vessels. Clark et al. have introduced the concept that distribution of blood flow in nutritive compared with non-nutritive vessels, independent of total muscle flow, may affect insulin-mediated glucose uptake [4]. Using studies in rats, applying different approaches to measure capillary recruitment (1-methylxanthine metabolism) and microvascular perfusion [CEU (contrast-enhanced ultrasound) and laser Doppler flowmetry], it could be demonstrated that insulin mediates changes in muscle microvascular perfusion consistent with capillary recruitment [4]. This capillary recruitment relates to changes in skeletal muscle glucose uptake independently of changes in total blood flow, requires lower insulin concentrations, and precedes muscle glucose disposal [4,17]. This has led to the hypothesis that insulin, possibly by reducing precapillary arteriolar tone and/or altering arteriolar vasomotion, redirects blood flow from non-nutritive vessels to nutritive capillary beds, resulting in an increased and more homogeneous overall capillary perfusion termed 'functional capillary recruitment'. The latter would enhance the access of insulin and glucose to a greater mass of muscle for metabolism. Consistent with such a mechanism in humans, insulin increases microvascular blood volume as measured with CEU or positron emission tomography and enhances the distribution volume of glucose in human muscle [3,17]. We have shown, by directly visualizing capillaries in human skin, that systemic hyperinsulinaemia is capable of increasing the number of perfused capillaries [7,16]. This insulin-dependent capillary recruitment is impaired in obese insulin-resistant subjects [7,18]. Moreover, it is associated with the number of capillaries recruited during post-occlusive reactive hyperaemia without insulin infusion, a measure of capillary recruitment which has been shown to be related to insulin-mediated whole body glucose uptake [2,6,7] and to be decreased in insulin-resistant hypertensive and obese subjects [6,7]. Making use of iontophoresis and laser Doppler flowmetry, we could also demonstrate that locally applied insulin induced microvascular vasodilation in human skin, independently of insulin's systemic effects [16]. Furthermore, we could demonstrate that systemic hyperinsulinaemia influences microvascular vasomotion in human skin [16] and muscle [19].

Vasomotion, the rhythmic fluctuations of microvascular blood flow, may be an important determinant of the spatial and temporal heterogeneity of microvascular perfusion and, therefore, of the number of perfused capillaries [19]. The origin and control of microvascular vasomotion is still a matter of debate. A central neurogenic regulatory mechanism is suggested by synchronicity on contralateral limbs and by the suppressive effect of central sympathectomy. However, local administration of vasoactive substances such as acetylcholine and sodium nitroprusside directly influences vasomotion. Furthermore, vasomotion has been shown in isolated small arteries, indicating a local regulatory mechanism. In view of these considerations, it can be suggested that vasomotion is regulated by both local vasoactive substances and influences of the central nervous system. The contribution of different regulatory mechanisms can be investigated by analysing the contribution of different frequency intervals to the variability of the laser Doppler signal. Our data suggest that an insulin-mediated effect on microvascular vasomotion occurs by increasing endothelial and neurogenic activity [16,19].

Further insight into the complex relationships among vasodilation, blood flow velocity and capillary recruitment was gained through measurement of the PS (capillary permeability-surface area product) for glucose and insulin. The PS for a substance describes its capacity to reach the interstitial fluid. This depends on the permeability and the capillary surface area, which in turn depends on the extent of capillary recruitment.

A recent investigation employing direct measurements of muscle capillary permeability showed that PS for glucose increased after an oral glucose load, and a further increase was demonstrated during an insulin infusion [20]. The increase of PS was exerted without any concomitant change in total blood flow. It was concluded that the insulin-mediated increase in PS seen after oral glucose is important for the glucose uptake rate in normal muscle [20].

Interestingly, PS for glucose is subnormal under steady-state insulin clamp conditions in insulin-resistant type 2 diabetic subjects [20]. Moreover, a close and positive correlation was demonstrated between the rate of muscle glucose uptake and PS for glucose. A stimulated uptake of glucose and insulin in the absence of an increased PS would, hypothetically, lead to depletion of these substances and a lowered interstitial concentration. Importantly, at steady state levels, the interstitial muscle insulin and glucose concentrations nevertheless were normal in the type 2 diabetes group. The concomitant cellular insulin resistance leading to a subnormal glucose uptake rate may balance the low transcapillary transport rate of glucose and insulin so that the interstitial fluid concentrations stay normal [20]. The importance of the perturbed capillary recruitment for the reduction in glucose uptake is evident, however, because a normal increase in PS in type 2 diabetes muscle would lead to supernormal interstitial concentrations [20].

Another aspect of insulin resistance is a delay in insulin action [21]. Previously it has been reported that the time of onset of insulin action is delayed in insulin-resistant obese, type 2 diabetic and hypertensive subjects. A delayed transcapillary insulin transport in insulin-resistant states has been reported from *in vitro* studies and some human *in vivo* studies. Moreover, in obese subjects, this delay in insulin action was accompanied by a slow delivery of insulin to the muscle interstitial fluid during insulin/glucose infusion [21].

These data illustrate the importance of the microcirculation in regulating nutrient and hormone access to muscle, and raise the possibility that any impairment in capillary recruitment may cause an impairment in glucose uptake by muscle.

Mechanisms involved in impairment of insulin-mediated capillary recruitment

Vascular insulin resistance

Insulin-stimulated glucose uptake in skeletal muscle and adipose tissue is mediated by translocation of the insulin-responsive glucose transporter GLUT4 to the cell surface. This requires PI3K (phosphatidylinositol 3-kinase)-dependent signalling pathways that involve the insulin receptor, IRS-1 (insulin receptor substrate-1), PI3K, PDK1 (phosphoinositide-dependent kinase 1) and Akt (protein kinase B) [22]. Ras/MAPK (mitogen-activated protein kinase) pathways do not contribute significantly to insulin-stimulated translocation of GLUT4, but are important for insulin-mediated regulation of growth and mitogenesis [23,24]. Interestingly, the vascular actions of insulin that stimulate the production of NO (nitric oxide) require PI3K-dependent insulin-signalling pathways that bear striking similarities to metabolic insulin-signalling pathways (Figure 2). Moreover, the MAPK branch of insulin signalling controls secretion of ET-1 (endothelin-1), a strong vasoconstrictor, by the endothelium [22–24]. Insulin has therefore opposing haemodynamic actions on vessels. In vessels from healthy rats, insulin has no net effect on vessel diameter, because of a balance between the stimulation of two pathways, NO-mediated vasodilation and ET-1-mediated vasoconstriction. Insulin stimulates activation of endothelial NO synthase: the signalling pathway is through IRS-1, PI3K and Akt [22]. However, if this pathway is inhibited, the arteriole constricts, a response mediated by ET-1 through the Ras/MAPK and ERK1/2 (extracellular signal-related kinase-1/2) pathway [24]. These observations imply a dual insulin signalling mechanism in vessels, one pathway stimulating the synthesis of NO, the other stimulating ET-1 release. In obese rats, these signalling pathways are selectively impaired: insulin-mediated activation of the ET-1 pathway is impaired, but insulin-mediated activation of ERK1/2 is intact [25]. In line with this evidence, we have recently found insulin-induced, ET-1-dependent vasoconstriction in skeletal muscle arterioles of obese rats (E.C. Eringa, C.D.A. Stehouwer, M.H. Roos, N. Westerhof and P. Sipkema, unpublished work). In addition, insulin resistance in spontaneously hypertensive rats is associated with endothelial dysfunction characterized by an imbalance between NO and ET-1 production [26]. Moreover, obese, hypertensive individuals show an insulin-induced vasoconstriction and increased ET-1-dependent vasoconstrictor tone and decreased NO-dependent vasodilator tone at the level of the resistance arteries [27]. Thus, shared insulin-signalling pathways in metabolic and vascular target tissues with complementary functions may provide a mechanism to couple the regulation of glucose and haemodynamic homoeostasis. The net haemodynamic action of insulin is dependent on a balance between its vasodilator and vasoconstrictor effects. An imbalance between NO and ET-1 production may explain insulin resistance-related hypertension.

Obesity-related endocrine signalling

The close association between measures of adiposity and microvascular function necessitates communicative pathways between adipose tissue and the microvasculature. Adipose tissue and in particular visceral adipose tissue cells secrete a variety of bioactive substances called adipokines such as NEFAs (non-esterified fatty acids), adiponectin, leptin, resistin, angiotensinogen and TNF-α (tumour necrosis factor-α). In the next section we will focus on the role of NEFAs and TNF-α.

Using magnetic resonance spectroscopy, NEFA-induced insulin resistance in humans has been shown to result from a significant reduction in the intramyocellular glucose concentration, suggestive of glucose transport as the affected rate-limiting step [15]. The current hypothesis, supported by data from PKC-θ (protein kinase Cθ) knockout mice, proposes that fatty acids upon entering the muscle cell activate PKC-θ as either fatty acyl-CoA or diacylglycerol. The PKC-θ activates a serine kinase cascade leading to the phosphorylation

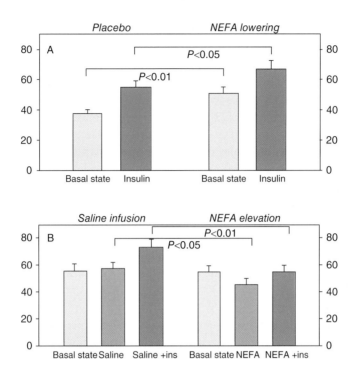

Figure 1. Capillary recruitment (%) before and during hyperinsulinaemia in obese women
Effects of NEFA lowering versus placebo **(A)**. Capillary recruitment (%) before and during hyper-insulinaemia in lean women. Effects of NEFA elevation versus saline infusion (control) **(B)**.

and inactivation of IRS-1 by preventing its activation by tyrosine phosphorylation [23]. Since the technique of magnetic resonance spectroscopy only identifies a gradient from extracellular to intracellular glucose in muscle cells, it remains to be proven that the gradient did not occur between the plasma and interstitial glucose and thus reflects a rate limiting step of glucose delivery induced by fatty acids. Interestingly, studies suggest that glucose delivery contributes to sustaining the transmembrane glucose gradient and, therefore, is a determinant of glucose transport [28]. This would be consistent with the finding in rats that NEFA elevation concomitantly impairs insulin-mediated muscle capillary recruitment and glucose uptake [4,17]. In addition, we could demonstrate that in lean individuals, NEFA elevation induces skin microvascular dysfunction and reduces whole body glucose uptake, while in obese individuals NEFA lowering has the opposite effect (Figure 1) [18]. Moreover, changes in capillary recruitment statistically explained approx. 29% of the association between changes in NEFA levels and insulin-mediated glucose uptake. A defect involving fatty-acid-induced impaired insulin signalling through the same PKC-θ mechanism in endothelial cells, which in turn may negatively influence the balance between insulin-mediated vasodilation and vasoconstriction, may be responsible for the impaired capillary recruitment.

Increased production of the proinflammatory cytokine TNF-α is associated with obesity-related insulin resistance [29] as well as obesity-related hypertension [30]. In rats, TNF-α elevation concomitantly impairs insulin-mediated muscle capillary recruitment and glucose uptake [4,17]. In addition, in humans, circulating TNF-α levels are associated with reduced whole body glucose uptake and skin capillary recruitment [29]. In isolated skeletal muscle resistance arteries, we could demonstrate that TNF-α impairs the vasodilator effects but not the vasoconstrictor effects of insulin through activation of the intracellular enzyme JNK (c-Jun N-terminal kinase) and impairment of insulin-mediated activation of Akt [31]. This selective inhibition of the vasodilator effects of insulin results in insulin-mediated vasoconstriction in the presence of TNF-α. JNK has been shown to regulate whole-body insulin sensitivity as well as insulin-mediated cell signalling [32]. In conclusion, both NEFA and TNF-α are likely candidates to link visceral adipose tissue with defects in microvascular function, at least in part by influencing insulin signalling and thereby insulin's vascular effects.

Vasocrine signalling

We have recently hypothesized an alternative communicative pathway [33]. Obese Zucker rats are characterized by a well-circumscribed depot of fat cells around the origin of the nutritive arteriole supplying the cremaster muscle whereas lean rats are not. Adipokines released by these fat cells may directly inhibit vasodilatory pathways distal in the arteriole and thereby cause loss of blood flow in the nutritive capillary network supplied by this arteriole (Figure 2).

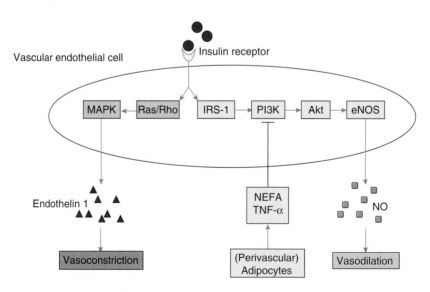

Figure 2. Mechanisms of insulin-mediated NO and ET-1 production leading to vasodilation and vasoconstriction respectively
Adipokines secreted by (perivascular) adipocytes inhibit the PI3K pathway of insulin signalling. eNOS, endothelial nitric oxide synthase.

In this hypothesis, which remains to be tested, adipokines released from periarteriolar fat depots have a local rather than a systemic vasoregulatory effect, which we named 'vasocrine'.

Conclusion

The metabolic syndrome defines a clustering of metabolic risk factors that confers an increased risk for type 2 diabetes and cardiovascular disease. The metabolic syndrome seems to have multiple etiological factors. A complex interaction between microvascular function, intracellular insulin signalling pathways and obesity-related endocrine signalling molecules may be one potential factor explaining the clustering of multiple metabolic risk factors such as hypertension, obesity, insulin resistance and glucose intolerance. A better understanding of the pathophysiology underlying the clustering of risk factors may lead to new therapeutic approaches that specifically target underlying causes of the metabolic syndrome. Microvascular dysfunction may play a central role by increasing not only peripheral vascular resistance and blood pressure, but also decreasing insulin-mediated glucose uptake in target cells (Figure 3).

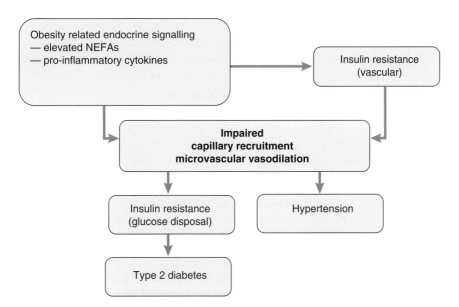

Figure 3. Microvascular dysfunction: postulated causative role in the association between hypertension, insulin resistance and the metabolic syndrome
Microvascular dysfunction of any cause may play a central role by increasing not only peripheral vascular resistance and blood pressure, but also decreasing insulin-mediated glucose uptake in target cells.

Summary

- *The metabolic syndrome defines a clustering of metabolic risk factors that confers an increased risk for type 2 diabetes and cardiovascular disease.*
- *Microvascular dysfunction, may be one potential factor explaining part of this clustering of multiple metabolic risk factors including hypertension, obesity and insulin resistance.*
- *Microvascular abnormalities such as vascular rarefaction can cause an increase in peripheral resistance and might initiate the pathogenic sequence in hypertension.*
- *Insulin has direct effects (increasing glucose uptake in skeletal muscle) and substantial indirect effects (promoting glucose disposal by redistributing blood flow from non-nutritive to nutritive vessels). This cross-talk between metabolic and vascular tissues is important for coupling glucose homoeostasis and (micro)vascular function.*
- *Shared insulin-signalling pathways in metabolic and vascular target tissues may provide a mechanism to couple the regulation of glucose and haemodynamic homoeostasis. Metabolic insulin resistance is characterized by pathway-specific impairment in PI3K-dependent signalling, which in endothelium may cause imbalance between production of NO and secretion of ET-1, leading to decreased microvascular perfusion and an impairment in glucose uptake.*
- *NEFAs and proinflammatory cytokines including TNF-α may contribute to impairment of insulin's metabolic and vascular actions by modulating insulin signalling and transcription.*

References

1. Grundy, S.M., Brewer, Jr, H.B., Cleeman, J.I., Smith, Jr, S.C., & Lenfant, C. (2004) Definition of metabolic syndrome: Report of the National Heart, Lung, and Blood Institute/American Heart Association conference on scientific issues related to definition. *Circulation* **109**, 433–438
2. Serné, E.H., Stehouwer, C.D., ter Maaten, J.C., ter Wee, P.M., Rauwerda, J.A., Donker, A.J. & Gans, R.O. (1999) Microvascular function relates to insulin sensitivity and blood pressure in normal subjects. *Circulation* **99**, 896–902
3. Levy, B.I., Ambrosio, G., Pries, A.R. & Struijker-Boudier, H.A. (2001) Microcirculation in hypertension: a new target for treatment? *Circulation* **104**, 736–741
4. Clark, M.G., Wallis, M.G., Barrett, E.J., Vincent, M.A., Richards, S.M., Clerk, L.H. & Rattigan, S. (2003) Blood flow and muscle metabolism: a focus on insulin action. *Am. J. Physiol. Endocrinol. Metab.* **284**, E241–E258
5. Serné, E.H., Gans, R.O., ter Maaten, J.C., Tangelder, G.J., Donker, A.J. & Stehouwer, C.D. (2001) Impaired skin capillary recruitment in essential hypertension is caused by both functional and structural capillary rarefaction. *Hypertension* **38**, 238–242
6. Serné, E.H., Gans, R.O., ter Maaten, J.C., ter Wee, P.M., Donker, A.J. & Stehouwer, C.D. (2001) Capillary recruitment is impaired in essential hypertension and relates to insulin's metabolic and vascular actions. *Cardiovasc. Res.* **49**, 161–168

7. de Jongh, R.T., Serné, E.H., IJzerman, R.G., de Vries, G. & Stehouwer, C.D. (2004) Impaired microvascular function in obesity: implications for obesity-associated microangiopathy, hypertension and insulin resistance. *Circulation* **109**, 2529–2535

8. Hedman, A., Reneland, R. & Lithell, H.O. (2000) Alterations in skeletal muscle morphology in glucose-tolerant elderly hypertensive men: relationship to development of hypertension and heart rate. *J. Hypertens.* **18**, 559–565

9. Wong, T.Y., Klein, R., Sharrett, A.R., Duncan, B.B., Couper, D.J., Klein, B.E., Hubbard, L.D. & Nieto, F.J. (2004) Retinal arteriolar diameter and risk for hypertension. *Ann. Intern. Med.* **140**, 248–255

10. Johnson, R.J., Herrera-Acosta, J., Schreiner, G.F. & Rodriguez-Iturbe, B. (2002) Subtle acquired renal injury as a mechanism of salt-sensitive hypertension. *N. Engl. J. Med.* **346**, 913–923

11. le Noble, F.A., Stassen, F.R., Hacking, W.J. & Struijker Boudier, H.A. (1998) Angiogenesis and hypertension. *J. Hypertens.* **16**, 1563–1572

12. Galletti, F., Strazzullo, P., Ferrara, I., Annuzzi, G., Rivellese, A.A., Gatto, S. & Mancini, M. (1997) NaCl sensitivity of essential hypertensive patients is related to insulin resistance. *J. Hypertens.* **15**, 1485–1491

13. Wright, D.L. & Sonnenschein, R.R. (1965) Relations among activity, blood flow and vascular state in skeletal muscle. *Am. J. Physiol.* **208**, 782–789

14. Ellis, C.G., Wrigley, S.M. & Groom, A.C. (1994) Heterogeneity of red blood cell perfusion in capillary networks supplied by a single arteriole in resting skeletal muscle. *Circ. Res.* **75**, 357–368

15. Shulman, G.I. (2004) Unraveling the cellular mechanism of insulin resistance in humans: new insights from magnetic resonance spectroscopy. *Physiology* **19**, 183–190

16. Serné, E.H., IJzerman, R.G., Gans, R.O., Nijveldt, R., de Vries, G., Evertz, R., Donker, A.J. & Stehouwer, C.D. (2002) Direct evidence for insulin-induced capillary recruitment in skin of healthy subjects during physiological hyperinsulinemia. *Diabetes* **51**, 1515–1522

17. Vincent, M.A., Clerk, L.H., Rattigan, S., Clark, M.G. & Barrett, E.J. (2005) Active role for the vasculature in the delivery of insulin to skeletal muscle. *Clin. Exp. Pharmacol. Physiol.* **32**, 302–307

18. de Jongh, R.T., Serné, E.H., IJzerman, R.G., de Vries, G. & Stehouwer, C.D. (2004) Free fatty acid levels modulate microvascular function: relevance for obesity-associated insulin resistance, hypertension and microangiopathy. *Diabetes* **53**, 2873–2882

19. de Jongh, R.T., Clark, A.D., IJzerman, R.G., Serné, E.H., de Vries, G. & Stehouwer, C.D. (2004) Physiological hyperinsulinaemia increases intramuscular microvascular reactive hyperaemia and vasomotion in healthy volunteers. *Diabetologia* **47**, 978–986

20. Gudbjornsdottir, S., Sjostrand, M., Strindberg, L. & Lonnroth, P. (2005) Decreased muscle capilary permeability surface area in type 2 diabetic subjects. *J. Clin. Endocrinol. Metab.* **90**, 1078–1082

21. Sjostrand, M., Gudbjornsdottir, S., Holmang, A., Lonn, L., Strindberg, L. & Lonnroth, P. (2002) Delayed transcapillary transport of insulin to muscle interstitial fluid in obese subjects. *Diabetes* **51**, 2742–2748

22. Eringa, E.C., Stehouwer, C.D., Merlijn, T., Westerhof, N. & Sipkema, P. (2002) Physiological concentrations of insulin induce endothelin-mediated vasoconstriction during inhibition of NOS or PI3-kinase in skeletal muscle arterioles. *Cardiovasc. Res.* **56**, 464–471

23. Kim, J.A., Montagnani, M., Koh, K.K. & Quon, M.J. (2006) Reciprocal relationships between insulin resistance and endothelial dysfunction: molecular and pathophysiological mechanisms. *Circulation* **113**, 1888–1904

24. Eringa, E.C., Stehouwer, C.D., Nieuw Amerongen, G.P., Ouwehand, L., Westerhof, N. & Sipkema, P. (2004) Vasoconstrictor effects of insulin in skeletal muscle arterioles are mediated by ERK1/2 activation in endothelium. *Am. J. Physiol. Heart Circ. Physiol.* **287**, H2043–H2048

25. Jiang, Z.Y., Lin, Y.W., Clemont, A., Feener, E.P., Hein, K.D., Igarashi, M., Yamauchi, T., White, M.F. & King, G.L. (1999) Characterization of selective resistance to insulin signaling in the vasculature of obese Zucker (fa/fa) rats. *J. Clin. Invest.* **104**, 447–457

26. Potenza, M.A., Marasciulo, F.L., Chieppa, D.M., Brigiani, G.S., Formoso, G., Quon, M.J. & Montagnani, M. (2005) Insulin resistance in spontaneously hypertensive rats is associated with endothelial dysfunction characterized by imbalance between NO and ET-1 production. *Am. J. Physiol. Heart Circ. Physiol.* **289**, H813–H822

27. Cardillo, C., Campia, U., Iantorno, M. & Panza, J.A. (2004) Enhanced vascular activity of endogenous endothelin-1 in obese hypertensive patients. *Hypertension* **43**, 36–40

28. Kelley, D.E., Williams, K.V. & Price, J.C. (1999) Insulin regulation of glucose transport and phosphorylation in skeletal muscle assessed by PET. *Am. J. Physiol.* **277**, E361–E369

29. IJzerman, R.G., Voordouw, J.J., van Weissenbruch, M.M., Yudkin, J.S., Serné, E.H., Delemarre-van de Waal, H.A. & Stehouwer, C.D. (2005) TNF-α levels are associated with skin capillary recruitment in humans: a potential explanation for the relationship between TNF-α and insulin resistance. *Clin. Sci.* **110**, 361–368

30. Pausova, Z., Deslauriers, B., Gaudet, D., Tremblay, J., Kotchen, T.A., Larochelle, P., Cowley, A.W. & Hamet, P. (2000) Role of tumor necrosis factor-α gene locus in obesity and obesity-associated hypertension in French Canadians. *Hypertension* **36**, 14–19

31. Eringa, E.C., Stehouwer, C.D., Walburg, K., Clark, A.D., Nieuw Amerongen, G.P., Westerhof, N. & Sipkema, P. (2006) Physiological concentrations of insulin induce endothelin-dependent vasoconstriction of skeletal muscle resistance arteries in the presence of tumor necrosis factor-α dependence on c-Jun N-terminal kinase. *Arterioscler. Thromb. Vasc. Biol.* **26**, 274–280

32. Hirosumi, J., Tuncman, G., Chang, L., Gorgun, C.Z., Uysal, K.T., Maeda, K., Karin, M. & Hotamisligil, G.S. (2002) A central role for JNK in obesity and insulin resistance. *Nature* **420**, 333–336

33. Yudkin, J.S., Eringa, E. & Stehouwer, C.D. (2005) "Vasocrine" signalling from perivascular fat: a mechanism linking insulin resistance to vascular disease. *Lancet* **365**, 1817–1820

13

Exercise, genetics and prevention of type 2 diabetes

Gang Hu*†[1], Jesús Rico-Sanz‡, Timo A. Lakka§ and Jaakko Tuomilehto*† ||

Department of Epidemiology and Health Promotion, National Public Health Institute, Helsinki, Finland, †Department of Public Health, University of Helsinki, Helsinki, Finland, ‡Laboratory of Internal Medicine, Department of Medicine, University of Kuopio, Kuopio, Finland, §Institute of Biomedicine, Department of Physiology, University of Kuopio, and Kuopio Research Institute of Exercise Medicine, Kuopio, Finland, and || South Ostrobothnia Central Hospital, Seinäjoki, Finland

Abstract

Type 2 diabetes is one of the fastest growing public health problems in both developed and developing countries. Cardiovascular disease is the most prevalent complication of type 2 diabetes. In the past decade, the associations of physical activity, physical fitness and changes in the lifestyle with the risk of type 2 diabetes have been assessed by a number of prospective studies and clinical trials. A few studies have also evaluated the joint associations of physical activity, body mass index and glucose levels with the risk of type 2 diabetes. The results based on prospective studies and clinical trials have shown that moderate or high levels of physical activity or physical fitness and changes in the lifestyle (dietary modification and increase in physical activity) can prevent type 2 diabetes.

[1]To whom correspondence should be addressed (email hu.gang@ktl.fi).

Introduction

It has been estimated that the number of individuals with diabetes among adults 20 or more years of age will double from the current 171 million in 2000 to 366 million in 2030 [1]. Both genetic and environmental factors are involved in the etiology of type 2 diabetes [2]. Results from prospective cohort studies and clinical trials have shown that moderate or high levels of physical activity or physical fitness, and changes in lifestyle (dietary modification, increase in physical activity and weight loss) can prevent type 2 diabetes. Despite sedentary lifestyle and obesity being the two important lifestyle risk factors for type 2 diabetes [3], few studies have been conducted on the interactions between exercise and genetic markers on type 2 diabetes and related metabolic traits in humans. It would be important to understand which genotypes are well and which are poorly responsive to diverse physical activity levels or exercise training programmes; that is, they may or may not result in favourable modifications in disease progression or outcome. In this chapter, we summarize the current evidence regarding the role of physical activity, physical fitness and the interactions between physical activity and the genotype in the primary prevention of type 2 diabetes.

Physical activity and type 2 diabetes: data from prospective cohort studies

The association between physical activity and the risk of type 2 diabetes was studied in 5990 male alumni from the University of Pennsylvania [4]. Leisure-time physical activity was inversely associated with the risk of type 2 diabetes. For each 500 kcal/week increment in leisure-time physical activity, the age-adjusted risk of developing diabetes decreased by 6%, even after adjustment for obesity, hypertension and parental history of diabetes. Two large studies confirmed these findings. The Nurses' Health Study and the Health Professionals' Follow-up Study found a progressive reduction in the multivariable-adjusted relative risk of type 2 diabetes across increasing quintiles of leisure-time physical activity, with risks being 26%–38% lower in the highest versus the lowest quintile [5,6]

Subsequently, the inverse relation between physical activity and type 2 diabetes has also been observed in prospective studies from several different countries. The results from the British Regional Heart Study indicated that men who engaged in moderate levels of physical activity had a 60% reduced risk of type 2 diabetes compared with physically inactive men, after adjustment for BMI (body mass index) and other confounding factors [7]. In Japanese male office workers, aged 35–59 years, who were free of diabetes, impaired fasting glucose, hypertension and cardiovascular disease at baseline, found that physical activity in daily life, expressed in terms of daily energy expenditure, was inversely associated with the risk of developing impaired fasting glucose or type 2 diabetes after adjustment for BMI and other potential confounding factors [8]. The MONICA/KORA Augsburg Cohort Study examined sex-specific associations between leisure-time physical activity and incidence of type 2 diabetes among 4069 German men and 4034 women 25–74 years of age, who were followed for 7.4 years [9]. A significant inverse association between leisure-time physical activity and incidence of type 2 diabetes was found in both men and women, but more consistently in women, after adjustment for BMI and other confounding factors.

We recently investigated 6898 Finnish men and 7392 women 35–64 years of age without a history of stroke, coronary heart disease or diabetes at base-line [10]. During a mean follow-up of 12 years, there were 373 incident cases of drug-treated or clinically diagnosed type 2 diabetes. A moderate level of physical activity at work was associated with a 30% reduction in the risk of type 2 diabetes compared with a low level, whilst a high level of physical activity at work was associated with a 26% reduction in the risk (Table 1). For moderate and high levels of leisure-time physical activity, the risk reductions were 19% and 16% respectively, compared with low levels. Daily walking or cycling to and from work for more than 30 min was also inversely associated with the risk. These associations were independent of BMI and other factors. We also evaluated the independent and joint associations of physical activity, BMI and plasma glucose levels on the risk of type 2 diabetes [11]. We classified participants into three levels of physical activity: (i) low occupational, leisure-time and commuting physical activity, (ii) moderate to high physical activity for only one kind of activity, and (iii) moderate to high physical activity for at least two kinds of activity. Level 2 physical activity was associated with a 15% reduction and level 3 with a 57% decrease in the risk of type 2 diabetes compared with level 1. The inverse association was observed both among individuals with BMI <30 kg/m^2 and ≥30 kg/m^2, and among those with normal and impaired glucose homoeostasis (Figures 1A and 1B). We also examined the joint relations among physical activity, BMI, plasma glucose and risk of type 2 diabetes (Figure 2). Obese individuals with low physical activity and impaired glucose homoeostasis had a 30-fold risk compared with non-obese persons with high physical activity and normal glucose.

These prospective studies, conducted among different populations and assessing different domains of activity, indicate that regular physical activity at work or during commuting, leisure time or daily life reduces the risk of type 2 diabetes by 15%–60%, with most studies showing a 30%–50% reduction in the risk. The benefit of physical activity is apparent in both men and women, and independent of age and other factors. Nevertheless, residual confounding due to unmeasured factors may still be present. In addition, questionnaires that are typically used in these studies are imprecise measurements of habitual physical activity. Random misclassification of physical activity, particularly over-report of the amount of physical activity, may have resulted in underestimation of the risk reduction between physical activity and type 2 diabetes. Studies assessing cardiorespiratory fitness, an objective indicator of physical activity level, provide additional information on the health effects of physical activity.

Table 1. Relative risks of type 2 diabetes according to different levels of occupational, commuting, and leisure-time physical activity among Finns

Model 1, adjusted for age, sex, and study year; Model 2, adjusted for the factors in Model 1, plus systolic blood pressure, smoking status, education, and the two other kinds of physical activity; Model 3, adjusted for the factors in Model 2, plus BMI. Data taken from [10].

Physical activity	No. of cases	Person-years	Relative risk (95% confidence interval)		
			Model 1	Model 2	Model 3
Occupational physical activity					
Light	199	67250	1.00	1.00	1.00
Moderate	63	48184	0.57 (0.43–0.76)	0.66 (0.49–0.90)	0.70 (0.52–0.96)
Active	111	55695	0.76 (0.60–0.97)	0.73 (0.56–0.94)	0.74 (0.57–0.95)
P value for trend			<0.001	0.008	0.020
Walking or cycling to/from work					
0 min/day	242	81556	1.00	1.00	1.00
1–29 min/day	93	54576	0.75 (0.59–0.96)	0.88 (0.68–1.15)	0.96 (0.74–1.25)
≥ 30 min/day	38	34998	0.42 (0.30–0.59)	0.54 (0.38–0.77)	0.64 (0.45–0.92)
P value for trend			<0.001	0.003	0.048
Leisure-time physical activity					
Low	173	56387	1.00	1.00	1.00
Moderate	166	88350	0.63 (0.50–0.78)	0.67 (0.53–0.84)	0.81 (0.64–1.02)
Active	34	26392	0.52 (0.36–0.75)	0.61 (0.41–0.90)	0.84 (0.57–1.25)
P value for trend			<0.001	0.001	0.186

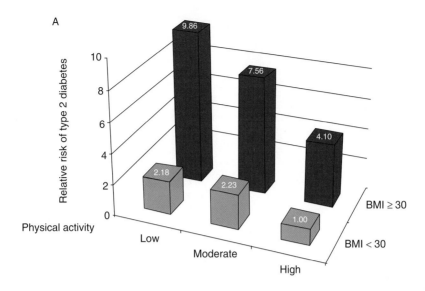

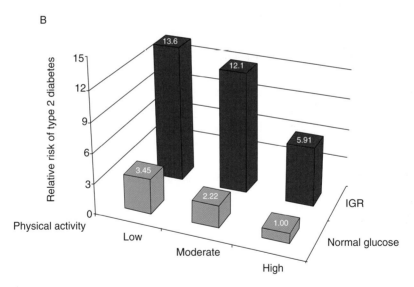

Figure 1. Relative risks of type 2 diabetes according to different levels of (a) physical activity and BMI (< 30 kg/m² and ≥ 30 kg/m²) and (b) physical activity and glucose (normal glucose, IGR)
Adjusted for age, sex, study year, systolic blood pressure, smoking status, education and BMI. IGR, impaired glucose regulation. Reproduced with permission from the American Medical Association. Source: Hu et al. (2004) Arch. Intern. Med. **164**, 892–896.

How much physical activity is required for a reduction in risk of type 2 diabetes? Whilst the data are sparse, it appears that even 30 min of moderate intensity physical activity per day is sufficient to reduce the risk. Additional benefits will

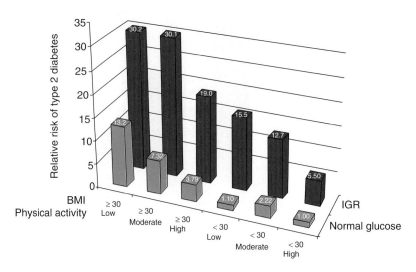

Figure 2. Relative risks of type 2 diabetes according to joint levels of physical activity, BMI and glucose homoeostasis
Adjusted for age, sex, study year, systolic blood pressure, smoking status and education. IGR, impaired glucose regulation. Reproduced with permission from the American Medical Association. Source: Hu et al. (2004) Arch. Intern. Med. **164**, 892–896.

likely be derived if activity levels exceed this level. Several studies found that the magnitude of the inverse association between walking and the risk of type 2 diabetes was similar to that between vigorous leisure activity and risk [5,6,8]. Perhaps some 30 min/day of brisk walking is sufficient. Additionally, sedentary behaviours, especially television watching, were associated with significantly elevated risk of type 2 diabetes [6]. Each 2 h increment in television watching per day was shown to be associated with a 14%–20% increase in the risk of type 2 diabetes [6].

Physical fitness and type 2 diabetes: data from prospective cohort studies

There is a much smaller body of evidence on the role of physical fitness in preventing type 2 diabetes. In the Aerobics Center Longitudinal Study comprising 8633 U.S. men aged 30–79 years men with low cardiorespiratory fitness (the least fit 20%) had a 3.7-fold risk of developing type 2 diabetes compared with men with high fitness (the most fit 40%) [12]. The CARDIA (Coronary Artery Risk Development in Young Adults) Study among 4487 U.S. men and women 18–30 years of age assessed whether low fitness, estimated by a short duration on a maximal treadmill test, predicted the development of type 2 diabetes or the metabolic syndrome, and whether improving fitness (increase in treadmill test duration between examinations) was associated with risk reduction [13]. After adjustment for BMI and other factors, participants with low fitness (bottom 20%) were about twice as likely to develop type 2 diabetes or the metabolic syndrome as those with high fitness (top 40%). Moreover, increasing fitness level during the 7 year study was associated with a 60% reduction in risk of type 2 diabetes and 50% reduction in risk of the metabolic syndrome [13].

These studies of physical fitness, primarily in men, show similar findings to the studies of physical activity, but with generally larger magnitudes of association. One explanation for this may be that measures of fitness are less prone to measurement error and misclassification than measures of physical activity. Additionally, factors other than physical activity may influence both physical fitness and health through related biological factors [14].

Change in lifestyle and type 2 diabetes: data from clinical trials

In recent years, several clinical trials have assessed whether regular physical activity, with or without dietary intervention, can reduce progression to type 2 diabetes among adults with impaired glucose tolerance [15–19].

The Malmö Study from Sweden targeted increased physical activity and weight loss as major intervention strategies to prevent and delay type 2 diabetes in a non-randomized clinical trial conducted among participants with impaired glucose tolerance [15]. Subjects participating in the exercise programme had less than half the risk of developing type 2 diabetes during a 5 year follow-up, compared with those who did not participate. In the Chinese study from Da Qing, 577 individuals with impaired glucose tolerance were randomized, by clinic, into one of the four groups: exercise only, diet only, diet plus exercise, and a control group [16]. The cumulative incidence of type 2 diabetes during 6 years was significantly lower in the exercise group (41%), diet group (44%), and diet plus exercise group (46%), compared with the control group (68%), and remained significant even after adjusting for differences in baseline body mass index and fasting glucose.

In the Finnish Diabetes Prevention Study (DPS), 522 middle-aged men (33%) and women (67%), who were overweight (mean BMI 31 kg/m^2) and had impaired glucose tolerance, were randomized either to an intensive lifestyle intervention group or a control group [17]. The participants in the intervention group had frequent consultation visits with a nutritionist. They received individual advice about how to achieve the intervention goals, which were: (i) reduction in body weight of 5% or more, (ii) total fat intake less than 30% of energy consumed, (iii) saturated fat intake less than 10% of energy consumed, (iv) fibre intake of at least 15 g per 1000 kcal, and (v) moderate exercise for at least 30 min per day. After the intensive intervention period, there was a maintenance phase that included a counselling session every three months. At each of these counselling sessions, exercise habits were discussed, and all kinds of physical activity were strongly recommended. Endurance exercise, including walking, jogging, swimming, aerobic ball games and skiing, was recommended to increase aerobic capacity and cardiorespiratory fitness. Participants were also offered an opportunity to attend supervised, progressive, individually tailored circuit-type resistance training sessions. The mean amount of weight lost between baseline and the end of year two was 3.5 kg in the intervention group and 0.8 kg in the control group. The cumulative incidence of type 2 diabetes after four years was 11% in the intervention group and 23% in the control group ($P<0.001$). During the entire trial, the risk of diabetes was reduced by 58% in the intervention group ($P<0.001$). The reduction in the incidence of diabetes was directly associated with changes in lifestyle; there was a strong inverse correlation between the number of intervention goals achieved (zero to five) and the incidence of diabetes. In fact, none of the participants achieving four or five of the five intervention goals developed diabetes.

A similar randomized clinical trial of lifestyle change and the risk of developing type 2 diabetes among persons at high risk, the DPP (Diabetes Prevention Program), was conducted in the U.S. Non-diabetic persons with elevated fasting and post-load plasma glucose concentrations were randomized to a placebo group, a group assigned metformin, or a group assigned to a lifestyle-modification program with the goals of at least a 7% weight loss and at least 150 min of physical activity per week [18]. The physical activity intervention emphasized brisk walking, but other activities with equivalent intensity were also recommended. Participants were advised to distribute their physical activity throughout the week, with sessions lasting at least 10 min. Voluntary, supervised physical activity sessions were offered at least twice per week throughout the study, including group walks, aerobic classes, and one-to-one personal training. After an average follow-up of 2.8 years, the incidence of diabetes was 11.0, 7.8 and 4.8 cases per 100 person-years in the placebo, metformin and lifestyle groups respectively. The lifestyle intervention reduced the incidence by 58% (95% confidence interval, 48%–66%) and metformin by 31% (95% confidence interval 17%–43%), compared with placebo. Noteworthy was the finding that the lifestyle intervention was significantly more effective than metformin in the prevention of type 2 diabetes.

Recently, in the Indian Diabetes Prevention Programme, 531 individuals with impaired glucose tolerance were randomized into four groups: a group assigned metformin, a group assigned to a lifestyle-modification, a group assigned to both lifestyle-modification and metformin, and a control group [19]. The cumulative incidence of type 2 diabetes during the median follow-up period (30 months) was significantly lower in the lifestyle-modification group (39%), the metformin group (41%), and the lifestyle-modification plus metformin group (40%), compared with the control group (55%).

Gene: physical activity interactions and diabetes risk

Genome-wide linkage scans
Genome-wide linkage scans provide useful information about regions of the genome that might be linked to a quantitative trait. Two genomic scans have been reported for the changes in quantitative metabolic traits related to type 2

diabetes in response to endurance exercise training of three bouts a week for 20 weeks in sedentary healthy individuals [20,21]. A linkage for the changes in fasting insulin in response to exercise training was found with a marker in the leptin gene on chromosome 7q31 in whites [21]. Linkage for insulin sensitivity in response to exercise training was found on 20q13 and 22q11–12, and for acute insulin response to glucose on chromosomes 15q15 and 18q12 in African Americans [20]. The changes in the disposition index after exercise training were linked to markers on chromosomes 1p35, 3q25, 6p21–22, 7q21, 1p13 and 12q24 in Caucasians, and on 6p22 and 13q14 in African Americans [20]. For the response of glucose effectiveness to exercise training the linkage was found with markers on chromosomes 1p31, 1q44, 2p22–21, 10p12, 10q23, 12q13, 15q26 and 19q13 in African Americans [20]. Genes that are harboured in these genomic regions may modify the effects of a standardized endurance exercise training programme on diabetes related traits.

Association studies

In previous studies, several candidate genes have been tested. Of the genes encoding for the two subunits of the ATP-sensitive potassium channels in pancreatic β-cells (SUR1 and Kir6.2 genes) the Finnish DPS showed that a haplotype in the SUR1 gene was associated with the risk for conversion to type 2 diabetes in the control group, but not in the group receiving an intensive exercise and diet intervention, indicating potential benefits for exercise in subjects at a high risk of diabetes [22].

The common polymorphism Ala23Thr, in linkage disequilibrium with the class III VNTR (variable number of tandem repeat) allele, in the insulin gene, as well as the polymorphisms K121Q in the PC-1 gene and the M326I in the PI3K gene did not regulate body mass or conversion to diabetes during the intervention period in the Finnish DPS [23]. The VNTR variation in the insulin gene modified the association between physical activity and the insulin area under the curve during an oral glucose tolerance test in healthy men [24].

Allelic variations in the VDR (vitamin D receptor) gene have been associated with body weight, glucose homoeostasis, diabetes and its vascular complications [25]. Men homozygous for the B allele of the BsmI VDR gene polymorphism had higher fasting glucose levels than the B allele carriers in those with low physical activity (≤3 h per week), but not in those with high physical activity [26].

PPAR-γ2 (peroxisome proliferator-activated receptor γ2) gene is a transcription factor that regulates adipocyte differentiation, fat-specific gene expression and insulin action [27], and is a major candidate gene for type 2 diabetes [28]. The interaction of the Pro12Ala gene variant and physical activity has been examined in a number of studies. In a study in patients with diabetes, the alanine carriers had a larger decrease in fasting plasma glucose after endurance or resistance exercise training [29]. In individuals with impaired glucose tolerance of the Finnish DPS, Ala[12] homozygotes lost more weight compared to the Pro[12] carriers after a lifestyle intervention and none of the Ala[12] homozygotes developed diabetes [30]. In offspring of patients with type 2 diabetes, body weight decreased more in the Ala[12] allele carriers than in the Pro[12] homozygotes after a ten week training programme [31]. In healthy Japanese men, the alanine allele was associated with improvement in insulin resistance after exercise training [32]. In sedentary subjects, endurance training resulted in a greater improvement in insulin area under the curve during an oral glucose tolerance test in the Pro12Ala heterozygotes than in the Pro[12] homozygotes among men [33].

Among individuals in the Finnish DPS, the risk for developing type 2 diabetes in the Lys[109] homozygotes of the Lys109Ala polymorphism and in the Gln[223] homozygotes of the Gln223Arg polymorphism in the LEPR (leptin receptor) gene was more pronounced in the control group compared with the lifestyle intervention group [34]. In sedentary Caucasians without diabetes, endurance exercise training increased insulin sensitivity and disposition index in the alanine allele carriers, increased glucose disappearance index more in alanine homozygotes, and decreased fasting glucose only in the Arg[109] allele carriers of the Lys109Ala polymorphism of the LEPR gene [35]. An interaction was found in the leptin gene and the LEPR gene after training; the decrease in insulin was strongest in the Ala109Ala homozygotes of the LEP gene who carried the Ala[109] allele in the LEPR gene [35].

α2-, β2- and β3-ADR (α2-, β2-, and β3-adrenergic receptor) genes are activated by cathecholamines and play a major role in the regulation of lipolysis. In the Finnish DPS, the carriers of the Glu[9] allele for the 12 Glu[9] polymorphism in the α2B-ADR (ADRA2B) gene in the intensive lifestyle intervention group had impaired first-phase insulin secretion and an increased risk of developing type 2 diabetes [36]. Adrenaline and noradrenaline bind to the β2-ADR and stimulate lipolysis. The elevation of plasma NEFAs (non-esterified fatty acids) during lipolysis is associated with insulin resistance and the development of type 2 diabetes [37]. In non-diabetic people physical activity modified the effect of the Arg16Arg genotype of the Gly16Arg polymorphism of the β2-ADR gene on the suppression of NEFA levels after an oral glucose load [38]. Also, men with low physical activity levels who were homozygous for the Gln[27] allele of the Gln27Glu polymorphism in the β2-ADR gene were more obese, but this was not the case in men who were regularly physical active [39]. The Arg[64] allele of the Trp64Arg polymorphism of the β3-ADR gene has been associated with an earlier onset of type 2 diabetes [40]. In the Finnish DPS, people in the lifestyle intervention group who possessed the Arg[64] allele in the β3-ADR gene tended to have a higher incidence of type 2 diabetes [41].

The ACE (angiotensin I-converting enzyme) gene catalyses the conversion of angiotensin I to angiotensin II [42]. In hypertensive individuals with an average age of 63 years old, an aerobic exercise programme resulted in a greater increase in insulin sensitivity and a decrease in acute insulin response to glucose in the I/I homozygotes of the Insertion (I)/Deletion (D) polymorphism in intron 16 of the ACE gene [43]. In sedentary individuals, carriers of the I allele had a trend for a greater reduction in insulin response to an oral glucose tolerance test after a strength training programme [44]. It has been proposed that the ACE genotype might modify the potential to become physically active and to achieve higher physical fitness. In a population-based Finnish study, however, there were no differences in physical activity patterns by the ACE genotype [45].

Nitric oxide is released from endothelial cells and muscle, and appears to be involved in glucose uptake in muscle [46]. A significant interaction between energy expenditure and a haplotype in the endothelial nitric oxide synthase gene on glucose intolerance was found in Caucasians [47].

A promoter region Gly174Cys polymorphism in the IL-6 (interleukin-6) gene has been associated with the risk of type 2 diabetes [48]. In sedentary men and postmenopausal women, the Gly174Cys polymorphism modified the training induced changes in glucose levels. A significant decrease after six months of aerobic exercise training occurred only in individuals with the GG genotype [49]. In the Finnish DPS, there was no interaction between the intervention group and the IL-6 genotype [50].

A promoter region Gly308Ala polymorphism in the TNF-α (tumour necrosis factor-α) gene has been shown to have an effect on TNF-α transcription and plasma levels by which it may affect insulin signalling and secretion [51]. Among individuals with glucose intolerance in the Finnish DPS, those with the A^{308} allele had higher conversion to type 2 diabetes in the exercise and diet intervention group [50].

The HL (hepatic lipase) gene regulates lipoprotein metabolism, and the Gly250Ala polymorphism in the promoter region of the HL gene has been associated with insulin resistance [52]. Exercise-induced improvement in insulin sensitivity was greater in the CC homozygotes in sedentary Caucasians and African Americans [53]. In the Finnish DPS, the proportion of people with the GG genotype of the Gly250Ala polymorphism, who converted to diabetes in the exercise and diet intervention group was higher than the proportion of individuals with the A^{250} allele [54].

Conclusions

The Centers for Disease Control and Prevention, the American College of Sports Medicine [55], and the National Institutes of Health [56] in the U.S. and the World Health Organization [57] have recommended that every adult should have at least 30 min of moderate-intensity physical activity (such as brisk walking, cycling, swimming, home repair and yard work) on most, preferably all, days of the week. Based on the scientific evidence to date, a level of physical activity consistent with these recommendations, at least 30 min per day of moderate-to-vigorous physical activity, is effective in preventing type 2 diabetes. Regular physical activity should be an important component of a healthy lifestyle for everyone. Health benefits regarding diabetes prevention from physical activity may vary, depending on the genotype. Even though gene-activity interactions seem to exist according to the results from several observational and a few intervention studies, it is too early at the present to make any specific recommendations regarding genetic testing in this respect. Public health messages, health care professionals, and the health care system should more intensively promote leisure-time, commuting and occupational physical activity in everyday life.

Summary

- *Data from prospective studies have shown that at least 30 min per day of moderate-to-vigorous physical activity can prevent type 2 diabetes.*
- *Moderate or high levels of physical fitness are effective in preventing type 2 diabetes.*
- *Results from clinical trials have shown that lifestyle changes, including dietary modification and an increase in physical activity, can prevent type 2 diabetes.*
- *It is likely that certain genotypes can modify the health effects of physical activity, and the potential for the prevention of type 2 diabetes.*
- *Genome scans and association studies show that genetic variations appear to modify the changes observed in type 2 diabetes-related phenotypes after intervention.*

The contribution of the Finnish Diabetes Prevention Study Group is appreciated. The members of the Finnish Diabetes Prevention Study Group are S. Aunola, Z. Cepaitis, J. Eriksson, M. Hakumäki, K. Hemiö, H. Hämäläinen, P. Härkönen, P. Ilanne-Parikka, A. Ilmanen, S. Keinänen-Kiukaanniemi, K. Kettunen, Mauri Laakso, Markku Laakso, T. Lakka, J. Lindström, A. Louheranta, M. Mannelin, P. Nyholm, M. Peltonen, A. Putila, M. Rastas, V. Salminen, J. Sundvall, J. Tuomilehto, M. Uusitupa and T. Valle. The Finnish Diabetes Prevention Study Group has been financially supported by Finnish Academy (grants 8473/2298, 40758/5767, 38387/54175, 46558), Ministry of Education, Novo Nordisk Foundation, Yrjö Jahnsson Foundation, Juho Vainio Foundation, Finnish Diabetes Research Foundation, and EVO funds from Tampere and Kuopio University Hospitals.

References

1. Wild, S., Roglic, G., Green, A., Sicree, R. & King, H. (2004) Global prevalence of diabetes: estimates for the year 2000 and projections for 2030. *Diabetes Care.* **27**, 1047–1053
2. Uusitupa, M. (2005) Gene-diet interaction in relation to the prevention of obesity and type 2 diabetes: evidence from the Finnish Diabetes Prevention Study. *Nutr. Metab. Cardiovasc. Dis.* **15**, 225–233
3. Wing, R.R., Goldstein, M.G., Acton, K.J., Birch, L.L., Jakicic, J.M., Sallis, Jr, J.F., Smith-West, D., Jeffery, R.W. & Surwit, R.S. (2001) Behavioral science research in diabetes: lifestyle changes related to obesity, eating behavior and physical activity. *Diabetes Care.* **24**, 117–123

4.   Helmrich, S.P., Ragland, D.R., Leung, R.W. & Paffenbarger, Jr, R.S. (1991) Physical activity and reduced occurrence of non-insulin-dependent diabetes mellitus. *N. Engl. J. Med.* **325**, 147–152

5.   Hu, F.B., Sigal, R.J., Rich-Edwards, J.W., Colditz, G.A., Solomon, C.G., Willett, W.C., Speizer, F.E. & Manson, J.E. (1999) Walking compared with vigorous physical activity and risk of type 2 diabetes in women: a prospective study. *J. Am. Med. Assoc.* **282**, 1433–1439

6.   Hu, F.B., Leitzmann, M.F., Stampfer, M.J., Colditz, G.A., Willett, W.C. & Rimm, E.B. (2001) Physical activity and television watching in relation to risk for type 2 diabetes mellitus in men. *Arch. Intern. Med.* **161**, 1542–1548

7.   Perry, I.J., Wannamethee, S.G., Walker, M.K., Thomson, A.G., Whincup, P.H. & Shaper, A.G. (1995) Prospective study of risk factors for development of non-insulin dependent diabetes in middle aged British men. *Br. Med. J.* **310**, 560–564

8.   Nakanishi, N., Takatorige, T. & Suzuki, K. (2004) Daily life activity and risk of developing impaired fasting glucose or type 2 diabetes in middle-aged Japanese men. *Diabetologia* **47**, 1768–1775

9.   Meisinger, C., Lowel, H., Thorand, B. & Doring, A. (2005) Leisure time physical activity and the risk of type 2 diabetes in men and women from the general population. The MONICA/KORA Augsburg Cohort Study. *Diabetologia* **48**, 27–34

10. Hu, G., Qiao, Q., Silventoinen, K., Eriksson, J.G., Jousilahti, P., Lindstrom, J., Valle, T.T., Nissinen, A. & Tuomilehto, J. (2003) Occupational, commuting, and leisure-time physical activity in relation to risk for type 2 diabetes in middle-aged Finnish men and women. *Diabetologia* **46**, 322–329

11. Hu, G., Lindstrom, J., Valle, T.T., Eriksson, J.G., Jousilahti, P., Silventoinen, K., Qiao, Q. & Tuomilehto, J. (2004) Physical activity, body mass index, and risk of type 2 diabetes in patients with normal or impaired glucose regulation. *Arch. Intern. Med.* **164**, 892–896

12. Wei, M., Gibbons, L.W., Mitchell, T.L., Kampert, J.B., Lee, C.D. & Blair, S.N. (1999) The association between cardiorespiratory fitness and impaired fasting glucose and type 2 diabetes mellitus in men. *Ann. Intern. Med.* **130**, 89–96

13. Carnethon, M.R., Gidding, S.S., Nehgme, R., Sidney, S., Jacobs, Jr, D.R. & Liu, K. (2003) Cardiorespiratory fitness in young adulthood and the development of cardiovascular disease risk factors. *J. Am. Med. Assoc.* **290**, 3092–3100

14. Blair, S.N., Cheng, Y. & Holder, J.S. (2001) Is physical activity or physical fitness more important in defining health benefits? *Med. Sci. Sports Exerc.* **33**, S379–S399

15. Eriksson, K.F. & Lindgarde, F. (1991) Prevention of type 2 (non-insulin-dependent) diabetes mellitus by diet and physical exercise. The 6-year Malmö feasibility study. *Diabetologia* **34**, 891–898

16. Pan, X., Li, G., Hu, Y., Wang, J., Yang, W., An, Z., Hu, Z., Lin, J., Xiao, J., Cao, H. et al. (1997) Effects of diet and exercise in preventing NIDDM in people with impaired glucose tolerance. The Da Qing IGT and Diabetes Study. *Diabetes Care* **20**, 537–544

17. Tuomilehto, J., Lindstrom, J., Eriksson, J.G., Valle, T.T., Hamalainen, H., Ilanne-Parikka, P., Keinanen-Kiukaanniemi, S., Laakso, M., Louheranta, A., Rastas, M., Salminen, V. & Uusitupa, M. (2001) Prevention of type 2 diabetes mellitus by changes in lifestyle among subjects with impaired glucose tolerance. *N. Engl. J. Med.* **344**, 1343–1350

18. Knowler, W.C., Barrett-Connor, E., Fowler, S.E., Hamman, R.F., Lachin, J.M., Walker, E.A. & Nathan, D.M. (2002) Reduction in the incidence of type 2 diabetes with lifestyle intervention or metformin. *N. Engl. J. Med.* **346**, 393–403

19. Ramachandran, A., Snehalatha, C., Mary, S., Mukesh, B., Bhaskar, A.D. & Vijay, V. (2006) The Indian Diabetes Prevention Programme shows that lifestyle modification and metformin prevent type 2 diabetes in Asian Indian subjects with impaired glucose tolerance (IDPP-1). *Diabetologia* **49**, 289–297

20. An, P., Teran-Garcia, M., Rice, T., Rankinen, T., Weisnagel, S.J., Bergman, R.N., Boston, R.C., Mandel, S., Stefanovski, D., Leon, A.S. et al. (2005) Genome-wide linkage scans for prediabetes phenotypes in response to 20 weeks of endurance exercise training in non-diabetic whites and blacks: the HERITAGE Family Study. *Diabetologia* **48**, 1142–1149

21. Lakka, T.A., Rankinen, T., Weisnagel, S.J., Chagnon, Y.C., Rice, T., Leon, A.S., Skinner, J.S., Wilmore, J.H., Rao, D.C. & Bouchard, C. (2003) A quantitative trait locus on 7q31 for the

changes in plasma insulin in response to exercise training: the HERITAGE Family Study. *Diabetes* **52**, 1583–1587

22. Laukkanen, O., Pihlajamaki, J., Lindstrom, J., Eriksson, J., Valle, T.T., Hamalainen, H., Ilanne-Parikka, P., Keinanen-Kiukaanniemi, S., Tuomilehto, J., Uusitupa, M. & Laakso, M. (2004) Polymorphisms of the SUR1 (ABCC8) and Kir6.2 (KCNJ11) genes predict the conversion from impaired glucose tolerance to type 2 diabetes. The Finnish Diabetes Prevention Study. *J. Clin. Endocrinol. Metab.* **89**, 6286–6290

23. Laukkanen, O., Pihlajamaki, J., Lindstrom, J., Eriksson, J., Valle, T.T., Hamalainen, H., Ilanne-Parikka, P., Keinanen-Kiukaanniemi, S., Tuomilehto, J., Uusitupa, M. & Laakso, M. (2004) Common poly-morphisms in the genes regulating the early insulin signalling pathway: effects on weight change and the conversion from impaired glucose tolerance to Type 2 diabetes. The Finnish Diabetes Prevention Study. *Diabetologia* **47**, 871–877

24. Waterworth, D.M., Jansen, H., Nicaud, V., Humphries, S.E. & Talmud, P.J. (2005) Interaction between insulin (VNTR) and hepatic lipase (LIPC-514C>T) variants on the response to an oral glucose tolerance test in the EARSII group of young healthy men. *Biochim. Biophys. Acta* **1740**, 375–381

25. Ortlepp, J.R., Lauscher, J., Hoffmann, R., Hanrath, P. & Joost, H.G. (2001) The vitamin D receptor gene variant is associated with the prevalence of type 2 diabetes mellitus and coronary artery disease. *Diabet. Med.* **18**, 842–845

26. Ortlepp, J.R., Metrikat, J., Albrecht, M., von Korff, A., Hanrath, P. & Hoffmann, R. (2003) The vitamin D receptor gene variant and physical activity predicts fasting glucose levels in healthy young men. *Diabet. Med.* **20**, 451–454

27. Auwerx, J. (1999) PPARγ, the ultimate thrifty gene. *Diabetologia* **42**, 1033–1049

28. Florez, J.C., Hirschhorn, J. & Altshuler, D. (2003) The inherited basis of diabetes mellitus: implica-tions for the genetic analysis of complex traits. *Annu. Rev. Genomics Hum. Genet.* **4**, 257–291

29. Adamo, K.B., Sigal, R.J., Williams, K., Kenny, G., Prud'homme, D. & Tesson, F. (2005) Influence of Pro12Ala peroxisome proliferator-activated receptor γ2 polymorphism on glucose response to exercise training in type 2 diabetes. *Diabetologia* **48**, 1503–1509

30. Lindi, V.I., Uusitupa, M.I., Lindstrom, J., Louheranta, A., Eriksson, J.G., Valle, T.T., Hamalainen, H., Ilanne-Parikka, P., Keinanen-Kiukaanniemi, S., Laakso, M. & Tuomilehto, J. (2002) Association of the Pro12Ala polymorphism in the PPAR-γ2 gene with 3-year incidence of type 2 diabetes and body weight change in the Finnish Diabetes Prevention Study. *Diabetes* **51**, 2581–2586

31. Ostergard, T., Ek, J., Hamid, Y., Saltin, B., Pedersen, O.B., Hansen, T. & Schmitz, O. (2005) Influence of the PPAR-gamma2 Pro12Ala and ACE I/D polymorphisms on insulin sensitivity and training effects in healthy offspring of type 2 diabetic subjects. *Horm. Metab. Res.* **37**, 99–105

32. Kahara, T., Takamura, T., Hayakawa, T., Nagai, Y., Yamaguchi, H., Katsuki, T., Katsuki, K., Katsuki, M. & Kobayashi, K. (2003) PPARγ gene polymorphism is associated with exercise-mediated changes of insulin resistance in healthy men. *Metabolism* **52**, 209–212

33. Weiss, E.P., Kulaputana, O., Ghiu, I.A., Brandauer, J., Wohn, C.R., Phares, D.A., Shuldiner, A.R. & Hagberg, J.M. (2005) Endurance training-induced changes in the insulin response to oral glucose are associated with the peroxisome proliferator-activated receptor-γ2 Pro12Ala genotype in men but not in women. *Metabolism* **54**, 97–102

34. Salopuro, T., Pulkkinen, L., Lindstrom, J., Eriksson, J.G., Valle, T.T., Hamalainen, H., Ilanne-Parikka, P., Keinanen-Kiukaanniemi, S., Tuomilehto, J., Laakso, M. & Uusitupa, M. (2005) Genetic variation in leptin receptor gene is associated with type 2 diabetes and body weight: The Finnish Diabetes Prevention Study. *Int. J. Obes. (London)* **29**, 1245–1251

35. Lakka, T.A., Rankinen, T., Weisnagel, S.J., Chagnon, Y.C., Lakka, H.M., Ukkola, O., Boule, N., Rice, T., Leon, A.S., Skinner, J.S., Wilmore, J.H. et al. (2004) Leptin and leptin receptor gene polymor-phisms and changes in glucose homeostasis in response to regular exercise in nondiabetic indi-viduals: the HERITAGE family study. *Diabetes* **53**, 1603–1608

36. Siitonen, N., Lindstrom, J., Eriksson, J., Valle, T.T., Hamalainen, H., Ilanne-Parikka, P., Keinanen-Kiukaanniemi, S., Tuomilehto, J., Laakso, M. & Uusitupa, M. (2004) Association between

a deletion/insertion polymorphism in the α2B-adrenergic receptor gene and insulin secretion and Type 2 diabetes. The Finnish Diabetes Prevention Study. *Diabetologia* **47**, 1416–1424

37. Boden, G. & Laakso, M. (2004) Lipids and glucose in type 2 diabetes: what is the cause and effect? *Diabetes Care* **27**, 2253–2259

38. Meirhaeghe, A., Luan, J., Selberg-Franks, P., Hennings, S., Mitchell, J., Halsall, D., O'Rahilly, S. & Wareham, N.J. (2001) The effect of the Gly16Arg polymorphism of the β(2)-adrenergic receptor gene on plasma free fatty acid levels is modulated by physical activity. *J. Clin. Endocrinol. Metab.* **86**, 5881–5887

39. Meirhaeghe, A., Helbecque, N., Cottel, D. & Amouyel, P. (1999) β2-adrenoceptor gene polymorphism, body weight, and physical activity. *Lancet* **353**, 896

40. Walston, J., Silver, K., Bogardus, C., Knowler, W.C., Celi, F.S., Austin, S., Manning, B., Strosberg, A.D., Stern, M.P., Raben, N. & et al. (1995) Time of onset of non-insulin-dependent diabetes mellitus and genetic variation in the beta 3-adrenergic-receptor gene. *N. Engl. J. Med.* **333**, 343–347

41. Salopuro, T., Lindstrom, J., Eriksson, J.G., Valle, T.T., Hamalainen, H., Ilanne-Parikka, P., Keinanen-Kiukaanniemi, S., Tuomilehto, J., Laakso, M. & Uusitupa, M. (2004) Common variants in β2- and β3-adrenergic receptor genes and uncoupling protein 1 as predictors of the risk for type 2 diabetes and body weight changes. The Finnish Diabetes Prevention Study. *Clin. Genet.* **66**, 365–367

42. Wicklmayr, M., Dietze, G., Brunnbauer, H., Rett, K. & Mehnert, H. (1983) Dose-dependent effect of bradykinin on muscular blood flow and glucose uptake in man. *Hoppe Seylers Z. Physiol. Chem.* **364**, 831–833

43. Dengel, D.R., Brown, M.D., Ferrell, R.E., Reynolds, T.H.T. & Supiano, M.A. (2002) Exercise-induced changes in insulin action are associated with ACE gene polymorphisms in older adults. *Physiol. Genomics* **11**, 73–80

44. Hurlbut, D.E., Lott, M.E., Ryan, A.S., Ferrell, R.E., Roth, S.M., Ivey, F.M., Martel, G.F., Lemmer, J.T., Fleg, J.L. & Hurley, B.F. (2002) Does age, sex, or ACE genotype affect glucose and insulin responses to strength training? *J. Appl. Physiol.* **92**, 643–650

45. Fuentes, R.M., Perola, M., Nissinen, A. & Tuomilehto, J. (2002) ACE gene and physical activity, blood pressure, and hypertension: a population study in Finland. *J. Appl. Physiol.* **92**, 2508–2512

46. Roy, D., Perreault, M. & Marette, A. (1998) Insulin stimulation of glucose uptake in skeletal muscles and adipose tissues in vivo is NO dependent. *Am. J. Physiol.* **274**, E692–E699

47. Franks, P.W., Luan, J., Barroso, I., Brage, S., Gonzalez Sanchez, J.L., Ekelund, U., Rios, M.S., Schafer, A.J., O'Rahilly, S. & Wareham, N.J. (2005) Variation in the eNOS gene modifies the association between total energy expenditure and glucose intolerance. *Diabetes* **54**, 2795–2801

48. Vozarova, B., Fernandez-Real, J.M., Knowler, W.C., Gallart, L., Hanson, R.L., Gruber, J.D., Ricart, W., Vendrell, J., Richart, C., Tataranni, P.A. & Wolford, J.K. (2003) The interleukin-6 (−174) G/C promoter polymorphism is associated with type-2 diabetes mellitus in Native Americans and Caucasians. *Hum. Genet.* **112**, 409–413

49. McKenzie, J.A., Weiss, E.P., Ghiu, I.A., Kulaputana, O., Phares, D.A., Ferrell, R.E. & Hagberg, J.M. (2004) Influence of the interleukin-6 -174 G/C gene polymorphism on exercise training-induced changes in glucose tolerance indexes. *J. Appl. Physiol.* **97**, 1338–1342

50. Kubaszek, A., Pihlajamaki, J., Komarovski, V., Lindi, V., Lindstrom, J., Eriksson, J., Valle, T.T., Hamalainen, H., Ilanne-Parikka, P., Keinanen-Kiukaanniemi, S. et al. (2003) Promoter polymorphisms of the TNF-α (G-308A) and IL-6 (C-174G) genes predict the conversion from impaired glucose tolerance to type 2 diabetes: the Finnish Diabetes Prevention Study. *Diabetes* **52**, 1872–1876

51. Kroeger, K.M., Carville, K.S. & Abraham, L.J. (1997) The -308 tumor necrosis factor-α promoter polymorphism effects transcription. *Mol. Immunol.* **34**, 391–399

52. Pihlajamaki, J., Karjalainen, L., Karhapaa, P., Vauhkonen, I., Taskinen, M.R., Deeb, S.S. & Laakso, M. (2000) G-250A substitution in promoter of hepatic lipase gene is associated with dyslipidemia and insulin resistance in healthy control subjects and in members of families with familial combined hyperlipidemia. *Arterioscler. Thromb. Vasc. Biol.* **20**, 1789–1795

53. Teran-Garcia, M., Santoro, N., Rankinen, T., Bergeron, J., Rice, T., Leon, A.S., Rao, D.C., Skinner, J.S., Bergman, R.N., Despres, J.P. & Bouchard, C. (2005) Hepatic lipase gene variant -514C>T is associated with lipoprotein and insulin sensitivity response to regular exercise: the HERITAGE Family Study. *Diabetes* **54**, 2251–2255

54. Todorova, B., Kubaszek, A., Pihlajamaki, J., Lindstrom, J., Eriksson, J., Valle, T.T., Hamalainen, H., Ilanne-Parikka, P., Keinanen-Kiukaanniemi, S., Tuomilehto, J., Uusitupa, M. & Laakso, M. (2004) The G-250A promoter polymorphism of the hepatic lipase gene predicts the conversion from impaired glucose tolerance to type 2 diabetes mellitus: the Finnish Diabetes Prevention Study. *J. Clin. Endocrinol. Metab.* **89**, 2019–2023

55. Pate, R.R., Pratt, M., Blair, S.N., Haskell, W.L., Macera, C.A., Bouchard, C., Buchner, D., Ettinger, W., Heath, G.W., King, A.C. et al. (1995) Physical activity and public health. A recommendation from the Centers for Disease Control and Prevention and the American College of Sports Medicine. *J. Am. Med. Assoc.* **273**, 402–407

56. NIH Consensus Development Panel on Physical Activity and Cardiovascular Health. (1996) Physical activity and cardiovascular health. NIH Consensus Development Panel on Physical Activity and Cardiovascular Health. *J. Am. Med. Assoc.* **276**, 241–246

57. World Health Organisation. (2004) Global strategy on diet, physical activity, and health. Geneva.

14

Integration of the metabolic and cardiovascular effects of exercise

Anton J.M. Wagenmakers*†[1], Natal A.W. van Riel†, Michael P. Frenneaux‡ and Paul M. Stewart§

*Exercise Metabolism and Biochemistry Group, School of Sport and Exercise Sciences, University of Birmingham, U.K., †Eindhoven Systems Biology Group, Eindhoven University of Technology, The Netherlands, ‡Department of Cardiovascular Medicine, Medical School, University of Birmingham, U.K., and §Department of Medicine, Medical School, University of Birmingham, U.K.

Abstract

Most of the essays in this volume have adopted a reductionist approach and have focused on the biochemistry either in skeletal muscle or in the vascular wall. There is however a complex interaction between the biochemistry in the endothelium of the microvascular wall, the vascular smooth muscle and the skeletal muscle fibres involving signalling pathways in the three tissues and an intense exchange of signal molecules between them. In the present essay an integrative overview is given of this complex metabolic interaction and the impairments in it that lead to type 2 diabetes and cardiovascular disease. A reduced nitric oxide production by the (micro)vascular endothelium is identified as the key event and is reversible by regular exercise and a reduced

[1]To whom correspondence should be addressed (email a.wagenmakers@bham.ac.uk).

calorie intake. The chapter also contains a description of the complex metabolic network controlled by the inducible transcription factor nuclear factor-κB, that is activated in more advanced stages of the chronic diseases, and either leads to repair of the microvascular wall or to irreversible damage and the severe complications of end stage cardiovascular disease and type 2 diabetes.

Introduction

We will first summarize the wide variety of metabolic and functional benefits of regular exercise that occur at the level of the muscle and the (micro)vascular endothelium. Together they lead to maintenance of optimal health in trained individuals, who regularly perform a combination of endurance and resistance exercise. This will be followed by a discussion of the mal-adaptations in lean and obese sedentary subjects taking healthy, active man as the norm for reasons explained by Chakravarthy and Booth [1]. These impairments progress with ageing and are rapidly accelerated by obesity. Endothelial impairments seem to lead to a chronic underperfusion of skeletal muscle, resulting in suboptimal exposure of the muscle to nutrients, oxygen and hormones. In the period following meal ingestion this leads to disturbances in the distribution of nutrients between skeletal muscle, liver and adipose tissue, and large transient increases in the concentration of blood nutrient and insulin concentrations (loss of homoeostasis). During exercise the underperfusion (potentially affecting both skeletal muscle and the heart) leads to exercise limitations. In combination with the reduced maximal cardiac output and a low oxidative capacity of skeletal muscle (low content of mitochondria) this does not make exercise training into an attractive treatment option for affected patients. Atherosclerosis develops in feed and resistance arteries, but potentially also deep down into the microvasculature and probably contributes to the metabolic barriers and dysfunction of the (micro)vasculature. As all tissues in the body seem to suffer from this microvascular pathology, eventually tissue degeneration and multiple organ failure occurs and results in the severe complications of end stage diabetes and cardiovascular disease. NADPH oxidase and the complex metabolic network controlled by NF-κB (nuclear factor-κB) play important roles in the underlying mechanisms and make the final choice between tissue repair or destruction.

Biochemistry and function of the (micro)vasculature and skeletal muscle in healthy, physically active individuals

The combined essays in this volume carry the message that only a physically active lifestyle combining regular periods of both endurance and resistance exercise leads to optimal human health. As explained by Chakravarthy and Booth [1] this is in line with the lifestyle of our ancestors who existed as hunter-gatherers in the 50000–10000 BC period. It was in this period that evolution via the 'survival of the fittest' principal selected the genes that most of us still carry today [1]. Endurance exercise activates the signals that lead to a high oxidative capacity, that induce mitochondrial biogenesis and that lead to a dense capillary network around the muscle fibres (Chapters 1 and 2). Resistance exercise leads to muscle protein anabolism and maintenance of a large muscle mass and strength (Chapters 5 and 6). As the muscle is continuously in a post-exercise state in subjects performing moderate- to high-intensity exercise ≥3 times per week, the insulin signalling cascade remains activated (Chapters 3 and 6). Regular exercise also leads to activation of glycogen synthase because of a regular lowering of the muscle glycogen stores (Chapter 3) and, therefore, to an increased extraction rate of glucose from the blood following ingestion of carbohydrate-containing meals. Regular exercise in trained muscles also leads to lipolysis and oxidation of intramuscular triglycerides, which are stored as lipid droplets next to the mitochondria (Chapter 4). This increases the ability of the muscle to extract plasma fatty acids and lipids from the blood in the period following a meal and guarantees maintenance of a plasma lipid profile with a low cardiovascular and diabetes risk (Chapter 7). Also the concentration of long-chain fatty acyl-CoAs, diacylglycerols and ceramides (fatty acid metabolites suggested to lead to insulin resistance) is kept low (Chapter 4).

In periods after meal consumption the blood insulin concentration rises and leads to recruitment of an increased number of muscle fibre capillaries (Chapter 10; Figure 1) and ensures high rates of glucose and triglyceride clearance by the muscle. A physically active lifestyle will therefore prevent large post-meal excursions in blood glucose and lipid concentrations as seen in sedentary subjects and patients with diabetes and insulin resistance. An increased buffering capacity of adipose tissue for the daily lipid flux also keeps plasma triglycerides low [2]. The responsiveness of the vascular endothelium to shear stress and other physiological stimuli is optimal too, leading to efficient opening of terminal arterioles, larger arterioles, resistance arteries and feed arteries during moderate- and high-intensity exercise (Chapter 9 and 11). The trained muscle, therefore, can increase blood flow 100-fold during high intensity aerobic exercise and can sustain exercise at high intensities for prolonged periods [3]. The trained individual also has high NOS (nitric oxide synthase) activities in the vascular endothelium and a high endothelial NO (nitric oxide) production in response to insulin and shear stress (Chapter 9). This will reduce vascular tone via its effect on the VSM (vascular smooth muscle) and prevent the development of high blood pressure. It has also been suggested that a high endothelial NO production prevents binding of leucocytes and reduces inflammation leading to atherosclerosis, and enhances training/shear stress induced angiogenesis (Chapters 9, 11 and 12) [4–6].

When master athletes (seniors) are compared with sedentary healthy elderly people then it is clear that the aforementioned benefits of regular exercise are maintained. However, ageing is inherently attended by a loss of muscle oxidative capacity and a slow progressive loss of muscle mass (sarcopenia). Reductions in both can be kept to a minimum when the frequency and duration of the exercise is maintained at appropriate intensities. Continued exercise in elderly subjects greatly improves independence, mobility, strength, quality of life and wellbeing (Chapter 6). A continued mixed exercise programme will also keep shifts in the plasma lipid profile, increases in percentage body fat, loss of muscle fibre capillaries, endothelial (micro)vascular impairments, increases in blood pressure, atherosclerosis and increases in fasting blood insulin and glucose concentration to a minimum (Chapter 6). Rises in proinflammatory cytokines are also an important cause of insulin resistance in the elderly and will be reduced by exercise and potentially counteracted by the increased IL-6 (interleukin-6) production of the exercising muscles (Chapter 8).

The consequences of the switch to a sedentary lifestyle in the second half of the 20th century

As explained in the introduction, a major shift in physical activity has occurred in the second half of the 20th century with most adults and children today leading a sedentary lifestyle. A sedentary lifestyle seems to be compatible with an acceptable health in those individuals who manage to keep caloric intake low despite the challenges of today's food quality and affluence. However, a major proportion of today's world population combines the sedentary lifestyle with a positive energy balance, eating more calories than their energy expenditure, and consuming food with a high fat content. This abrupt change in lifestyle is regarded as the primary cause for the dramatic increase in obesity and chronic diseases in the last 20 years [7] (Chapters 8 and 13 for epidemiological evidence). The physiological consequences for human metabolism of being sedentary are the exact reverse of the benefits described for the physically active lean individuals with faster and bigger metabolic and functional changes occurring in obese than in lean subjects.

Metabolic and functional abnormalities in obese sedentary subjects and the metabolic syndrome

Obese subjects with normal fasting plasma glucose, were recently shown to have a blunted insulin-mediated microvascular recruitment in muscle (Chapter 10). Infusion of intralipid plus heparin (leading to high plasma fatty acid concentrations) and of TNF-α (tumour necrosis factor-α), an inflammatory cytokine that is high in obese subjects, elderly people and patients with type 2 diabetes (Chapter 8), also leads to an acute blunting of the insulin-mediated microvascular recruitment (Chapter 10). In healthy individuals a 40–50% increase in the number of perfused or recruited muscle capillaries is seen in response to low physiological increases in insulin concentration (Chapter 10). This will lead to an increase in the capillary permeability surface area, which is a prerequisite for an insulin-induced increase in the transport of both insulin and glucose from the capillary lumen into the interstitium of the muscle [8,9] and, therefore, for insulin induced increases in muscle glucose uptake.

The mechanism which has been proposed for the insulin induced recruitment of muscle capillaries is that insulin binds to the insulin receptor on the endothelial cells of terminal arterioles leading to activation of Akt (protein kinase B) and eNOS (endothelial NOS) and increased NO production. NO then diffuses to the VSM in the terminal arteriolar wall leading to opening of the terminal arterioles and recruitment of additional muscle capillaries further downstream in the vascular tree (Figures 1 and 2 in Chapter 10).

Failure of insulin to increase the number of perfused muscle capillaries has not only been observed in humans with uncomplicated obesity, but also in obese Zucker rats, an animal model of the metabolic syndrome. The metabolic syndrome is a transition state with a high risk for type 2 diabetes (see Chapter 11 for an exact definition). In type 2 diabetic patients insulin failed to increase glucose uptake and the capillary permeability surface area [10].

Failure of insulin to increase the number of perfused muscle capillaries reduces the total amount of insulin and glucose that enters the muscle capillaries, reduces transport through the endothelial cell layer covering the capillary wall, and thus limits uptake in the interstitial fluid that surrounds the skeletal muscle fibres (Figure 1). This then leads to a reduced insulin and glucose concentration in the external milieu of the muscle fibres and a reduced activation of the insulin signalling cascade in muscle fibres. These recent discoveries have important implications for our understanding of the mechanisms leading to insulin resistance as (i) insulin resistance may simultaneously occur at the level of the microvascular endothelium and in the muscle fibres; (ii) a defect in muscle capillary recruitment occurs in clinically uncomplicated obese subjects and thus seems to be an early event in the pathogenesis leading to insulin resistance and type 2 diabetes; and (iii) this defect reduces the insulin concentration seen by the insulin receptor in the muscle plasma membrane and thus prevents activation of the insulin signalling cascade in the skeletal muscle fibres.

Further metabolic implications of impaired capillary recruitment by insulin

The supply of amino acids, fatty acids and triglycerides (to be split by lipoprotein lipase present on the endothelium of the muscle capillary bed; Figure 1) are also reduced by impaired insulin induced capillary recruitment. Therefore hyperaminoacidaemia and hypertriglyceridaemia result because of a failure of muscle clearance of meal-derived amino acids and triglycerides from the circulation (Chapter 7). A muscle capillary recruitment defect may also explain the reduction of diet-induced thermogenesis in obese subjects and patients with type 2 diabetes and the reduced insulin-induced increase in

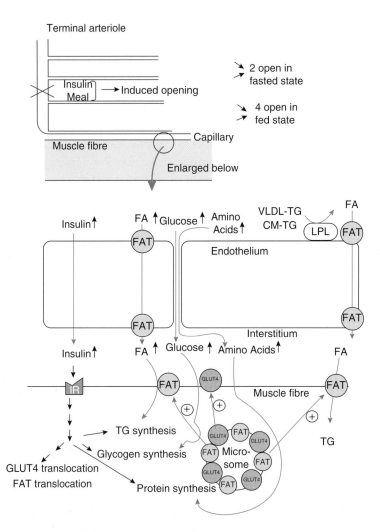

Figure 1. Insulin induced opening of terminal arterioles leads to recruitment of more muscle capillaries in the period following meal ingestion (top of Figure 1)

As a consequence more insulin, glucose, amino acids and fatty acids (FA) will be transported over the endothelial layer of the muscle capillaries and penetrate into the interstitial fluid surrounding the muscle fibres. This then leads to increased uptake of these nutrients in the muscle. The higher concentration of insulin activates the insulin signalling cascade in muscle and leads to translocation of GLUT4 (Chapters 5 and 6) and FAT (fatty acid translocase; Chapter 4), and higher rates of amino acid uptake. The higher insulin concentration also leads to an increased stimulation of glycogen synthesis, protein synthesis and triglyceride synthesis. Failure of this opening mechanism in insulin resistant states (obesity, type 2 diabetes and cardiovascular disease) leads to high blood concentrations of glucose, triglycerides, amino acids and insulin in the postprandial period (following ingestion of mixed meals). Note that capillary recruitment increases the access of VLDL-TG (very low density lipoprotein-triglyceride) and CM-TG (chylomicron-TG) to muscle capillary LPL (lipoprotein lipase). Also note that insulin in contrast with exercise does not increase the rate at which red blood cells travel through individual capillaries and does not increase total muscle blood flow (see Chapter 10 for detailed explanation). The latter may increase 100-fold during high-intensity exercise [3].

muscle ATP turnover that has recently been observed in the offspring of type 2 diabetic parents [11,12]. Reduced recruitment of muscle capillaries will prevent insulin and other anabolic hormones and growth factors reaching the muscle plasma membrane and will reduce escape of locally produced hormones (e.g. cortisol and noradrenalin) into the circulation. This will acutely change muscle metabolism (e.g. reduced protein synthesis, increased protein degradation and increased lipolysis). A long-term change of the external milieu of the muscle fibres is likely to change the expression of genes and the protein profile and to contribute to the molecular adaptation and tissue degeneration that is observed in the chronic diseases.

The metabolic network leading to insulin resistance in endothelial cells and skeletal muscle fibres

The molecular mechanisms that have been proposed to lead to insulin resistance in the microvascular endothelium and in skeletal muscle fibres are initiated by the same signals and seem to involve the same pathways [13–16]. A high flux of fatty acids (Chapters 4 and 7) originating from enlarged adipose tissue stores is assumed to lead to increases in long-chain fatty acylCoA and diacylglycerol concentrations and to activate the PKC (protein kinase C) isomers β and θ (Figure 2). The PKC-isomers are serine kinases which are able to phosphorylate the insulin receptor and IRS-1 (insulin receptor substrate-1) on specific serine residues thus preventing insulin-induced tyrosine phosphorylation and activation of the insulin signalling cascade (Chapter 4). PKC-β is chronically activated in the muscle of obese subjects [13] and PKC-θ in patients with type 2 diabetes [14]. PKC-β can also be switched on in the muscle of healthy lean subjects by acute 5–6 h infusions of intralipid plus heparin [15]. In skeletal muscle PKC activation leads to reduced GLUT-4 (glucose transporter 4) translocation (Chapters 3 and 4). In the vascular endothelium it leads to attenuation of insulin induced NO production and reduced recruitment of muscle capillaries (Figure 2) [16].

Activation of the inducible transcription factor NF-κB (see below) has also been implicated in serine phosphorylation of IRS-1, again both in the microvascular endothelium and the muscle [15,17–19]. NF-κB is activated in cultured endothelial cells by high fatty acid levels [18], high glucose concentrations [19] and inflammatory cytokines of the TNF superfamily [20,21].

Impairments in flow (shear stress)-mediated increases in muscle perfusion

Vasodilation of feed and resistance arteries and of larger arterioles is essential for the massive increase in total muscle blood flow seen during exercise [3]. Vasodilation of these larger vessels is in part achieved by the effects of shear stress (physical interaction of the high blood flow with

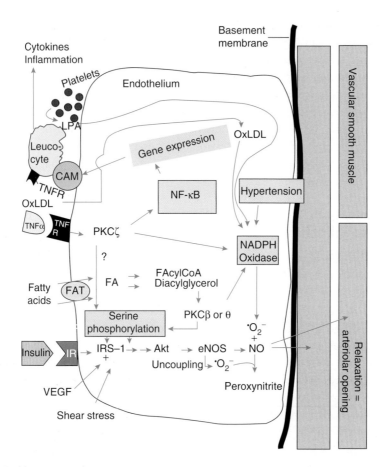

Figure 2. The mechanisms leading to reduced NO production in the endothelium of the microvasculature

Increases in insulin, VEGF (vascular endothelial growth factor) and shear stress stimulate endothelial NO production via activation of the insulin signalling cascade. High fatty acid levels lead to high intracellular concentrations of long chain fatty acylCoA's (FAcylCoA) and diacylglycerol. These fatty acid metabolites activate the protein kinase C isomers PKC-β or -θ, which then phosphorylate IRS-1 on specific serine residues preventing the normal activation of IRS-1 by tyrosine phosphorylation. This prevents eNOS phosphorylation by activated Akt and reduces NO production and smooth muscle cell relaxation. Activation of NADPH oxidase in the endothelium of patients with the chronic diseases leads to superoxide anion production which takes away NO via the formation of peroxynitrite. TNF-α and other members of the TNF superfamily activate NADPH oxidase via a direct mechanism involving activation of PKC-ζ and via a number of indirect mechanisms. TNF-α increases activity and nuclear translocation of NF-κB. This leads to the increased expression of cellular adhesion molecules (CAM) playing a role in the binding of leucocytes. Secondary cytokines produced by the leucocytes and macrophages lead to local inflammation processes in the (micro)vascular wall, attract platelets and destroy the normal endothelial barrier function among others leading to the uptake of oxLDL (oxidized low density lipoprotein), which contains lysophosphatidylcholine a known activator of NADPH oxidase. The platelets produce lysophosphatidic acid (LPA) another signal molecule that activates NADPH oxidase. Hypertension activates NADPH oxidase both via mechanisms involving increases in angiotensin II and increased strain. Finally the enzyme eNOS itself can produce oxygen free radicals via uncoupling due to a low availability of its cofactor tetrahydrobiopterin. IR, insulin receptor; TNFR, TNF-receptor; FAT, fatty acid translocase. Consulted sources [4,13–16,22,24] the endothelium)-mediated NO-dependent dilation (Chapters 9, 11 and 12). The mechanism is also assumed to involve eNOS activation and is mediated by the insulin-signalling cascade (Figure 2). This most likely implies that the same molecular mechanisms that impair insulin-induced NO-production in terminal arterioles also restrict shear stress-mediated dilation of feed and resistance arteries during exercise in obese subjects and patients with chronic diseases. This restriction is potentially present both in skeletal muscle and the heart and may contribute to the reduced work capacity of both tissues. In patients with hypertension there is also an increase in vasoconstrictor tone (Chapters 11 and 12) and a substantial decrease in muscle capillary density (also called rarefaction; Chapters 11 and 12), both of which restrict muscle perfusion during exercise. These mechanisms, in combination with other causes of cardiac failure, limitations in ventilation and a low oxidative capacity of skeletal muscle (reduced number of mitochondria) limit the exercise capacity of patients with type 2 diabetes and cardiovascular disease.

Loss of functional NO by superoxide anion production

The NADPH oxidases are an enzyme family activated in the vasculature in cardiovascular disease and are thought to play an important role in the initiation of microvascular impairments [22]. Many vascular stimuli, including all those known to lead to insulin resistance, activate NADPH oxidase via both increased gene expression and complex activation mechanisms [22]. NADPH oxidase activation, like IRS-1 serine phosphorylation, has been suggested to depend on prior PKC activation. NADPH oxidase leads to superoxide anion production ($^{\bullet}O_2^{-}$). Superoxide reacts with NO resulting in the formation of peroxynitrite, reducing the bioactive NO needed to dilate terminal arterioles, feed arteries and resistance arteries. Superoxide anion, peroxynitrite and other ROS (reactive oxygen species) also lead to pathology via peroxidation of proteins and lipids and via activation of redox-sensitive [depending on the NAD(P)H/NAD(P) ratio] signalling cascades and protein nitrosylation.

Another potential source of superoxide anion production in the vascular endothelium is the enzyme eNOS itself. *In vitro*, in the presence of low concentrations of its substrate (arginine) and of its main cofactor (tetrahydrobiopterin), eNOS acts on molecular oxygen to form superoxide anion [23]. This process is called eNOS uncoupling and has been suggested to be a major cause of hypertension [23,24]. Addition of tetrahydrobiopterin to microvascular endothelial cells reduces eNOS uncoupling [24,25], whereas infusion of tetrahydrobiopterin in patients with type 2 diabetes and coronary heart disease improves insulin sensitivity [26].

Consequences of reduced NO production

In summary, NO production in the microvascular endothelium is reduced in patients with the metabolic syndrome, type 2 diabetes and cardiovascular disease because of a reduced expression and activity of eNOS, reduced phosphorylation of eNOS via the insulin signalling cascade and removal of functional NO by superoxide anions produced by activation of NADPH oxidase and uncoupling of eNOS (Figure 2). This reduction in NO available for relaxation of the VSM cells also has been suggested to increase monocyte/macrophage adhesion to endothelial cells, to enhance platelet aggregation/thrombosis, to increase the degree of inflammation, atherosclerosis and VSM proliferation and hypertophy throughout the circulation (Chapters 9,11 and 12) [4]. The effect of chronic exercise on angiogenesis (an increase in capillary density with training) has been shown to depend on the original increase in shear stress-induced NO production in the pre-existent muscle capillaries, with less angiogenesis occurring when the NO production is reduced [6].

The role of inflammation and atherogenesis in the communication between endothelium and VSM

An important question when we consider the tissues and pathways activated by TNF-α and other members of the TNF superfamily (e.g. NADPH oxidase and the NF-κB network [21,22]) is whether the endothelial lining forms a barrier for these proinflammatory cytokines, other vascular metabolites and for monocytes and macrophages (Figure 3). If so, then the involved cytokines and immune cells could not exert direct effects on VSM and skeletal muscle fibres/cardiomyocytes. Suggestions have been made that TNF-α activates peripheral blood mononuclear cells to produce other cytokines that change the shape of endothelial cells and create large gaps between the cells [27]. Loss of the endothelial barrier function due to this local inflammatory process (Figure 3) will have large consequences for the interaction between the endothelium, the VSM and skeletal muscle fibres as the co-ordinated exchange of signal molecules will be lost. Loss of the endothelial barrier function probably also plays a role in the onset and progression of atherosclerosis and VSM hypertrophy.

Atherosclerosis is a slow progressive disease that may start in childhood and is dramatically accelerated by a sedentary lifestyle and obesity. The atherosclerotic process is still poorly understood but leads to a progressive deposition of fats, cholesterol, oxidized lipoproteins, platelets, macrophages, cellular debris, collagen and calcium in the wall of feed arteries and resistance arteries and is a major cause of arterial stiffness. The depositions are called atherosclerotic plaques. Eventually the diameter of the lumen of the artery will be reduced and less blood will flow to the downstream circulation and the oxygen supply to tissue beds will be reduced. Atherosclerotic plaques are present between the endothelial lining and the VSM cells and are a likely physical barrier for NO produced by the endothelium to reach the VSM and will thus further decrease NO availability.

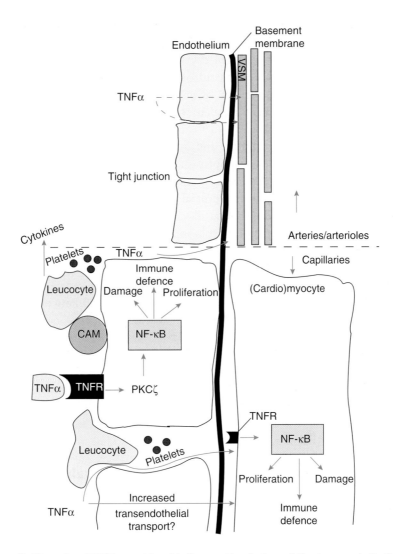

Figure 3. The role of TNF-α and local inflammation in loss of the transendothelial barrier, artherosclerosis and muscle cell degeneration

In the healthy state (top of the figure) the endothelial cells form a closed barrier for TNF-α and members of the TNF family. VSM cells in arteries and arterioles and (cardio)myocytes will not be exposed to the cytokines and NF-kB will not be activated. In a state of chronic inflammation (bottom of Figure 3) the events described in Figure 2 lead to local inflammation and make the endothelial cells permeable for cytokines, while simultaneously widening the tight junctions and allowing leucocyte/macrophage penetration into deeper tissue layers. As a result, cytokines can reach VSM cells and (cardio)myocytes and activate NF-κB and NADPH oxidase. Loss of the endothelial barrier function also speeds up the atherosclerotic process.

Dual role of the NF-κB network in tissue repair and tissue damage

NF-κB is a transcription factor, inducible in most cells of our body. The activation signals and pathways and the effector pathways (enzyme pathways expressed when NF-κB is activated) form an incredibly complex network with multiple overlapping processes and interaction/cross talk with many other signalling pathways [20,21,28,29]. Knowledge on gene expression and the signalling regulation network controlled by NF-κB is expanding rapidly (>5400 hits in PubMed in the last 18 months) but our understanding of its physiological role and the many regulatory mechanisms is still in a rudimentary state. NF-κB (among other factors) activates the expression of groups of genes promoting and regulating immune and inflammatory responses, cell survival and growth, cell cycles and also apoptosis and necrosis.

It is clear today that damage and repair of the endothelial lining in the blood vessels of our body plays a crucial role in the long-term pathogenesis of type 2 diabetes and cardiovascular disease. It also is clear that the network controlled by NF-κB plays a key role in this process [20,21,28,29]. NF-κB activation leads to the expression of proteins involved in the binding of leucocytes, required to assist in these repair processes, but simultaneously able to produce severe damage among others by uncontrolled free radical production [28]. Once the endothelial barrier function is lost the NF-κB network seems to be able to extend its action to the VSM cells, (cardio)myocytes and most other tissues of our body (Figure 3). When the NF-κB network, with the help of the immune system, does not succeed in repairing these tissues, severe diabetic and cardiovascular complications will follow such as left ventricular hypertrophy [30,31], claudication, lower leg denervation [32], neurodegenerative diseases [33], retinopathy [34] and kidney disease [35]. However, we are a long way from understanding the exact regulatory mechanisms that lead to repair, and that decide on the balance between repair, apoptosis and necrosis.

Complexity of the networks involved: added value of systems biology

The picture that emerges above, shows a complex, intertwined network of many signalling pathways and metabolic networks in different cell types and tissues, operating at multiple scales in space and time (Figure 4). How these systems are interconnected and the sequence of events leading to metabolic dysregulation and pathology are largely unknown. A systems approach that combines comprehensive and accurate quantitative experimental work with a high temporal resolution and mechanism-based computational model is necessary to make progress in the understanding of these highly complex pathways and involves a rapidly growing body of literature comprising many thousands of publications per year. It is time to realize that the traditional integrative physiology/biochemistry approach is not enough in order to enhance our understanding of the biochemical and biological mechanisms leading to the chronic diseases and the effect of exercise upon it. We depend on the development of a new discipline called systems biology, which combines the expertise of molecular biologists and biochemists, integrative physiologists, computational biologists and control systems engineers with an interest in the

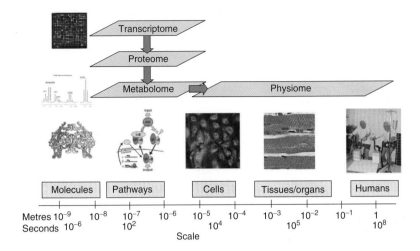

Figure 4. A multi-scale problem requires a multi-scale approach, both in space and time

Mathematics can be used to form integrative (across scales) models of human physiology and disease. However, different processes that operate on time and spatial scales that are 14 respectively 9 orders of magnitude apart can never be combined in full detail in a single simulation model. From an experimental point of view, it is a huge challenge to accurately measure a multitude of system components in time and space in response to well-defined physiological or pharmaceutical perturbations.

chronic diseases. Systems biology aims to understand physiology and disease from the level of molecular pathways, regulatory networks, cells, tissues, and organs upwards, ultimately, to the level of the whole organism (Figure 4). To understand complex, multi-factorial diseases the system cannot be restricted to intracellular pathways (which currently dominate the literature). It also needs to include larger-scale systems physiology to identify the important control points that are determinants of disturbed metabolism [36]. Mathematical models can be used to identify the most important components and interactions in a complex system using high-throughput genomic, proteomic and metabolomic data complemented with quantitative data obtained in functional assays providing information on changes in time and space in response to well defined physiological and/or pharmaceutical perturbations [37]. Models provide a platform for hypothesis-driven research and can assist in the optimization of new experiments and therapies. A continuous iterative cycle of prediction and experimental validation progressively strengthens the predictive power of the model and ultimately will lead to a full comprehension of the disease mechanism (Figure 5).

Does underperfusion of skeletal muscle and the heart lead to an energy deficit?

We have seen in this essay that there are many processes that might limit the supply of blood and the transport of fuels and oxygen from capillary blood

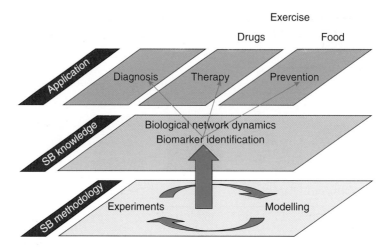

Figure 5. Systems biology (SB) uses a hypothesis-driven approach, in which the iterative cycle between experiment and model is exploited
This yields a quantitative understanding of network dynamics and regulation, which can be used to identify biomarkers and potential therapeutic targets. Socially and clinically relevant applications are in the areas of diagnosis, therapy and prevention of complex, multi-factorial, degenerative diseases. This figure was compiled by Natal van Riel and Jeroen Jeneson.

to the (cardio)myocytes. Therefore it might well be possible that a chronic energy deficit develops in skeletal muscle and the heart especially in the final stages of the chronic disease process. In line with this hypothesis, significantly lower PCr/ATP rates were indeed observed in the heart of patients with type 2 diabetes in the resting state [38]. This ratio was normal in skeletal muscle at rest, but the loss of PCr during exercise was faster in the type 2 diabetic individuals and the PCr recovery following exercise was slower. Lower ATP turnover rates have also been found in the offspring of parents with type 2 diabetes both in the fasted state and during a hyperinsulinaemic euglycaemic clamp all in line with a relative underperfusion [11,12]. Indications of a reduced skeletal muscle perfusion during exercise were also observed in obese Zucker rats in Chapter 10. A suboptimal perfusion of heart and skeletal muscle leading to an energy deficit or reduced ATP turnover rates is likely to contribute to a reduced contractility of these tissues or failure of other ATP requiring metabolic processes (maintenance of the Na^+/K^+ gradient or protein synthesis rates etc.).

The benefits of acute and regular exercise for patients

Acute exercise will open the muscle capillaries among others via adenosine and K^+-induced opening of the terminal arterioles [3]. As these metabolites are released by the contracting muscle fibres, this is an opening mechanism that does not depend on endothelial function or integrity. Obese subjects and patients with insulin resistance and other microvascular impairments may, therefore, experience acute benefits of exercise when they perform walking or resistance exercise in the period following meal ingestion. Exercise will help to recruit more muscle capillaries and will thus direct more insulin and meal-derived nutrients towards the muscle fibres, simulating the effect that insulin has in healthy individuals. Most of the benefits of regular exercise (≥3 times per week) that are seen in trained subjects do also occur in patients with the metabolic syndrome and advanced stages of type 2 diabetes and cardiovascular disease. However, due to the inherent lower exercise intensity, the effects will be smaller and it will take longer after the start of a physical activity increase before the benefits become significant and noticeable to the patient. This in part is due to the structural changes in the microvasculature, which prevent rapid improvement of the endothelial function and transendothelial oxygen and nutrient transport. An exhaustive description of all the benefits of regular exercise in healthy subjects and patients with chronic disease is given in previous chapters in this volume.

Recent studies in rats chronically increasing the coronary blood flow in hypertrophied hearts [5] and aortic blood flow [39] reveal large increases in expression of eNOS and the enzymes leading to the expression of its cofactor tetrahydrobiopterin. Brown et al. [5] also noted a marked increase in the density of the coronary capillary bed in hypertrophied hearts due to high rates of angiogenesis. These data suggest that the microvasculature in patients with left ventricular hypertrophy might benefit from regular bouts of exercise.

Conclusions

In recent years a major research effort worldwide has generated a massive amount of new information on the metabolic and vascular defects that lead to insulin resistance, type 2 diabetes and cardiovascular disease. In all these conditions, parallel biochemical pathways and mechanisms seem to be activated in many tissues, not only skeletal and cardiac muscle but also the central nervous system, peripheral nerves, the gut and the kidney. The comprehensive picture is far from complete though and therefore we cannot say at this moment in time what the primary event leading to tissue energy depletion and degeneration is. The working hypothesis of this and other essays in this volume is that people who avoid exercise in day-to-day to life and eat too much fatty foods and calories, first develop an unresponsiveness of the vascular endothelium to insulin (in terminal arterioles) and shear stress (arteries and larger arterioles) and that changes in metabolism and function of skeletal muscle, heart and other tissues are secondary. The combined essays in this volume provide hard evidence that both the (micro)vascular wall defects and the impairment at the (cardio)myocyte level can be prevented by lifestyle changes involving regular exercise and a more balanced nutrition.

Summary

- *In order to maintain optimal health, man should be physically active from birth to death.*
- *A sedentary lifestyle increases the risk for development of type 2 diabetes and cardiovascular disease, especially when combined with a high caloric intake.*
- *A reduction in vascular NO production is the key event leading to unresponsiveness of the vascular wall to insulin and shear stress.*
- *A reduced expression of eNOS, reduced activation of eNOS and increased superoxide anion production by NADPH oxidase and eNOS uncoupling all reduce the endothelial NO production.*
- *The reduction in NO production has a negative impact on atherosclerosis and angiogenesis.*
- *Changes in muscle metabolism and tissue degeneration are secondary to the changes in the microvascular wall.*
- *Activation of the metabolic network controlled by the transcription factor NF-κB originally seems to function to repair the endothelial lining and underlying tissues, but eventually leads to tissue destruction.*
- *The benefits of acute and regular exercise in patients are numerous and large and every GP should encourage patients to be as physically active as possible.*
- *More research is needed to investigate whether lifetime exercise interventions started in children prevent insulin resistance and the chronic diseases in adulthood.*

References

1.   Chakravarthy, M.V. & Booth, F.W. (2004) Eating, exercise, and 'thrifty' genotypes: connecting the dots toward an evolutionary understanding of modern chronic diseases. *J. Appl. Physiol.* **96**, 3–10
2.   Frayn, K.N. (2002) Adipose tissue as a buffer for daily lipid flux. *Diabetologia* **45**, 1201–1210
3.   Anderson, P. & Saltin, B. (1985) Maximal perfusion of skeletal muscle in man. *J. Physiol.* **366**, 233–249
4.   Landmesser, U., Hornig, B. & Drexler, H. (2004) Endothelial function: a critical determinant in atherosclerosis? *Circulation* **109**, 27–33
5.   Brown, M.D., Davies, M.K. & Hudlicka, O. (2005) Angiogenesis in ischaemic and hypertrophic hearts induced by long-term bradycardia. *Angiogenesis* **8**, 253–262
6.   Hudlicka, O., Brown, M.D., May, S., Zakrzewicz, A. & Pries, A.R. (2006) Changes in capillary shear stress in skeletal muscles exposed to long-term activity: role of nitric oxide. *Microcirculation* **13**, 249–259
7.   World Health Organization (2006) Global strategy on diet, physical activity and health: diabetes. Geneva: World Health Organization. Available: http://www.who.int/dietphysicalactivity/publications/facts/diabetes/en/index.html Accessed 23rd July 2006.
8.   Renkin, E.M. & Crone, C. (1996) Microcirculation and capillary exchange. In: *Comprehensive Human Physiology*, (Greger, R. & Windhorst, U., eds), pp 1965–1979, Berlin-Heidelberg Springer Verlag.

9.   Gudbjörnsdóttir, S., Sjöstrand, M., Strindberg, L., Wahren, J. & Lönnroth, P. (2003) Direct meas-
     urements of the permeability surface area for insulin and glucose in human skeletal muscle. *J. Clin.
     Endocrinol. Metab.* **88**, 4559–4564

10. Gudbjörnsdóttir, S., Sjöstrand, M., Strindberg, L. & Lönnroth, P. (2005) Decreased muscle capil-
     lary permeability surface area in type 2 diabetic subjects. *J. Clin. Endocrinol. Metab.* **90**, 1078–1082

11. Petersen, K.F., Dufour, S. & Shulman, G.I. (2005) Decreased insulin-stimulated rates of mitochon-
     drial ATP synthesis and phosphate transport in skeletal muscle of insulin-resistant offspring of
     type 2 diabetic patients. *PLoS Med* **2**, e233

12. Wagenmakers, A.J.M. (2005) Insulin resistance in the offspring of parents with type 2 diabetes.
     PLoS Med **2**, e289

13. Itani, S.I., Zhou, Q., Pories, W.J., MacDonald, K.G. & Dohm, G.L. (2000) Involvement of protein
     kinase C in human skeletal muscle insulin resistance and obesity. *Diabetes* **49**, 1353–1358

14. Itani, S.I., Pories, W.J., Macdonald, K.G. & Dohm, G.L. (2001) Increased protein kinase C-θ in
     skeletal muscle of diabetic patients. *Metabolism* **50**, 553–557

15. Itani, S.I., Ruderman, N.B., Schmieder, F. & Boden G. (2002) Lipid-induced insulin resistance in
     human muscle is associated with changes in diacylglycerol, protein kinase C and IκBα. *Diabetes*
     51, 2005–2011

16. Naruse, K., Rask-Madsen, C., Takahara, N., Ha, S.-W., Suzuma, K., Way, K.J., Jacobs, J.R.C.,
     Clermont, A.C., Ueki, K., Ohshiro, Y. et al. (2006) Activation of vascular protein kinase C-β
     inhibits Akt-dependent endothelial nitric oxide synthase function in obesity-associated insulin
     resistance. *Diabetes* **55**, 691–698

17. Yuan M., Konstantopoulos N., Lee J., Hansen L., Li Z.-W., Karin M. & Shoelson S.E. (2001)
     Reversal of obesity- and diet-induced insulin resistance with salicylates or targeted disruption of
     IKKβ. *Science* **293**, 1673–1677

18. Kim, F., Tysseling, K.A., Rice, J., Pham, M., Haji, L., Gallis, B.M., Baas, A.S., Paramsothy, P.,
     Giachelli, C.M., Corson, M.A. & Raines, E.W. (2005) Free fatty acid impairment of nitric oxide
     production in endothelial cells is mediated by IKKβ. *Arterioscler. Thromb. Vas. Biol.* **25**, 989–994

19. Kim, F., Tysseling, K.A., Rice, J., Gallis, B., Haji, L., Giachelli, C.M., Raines, E.W., Corson, M.A. &
     Schwartz, M.W. (2005) Activation of IKKβ by glucose is necessary and sufficient to impair insulin
     signaling and nitric oxide production in endothelial cells. *J. Mol. Cell. Cardiol.* **39**, 327–334

20. Jones, W.K., Brown, M., Wilhide, M., He, S. & Ren, X. (2005) NF-κB in cardiovascular disease:
     diverse and specific effects of a 'general' transcription factor. *Cardiovasc. Toxicol.* **5**, 183–202

21. Shen, H.M. & Pervaiz, S. (2006) TNF receptor superfamily-induced cell death: redox dependent
     execution. *FASEB J.* **20**, 1589–1598

22. Brandes, R.P. & Kreuzer, J. (2005) Vascular NADPH oxidases: molecular mechanisms of activa-
     tion. *Cardiovasc. Res.* **65**, 16–27

23. Xia, Y., Tsai, A.-L., Berka, V. & Zweier, J.L. (1998) Superoxide generation from endothelial
     nitric-oxide synthase. A Ca^{2+}/calmodulin-dependent and tetrahydrobiopterin regulatory process.
     J. Biol. Chem. **273**, 25804–25808

24. Landmesser, U., Dikalov, S., Price, S.R., McCann, L., Fukai, T., Holland, S.M., Mitch, W.E. &
     Harrison, D.G. (2003) Oxidation of tetrahydrobiopterin leads to uncoupling of endothelial cell
     nitric oxide synthase in hypertension. *J. Clin. Invest.* **111**, 1201–1209

25. Bevers, L.M., Braam, B., Post, J.A., van Zonneveld, A.J., Rabelink, T.J., Koomans, H.A., Verhaar,
     M.C., & Joles, J.A. (2006) Tetrahydrobiopterin, but not L-arginine, decreases NO synthase uncou-
     pling in cells expressing high levels of endothelial NO synthase. *Hypertension* **47**, 87–94

26. Nyström, T., Nygren, A. & Sjöholm, Å. (2004) Tetrahydrobiopterin increases insulin sensitivity in
     patients with type 2 diabetes and coronary heart disease. *Am. J. Physiol.* **287**, E919–E925

27. Seynhave, A.L., Vermeulen, C.E., Eggermont, A.M. & Ten Hagen, T.L. (2006) Cytokines and
     vascular permeability: an *in vitro* study on human endothelial cells in relation to tumor necrosis
     factor-α-primed peripheral blood mononuclear cells. *Cell. Biochem. Biophys.* **44**, 157–169

28. Hoffmann, A. & Baltimore, D. (2006) Circuitry of nuclear factor κB signaling. *Immunol. Rev.* **210**, 171–186

29. Campbell, K.J. & Perkins. N.D. (2006) Regulation of NF-κB function. *Biochem. Soc. Symp.* **73**, 165–180

30. Li, Y., Ha, T., Gao, X., Kelley, J., Williams, D.L., Browder, I.W., Kao, R.L. & Li, C. (2004) NF-κB activation is required for the development of cardiac hypertrophy *in vivo*. *Am. J. Physiol.* **287**, H1712–H1720

31. Smith, R.S., Agata, J., Xia, C.F., Chao, L. & Chao, J. (2005) Human endothelial nitric oxide synthase gene delivery protects against cardiac remodeling and reduces oxidative stress after myocardial infarction. *Life Sci.* **76**, 2457–2471

32. Jeffcoate, W.J., Game, F. & Cavanagh, P.R. (2005) The role of proinflammatory cytokines in the cause of neuropathic osteoarthropathy (acute Charcot foot) in diabetes. *Lancet* **366**, 2058–2061

33. Pizzi, M. & Spano P. (2006) Distinct roles of diverse nuclear factor-kappaB complexes in neuropathological mechanisms. *Eur. J. Pharmacol.* **545**, 22–28

34. Harada, C., Okumura, A., Namekata, K., Nakamura, K., Mitamura, Y., Ohguro, H., & Harada, T. (2006). Role of monocyte chemotactic protein-1 and nuclear factor-κB in the pathogenesis of proliferative diabetic retinopathy. *Diabetes Res. Clin. Pract.*, doi: 10.1016/J.diabres. 2006.04.017

35. Zoja, C., Abbate, M. & Remuzzi, G. (2006) Progression of chronic kidney disease: insights from animal models. *Curr. Opin. Neprol. Hypertens.* **15**, 250–257

36. Kitano H., Oda K., Kimura T. et al. (2004) Metabolic syndrome and robustness tradeoffs. *Diabetes* **53**, S6–S15

37. Butcher E.C., Berg E. L. & Kunkel E. J. (2004) Systems biology in drug discovery. *Nat. Biotech.* **22**, 1253–1259

38. Scheuermann-Freestone, M., Madsen, P.L., Manners D., Blamire, A.M., Buckingham, R.E., Styles, P., Radda, G.K., Neubauer, S. & Clarke, K. (2003) Abnormal cardiac and skeletal muscle energy metabolism in patients with type 2 diabetes. *Circulation* **107**, 3040–3046

39. Lam, C.-F., Peterson, T.E., Richardson, D.M., Croatt, A.J., d'Uscio, L.V., Nath, K.A. & Katusic, Z.S. (2006) Increased blood flow causes coordinated upregulation of arterial eNOS and biosynthesis of tetrahydriobiopterin. *Am. J. Physiol.* **290**, H786–H793

Subject index